Psychopathology in Adolescents and Adults with Autism Spectrum Disorders

Roberto Keller
Editor

Psychopathology in Adolescents and Adults with Autism Spectrum Disorders

Springer

Editor
Roberto Keller
Adult Autism Centre
Mental Health Department
Local Health Unit ASL Città di Torino
Turin
Italy

ISBN 978-3-030-26275-4 ISBN 978-3-030-26276-1 (eBook)
https://doi.org/10.1007/978-3-030-26276-1

This Springer imprint is published by the registered company Springer Nature Switzerland AG
The registered company address is: Gewerbestrasse 11, 6330 Cham, Switzerland

This book is dedicated to persons with autism, to their families who everyday stay with them along the life path, and to professionals who seriously work to improve their quality of life.

Roberto Keller

Preface

Autism spectrum disorder is a neurodevelopmental disorder that needs a lifetime support. Unfortunately, adolescents and adults are often not correctly diagnosed and don't receive the correct treatment and/or support.

A major concern is related to psychopathological co-occurrence that may worse autism functioning and quality of life of people with autism.

Bullying and mobbing could be a trigger for psychopathological co-occurrence, but also genetic vulnerability must be considered.

Clinicians must detect psychopathological disorders, and this book could help them in their work, especially when, as in intellectual disabilities and autism, the clinical symptoms could be different from general population.

Turin, Italy Roberto Keller

Contents

1 Diagnosing ASD in Adolescence and Adulthood

Roberto Keller, Stefania Bari, and Romina Castaldo

1.1 Introduction

Autism spectrum disorder (ASD) is a neurodevelopmental disorder with a broad phenotype, based on a complex genetic–epigenetic interaction. ASD diagnosis is highly stable over the lifetime and has a higher mortality rates, medical and psychiatric disorder comorbidity, and poorer overall outcome compared to general population [1, 2]. The correct diagnosis is the basis for a targeted treatment, family support, correct use, or not-use of drugs. Improvement of symptoms and social skill are the first step to offer capability to people with autism [3].

In accordance with the United Nations Convention on the Rights of Persons with Disabilities and the Charter for Persons with Autism (PWA) adopted by the European Parliament, a right to diagnostic clarification and treatment assistance applies across the entire autistic spectrum, including people with additional intellectual disability [4–6].

In this text, even if we use medical words and a clinical approach, we know that the definition of "person with autism" (PWA) is the right one. Other Associations prefer the definition "autistic person". Anyway, in this context, we are describing complex clinical situation and also severe form of autism with intellectual disability, epilepsy, language disorder, and psychiatric comorbidity, so medical terms are correctly allowed.

We propose comprehensive assessment based on a multistep model [7].

- Use of international validated diagnostic criteria
- Collecting clinical information from the family and the person with suspected ASD

R. Keller (✉) · S. Bari · R. Castaldo
Adult Autism Centre, Mental Health Department, Local Heath Unit ASL Città di Torino, Turin, Italy

R. Keller (ed.), *Psychopathology in Adolescents and Adults with Autism Spectrum Disorders*, https://doi.org/10.1007/978-3-030-26276-1_1

- Psychiatric and Neurological clinical examination
- Test evaluation
- Medical assessment
- Define a personalized project of treatment

1.2 Clinical Diagnosis and Diagnostic Criteria

The diagnosis of ASD is clinically based on the course of neurodevelopment and the individual's current symptoms [8], and tests could be useful but are only complementary pieces of the diagnostic puzzle [9].

Diagnostic criteria are defined in the current diagnostic manuals of the American Psychiatric Association (DSM) [10] and the World Health Organization (ICD) [11].

ASD in DSM-5 [10] is characterized by—as first and core criterion—persistent deficits in social communication and social interaction across contexts, not accounted for by general developmental delays, and manifested by deficits in social–emotional reciprocity, in nonverbal communicative behaviors used for social interaction, and in developing and maintaining relationships.

The second criterion is the presence of restricted, repetitive patterns of behavior, interests, or activities, manifested by at least two of the following: (1) stereotyped or repetitive speech, motor movements, or use of objects; (2) excessive adherence to routines, ritualized patterns of verbal or nonverbal behavior, or excessive resistance to change; (3) highly restricted, fixated interests that are abnormal in intensity or focus; (4) hyper- or hypo-reactivity to sensory inputs or unusual interest in sensory aspects of environment. Symptoms must be present in early childhood (but may not become fully manifest until social demands exceed limited capacities, and together limit and impair everyday functioning).

The DSM-5 defines ASD as a unique cluster of disorders [12] with a common clinical core that includes subtypes with large differences in functioning that could be caused by different neurobiological bases (genetic syndrome or not, autism with severe intellectual disability and language disorder, or high academic performance) [13, 14, 15].

Symptoms must be present in early childhood but may not become fully manifest until social demands exceed limited capacities (approximately age 8 and younger).

To not overdiagnose autism, we must remember that symptoms together must limit and impair everyday functioning.

DSM-5 describes three levels of ASD functioning that need more or less support [10]:

Level 1 is the higher level of functioning and includes high-functioning ASD and Asperger disorder. At this level of autism, "Requiring support," we observe that without supports in place, deficits in social communication cause impairments. PWA has difficulty in initiating social interactions and demonstrates clear examples of atypical or unusual or unsuccessful responses to social overtures of others and seems to have decreased interest in social interactions, especially with pairs. Rituals and repetitive behaviors cause interference with functioning in one or more contexts and PWA show opposite behavior when others try to interrupt rituals.

Level 2 is an intermediate level of functioning that requires "substantial support." PWA has marked deficits in verbal and nonverbal social communication skills and social impairments, even with supports in place. PWA has limited initiation of social interactions and reduced or abnormal response to social overtures from others.

Level 3 is the most severe type of autism, with higher comorbidity too (e.g., language disorder, epilepsy, and genetic and metabolic syndromes). This level "requires very substantial support" and has severe deficits in verbal and nonverbal social communication skills. Social interactions are very limited and with minimal response to social overtures from others. Rituals and/or repetitive behaviors markedly interfere with functioning and is very difficult to interrupt rituals.

During the clinical examination, we must notice deficits in social–emotional reciprocity that range from abnormal social approach and failure of normal back and forth conversation through reduced sharing of interests, emotions, and affect and response, to total lack of initiation of social interaction. We can observe an abnormal social approach during the first visit, when the person with autism (PWA) presents an intrusive touching or licking or sniffing. Especially in childhood or in intellectual disability, the PWA uses others as tools. There is a failure of normal back and forth conversation, and the PWA could not respond when the name is called or when spoken directly to or could not initiate conversation, not sharing interest to other people. We observe the same deficit in sharing emotions or affect or responsive social smile, but we can also observe PWA with an excess of showing emotions because the deficit is the appropriate response to the social context.

In PWA, deficits in nonverbal communicative behavior used for social interaction range from poorly integrated verbal and nonverbal communication, through abnormalities in eye contact and body language, or deficits in understanding and use of nonverbal communication, to total lack of facial expression or gestures. This condition reflects difficulties with nonverbal communication, so the PWA could show impairments in social use of eye contact and especially in understanding what a look can mean; the impairment could imply the use and understanding of body postures and gestures. The voice can present an abnormal volume, or pitch, or rhythm. A problem for the PWA is the inability to recognize or interpret other's nonverbal expressions and prosody.

Deficits are strictly related to deficits in developing and maintaining relationships appropriate to developmental level (beyond those with caregivers), ranging from difficulties adjusting behavior to suit different social contexts through difficulties in sharing imaginative play and in making friends. PWAs are unaware of social conventions/appropriate social behavior. They have difficulties in making friends, and even when they want to have friends, they lack in adequate social skill.

A repetitive pattern of behavior includes atypical speech, movements, and play. In speech, PWA can show echolalia (immediate or delayed repetition of words or phrases) or repetitive vocalizations such as repetitive guttural sounds, intonational noise-making, unusual squealing, and repetitive humming. The language can show neologisms or pronoun reversal (e.g., "You" for "I;" or refers to self by own name (does not use "I")).

Also motor movements can be stereotyped or we can observe repetitive movements as repetitive hand movements (e.g., clapping, finger flicking, flapping, and twisting). Stereotyped movement can be complex including whole body movements (e.g., foot-to-foot rocking, dipping, swaying, and spinning). PWA can show abnormalities of posture or unusual facial grimacing and excessive teeth grinding.

Also use of objects can be stereotyped or repetitive as nonfunctional playing with objects (waving sticks and dropping items) or alignment toys or objects or repetitively opening and closing doors or turning lights on and off.

PWA can show excessive adherence to routines and/or ritualized patterns of verbal or nonverbal behavior, or excessive resistance to change. This diagnostic criteria includes rituals and insistence on rigidly following specific routines. Ritualized patterns of verbal and nonverbal behavior or repetitive questioning about a particular topic or verbal rituals could be another item. PWA may have a rigid thinking or inability to understand humor/nonliteral aspects of speech such as irony or implied meaning or excessively rigid in behavior.

In PWA interests could be highly restricted, fixated, and abnormal in intensity or focus (e.g., focused on the same few objects, topics or activities), preoccupation with numbers, letters, symbols, being overly perfectionistic, attachment to unusual inanimate object (e.g., piece of string or rubber band) or unusual fears (e.g., afraid of people wearing earrings).

DSM-5 [10] new criteria concerning with hyper- or hypo-reactivity to sensory input or unusual interest in sensory aspects of environment is very useful for diagnosing and typically related to autism. On the one side PWA can show a high tolerance for pain, and on the other side PWA can have preoccupation with texture or touch that includes attraction/aversion to texture or could be uncomfortable to specific sound, smell, light, and taste.

Asperger's syndrome (AS) is a subtype of ASD level 1 described in DSM-5, with normal or higher cognitive functioning and restricted interests. AS in adolescence and adulthood is still insufficiently recognized. In particular, there is a lack of awareness of this condition. In childhood, AS is often considered as "little genius," and the lack of social skill is considered as a side effect to be more clever than other children. Adolescent and adult patients with AS come to the attention of Mental Health Services complaining of difficulties within their social context and interpersonal relationships, and especially of psychopathogical comorbidities (depressive disorder, anxiety, and psychosis). AS is the best candidate to be victim of bullying [16].

Teachers and clinicians must be careful in recognizing AS when an adolescent presents: psychological difficulties in changing situation (change of type of school), high discrepancy in good academic and in poor social skill especially in non-structured situation (school break), is social naïve, is a serious and lonely student, has poor social relations, and is bullied.

In female, AS diagnosis is more difficult: restricted interests are less unusual and bizarre and could be social-related (e.g., makeup), the autism is more "internalized" with high level of hypersensoriality, social deficit could be hidden by coping social skill of another girl; but the AS girl copies only the external behavior of another neurotypical girl and remains naïve inside and so could be exposed to high risk of sexual abuse.

Individuals with ASD display interest in sexual interactions and to engage in sexual behavior. Age appropriate sexual interest, limited sexual knowledge and experiences, and social skill deficits may drive adolescent and adult with ASD to an increased risk of sexual abuse [17].

Girls with ASD are at greater risk for anxiety, depression, suicidal ideation, and for psychiatric hospitalization than male and present more abnormalities in sensory profile [18]. Camouflage or pretending to be normal or putting on a mask is widespread in AS females, who use a prolonged autodidacticism based on careful observation of peers, reading novels and psychology books, imitating fictional characters. But camouflage cause a sense of exhaustion and confusion about individual's true identity [19, 20].

Inside the range of ASD level 1, from a clinical observation, AS is different from high-functioning autism (HFA). AS subjects have earlier language development, more appropriate intonation and pitch, and more pedantic speech and idiosyncratic vocabulary, while HFA subjects show more echolalia, pronoun reversal, and simple neologism. AS children also display more imitative social play, attention and help seeking, and reciprocal social interactions than HFA children. But superior linguistic and social skills of AS children do not translate into superior ability to make friends or engage in reciprocal conversation. Cognitively AS shows a nonverbal learning disability profile, with superior verbal performance and visual-spatial/perceptual/motor deficits; the opposite profile characterizes HFA. Motor clumsiness is present in both HFA and AS. AS subjects perform significantly better academically but not in term of independent living. Genetic is common to both AS and HFA and more linked to a general susceptibility shared by neurodevelopmental disorders. But the main point is that AS and HFA correspond to distinct developmental trajectories: HFA sign of a disorder is more evident in childhood, so the children can receive an early treatment and could improve; on the contrary, AS could be not recognized as a disorder and did not receive help in childhood, so they have a major risk of co-occurrence of psychiatric disorder and bullying [21].

In low-functioning ASD (especially level 3 of DSM-5), the intellectual disability may overshadow autism symptoms. The different presentation of psychiatric symptoms (especially irritability as symptom of depressive disorder) could lead to misdiagnosis. In the presence of intellectual disability, the impairment of social communication has to exceed the level of impairment which can be expected for a certain severity of intellectual disability to allow the additional diagnosis of ASD. Social reciprocity and nonverbal communication are especially valuable to distinguish an additional ASD from an intellectual disability alone, while verbal communication and stereotypic behaviors are of less value for this purpose [22, 23].

1.3 Collecting Clinical Information from the Family and the Person with Suspected ASD

Family is the center for both collecting clinical history and defining the personalized project of treatment. Only in Asperger syndrome, we could have a unique reference in the person with autism; but also in some adolescent/adult AS people, we need to collect information concerning with childhood, especially in differential diagnosis with the onset of psychosis.

In visiting the family of ASD, we have to first consider that most of the families of adults with ASD have been blamed to be the cause of ASD of their children (in the Bettelheim's theory of autism described in his book *The Empty Fortress* [24]) and that they did not receive a correct treatment for ASD of their children. During the 1970s, the psychogenic theory of the cause of autism was beginning to be rejected. So we have to explain now how we think about the pathogenesis of autism as related to a genetic–epigenetic basis and not to an incompetent mother–newborn relationship; otherwise, we must be careful not to blame parents as a direct hereditary origin of the disorder of their son. Genetic is not equivalent to hereditary.

We should collect information concerning with:

- Neurological and psychiatric disorders in parents or relatives
- Pregnancy and use of drugs, environmental situation, pollution, infections before and during pregnancy
- Birth
- Age of language development
- Age and way of walking
- Age of sphinteric control
- Social relationship with children in age 3–8 years
- Way of playing with other children in age 3–8 years
- Social relationship at school
- Educational ability and need of educational support
- High sensoriality level
- Repetitive games
- Motor control and repetitive movements in childhood
- Repetitive speech
- Self-harm
- Other medical and neurological disorders in childhood, infections
- Use of drugs and side effects
- Modification of the disorder during time

If possible (depending on the age of the parents), it could be useful to detect in the history of the suspected PWA the childhood "red flags" of autism as:

By 6 months:

- No social smiles or other warm, joyful expressions directed to people
- Limited or no eye contact, appropriate eye gaze

By 9 months:

- No sharing or vocal sounds, smiles, or other nonverbal communication

By 12 months:

- No babbling
- No use of gestures to communicate (e.g., waving, reaching, and pointing)
- No response to name when called

By 16 months, no words

By 24 months, no meaningful, two-word phrases

Any loss of any previously acquired speech, social skills, babbling

Deficit in social interactions in social context (especially nursery school) at 2–3 years old is a clear marker.

Presence of selective feeding in childhood, lack of response to name and sharing interest or enjoyment, unusual prosody (little variation in pitch, odd intonation, irregular rhythm, unusual voice quality), repetitive movement with objects, or repetitive posturing of body, arms, hands, or fingers

All symptoms must be shown in early childhood, e.g., before 8 years of age.

To detect AS, we must especially search the presence of social skill deficits with pairs and special interest in a child with a good cognitive functioning and good academic level.

Including the family and PWA since the first diagnosis step in building the personal project of treatment is a core point of our multistep model.

1.4 Psychiatric and Neurological Clinical Examination

The "focus of assessment should not only be on diagnosis but should also consider the person's physical, psychological and social functioning, and any risks that they might face" [25].

We must take care of the person with autism or suspected ASD.

So a milieu of human reception must be the basis to collect clinical information, to observe behavior, and to complete the psychopathological evaluation with a neurological examination.

During the visit, we observe how the persons enter in the ward, how they relate with us, the interpersonal distance, the mimic, the posture, the use and complexity of the language, and the movement of the body.

First, we explore the presence of special interest of the persons, and we use a *pairing* technique, to feel the persons being confident with us, speaking about their interest.

After that, if they are competent in the language, we evaluate the psychopathological status exploring form and content of thought, mood, presence of obsession, delusion, perception, feeding, sleeping, and impulse control.

Lifetime psychiatric Axis I comorbidity is very common in adolescence and adulthood, most notably mood (more than 50%) and anxiety disorder, but also ADHD (42%) and psychotic disorders (10%). Frequency of reading disorder in combination with disorder of written expression (i.e., dyslexia) is 14% and need appropriate assessment [26]. Research into the possible link between ASD (especially AS) and anorexia nervosa has shown potential links both in specific characteristics of the two disorders and in the prevalence rate of comorbidity or elevated levels of ASD traits within anorexia nervosa population [27]. Misdiagnosis of AS female could also be linked to ASD symptoms hidden behind anorexia nervosa symptoms, especially the restrictor type, with special interest linked to eating and body.

During the visit, we clinically define a supposed level of functioning to choose the most appropriate test in the next step.

We complete the visit with a neurological examination to detect a possible neurological disorder related to ASD (especially Wilson disease with late clinical onset).

Motor function is frequently impaired in ASD, and motor clumsiness is a diagnostic sign, and a motor neurological examination must be included in the medical assessment. A number of different motor deficits have been observed in ASD as clumsiness, postural instability, motor coordination, and, more in general, a widespread poorer performance on motor skills tests in comparison to people without ASD. These problems seem to be in part negatively correlated to language acquisition so that, for instance, adolescents with ASD who do not present any speech delay show poorer bimanual coordination in comparison with those with speech delay. Recent studies linked these motor deficits to a possible alteration of motor simulation processes in ASD. The theory behind motor simulation states that all sensorimotor information related to the execution of a movement is also used by other processes such as imitation, understanding of movements performed by other people and the skill to imagine one's own movements [28].

Altered motor coordination is also observed, and a dysfunction of motor imagery has been recently reported on implicit tasks. In a recent study, we employed a spatial bimanual task to concurrently assess motor coordination and explicit motor imagery in autism. Our results showed a significant and similar coupling effect in the bimanual condition values with respect to the unimanual condition in both controls and ASD participants. On the contrary, in the imagery condition, a significant coupling effect was found only in controls. Furthermore, adult controls showed a significantly higher imagery coupling effect in comparison to all the other groups. These results demonstrate that atypical motor imagery processes in ASD are not limited to implicit tasks and suggest that development of neural structures involved in motor imagery are immature in ASD [28].

Motor imagery and actual motor coordination are interrelated processes that, however, seem to be dissociated in ASD, where development of spatial coordination consolidates earlier in respect to motor imagery [29].

ASD must be differentiated from stereotypic movement disorder (SMD) that occurs in people without ASD or intellectual disability since childhood. Stereotypies are involuntary, patterned, repetitive, coordinated, rhythmic and non-reflexive behaviors that are suppressible by sensory stimuli or distraction. Repetitive movement are common in neurotypical infants and young children (over 60%). SMD movement patterns are not distinguishable from those in ASD solely by their motor description. Distinguished features are the presence of abnormalities in socialization and quality of communication in ASD [30, 31].

Stereotypies should be distinguished from tics, especially complex tics: there is a cluster of simple tics or a more coordinated sequence of intermittent movements (hop, jump, and knee bend); like stereotypies they are periodic, patterned, and exacerbated by stress, anxiety, and fatigue; in contrast, tics have a later onset (6–7 years versus 3 years), have more variable pattern, involve eye blinks, facial grimaces, head twists, and shoulder shrugs; they are less rhythmic, are associated with premonitory urges or desire to reduce an inner tension, and are briefly suppressible [31].

We must be careful to detect other neurological sign as extrapyramidal sign that could be side effects (especially antipsychotic drugs) but also sign of late onset of metabolic disorders [32].

1.5 Test Evaluation

In this section, we present a sample of test useful in ASD assessment; other tests are available in literature. No single diagnostic testing procedure can solely define the diagnostic decision. Tests are complementary to the clinical evaluation and could be useful to complete the assessment, but an incorrect use of a test could lead to a misdiagnosis, ASD over- or under-diagnosing. According to the current diagnostic manuals, such as the ICD-11 and the DSM-5, the final diagnostic decision is clinical, based on the core symptoms of ASD. Standardized instruments may help to detect autism and prompt a more comprehensive assessment but must be distinguished if they are instruments of screening or instruments for diagnosing or for evaluating the functioning. In adolescence and adulthood, test must be specific for the age and purpose and for the level of ASD and cognitive functioning. Some of the following tests are not translated in all languages and not validated in all countries, so the clinician must be careful to check these aspects and age of possible usage.

1. A cognitive assessment completes the clinical evaluation (WISC [33]; WAIS [34]; Leiter-r Raven Matrices or CPM [35]) and could help to choose properly the test for diagnosing ASD. WAIS IV is useful for verbal patients coming from the same country or culture; Raven matrices, for population from different country or difficulties in language [36]; CPM, for more severe ASD; Leiter-r, for nonverbal patients.
2. Test for ASD screening: they must not be used for diagnosing but only for screening or for research purpose.
   - AQ-autism quotient, EQ-empathy quotient (Baron-Cohen), self-report, useful for ASD level 1 DSM-5 and especially for Asperger disorder; ASD must have good awareness of their behavior [37, 38]. Usefulness of AQ in differentiating high-functioning ASD from schizophrenia is limited.
   - The *Autism Spectrum Disorder—Diagnosis Scale for Intellectually Disabled Adults* (ASD-DA [39]) is a structured interview that is used to screen for ASD in adults with intellectual disability.

- The *Social Communication Questionnaire* (SCQ [40]) is a third-party assessment tool developed for children and adolescents. In two versions, current or lifetime behavior is recorded. This questionnaire has been validated in a transcultural sample of 451 adults with ID [41]. The *Social Communication Questionnaire for Adults with ID* (SCQ-AID [42]) is specifically developed for adults with intellectual disability and consists of a core set of valid and adult-appropriate items.
- The *Autism Checklist* (ACL [4]) is a screening tool based on the ICD-10 research criteria. It facilitates a structured medical history and assessment in medical visits.
- The *Diagnostic Behavioral Assessment for ASD-Revised* (DiBAS-R [43]) is an ICD-10/DSM-5-based caregiver report screening tool that consists of 19 Likert-scaled items. Meanwhile, it is validated in a second independent sample.
- The *Psychiatric Instrument for the Intellectually Disabled Adult* (SPAID) is an Italian tool package for the diagnostic assessment in adults with ID. It consists of a general form and specific checklists for certain disorders, including ASD [44].
- The STA-DI is a structured interview that could be used to help the clinician during the screening of ASD in intellectual disability (ID), related to observation of the patient [45].

3. Test for ASD diagnosing
   - The *Autism Diagnostic Interview—Revised* (ADI-R, [46]) is a semi-structured parental interview assessing social reciprocity, communication, and restrictive, repetitive behaviors between the ages of 4 and 5 years. It consists of 93 Likert-scaled items, and a selection of these is adopted by the final algorithm, resulting in a classification of "autism" or "no autism." Is useful especially for typical autism but could be false negative in AS because symptoms are recognized later at the school time; another limit of its use is related to the age of the patient and particularly the age of the parents because the evaluation is based on the memory of first years of life and of the timing of the neurodevelopmental step.
   - The *Autism Diagnostic Observation Schedule* (ADOS [47]) is a semi-structured observation tool to assess social communication in persons suspected of having ASD. Depending on their verbal abilities, one of four modules can be applied, and generally module IV is used in adulthood. It is useful in typical form of autism but not in severe level of autism or in AS. In AS with high cognitive level (e.g., professor of university), the use of so a simple test that could also lead to false negative could be embarrassing. Otherwise, in psychotic patients with prevalent negative symptoms, ADOS could lead to a false-positive result, up to 30% among adults with psychosis. ADOS-2 is not designed to be used as a standalone diagnostic measure. Developmental history has often a key role in differential diagnosis of ASD or psychosis.

- The GARS is an interview used to assess ASD in comorbidity with moderate-severe ID when the level of intellectual disability does not allow the patient to collaborate during the clinical evaluation or to ADOS use [48].
- RAADS (Ritvo Autism Asperger Diagnostic Scale Revised), an assessment for Asperger disorder [49]; it is free of charge and available online, so a lot of patients come to clinical evaluation with this test already done as self-report. For a specialistic assessment must be used a clinical interview and not a self-report, asking several examples for each item and considering not only the total score but the single four subscales, too. The evaluation must be linked to clinical assessment of neurodevelopmental step of first years of life, and RAADS must not be used as the solely evaluation, that could lead to false positive in personality disorder and to false negative in AS without awareness of their autism and social skill deficit.
- Adult Asperger Assessment, a structured diagnostic interview [50].
- SRS-2, a clinical-functional evaluation that has the advantage that could be used from childhood to adulthood, and that is based on direct observation and reports from the others (e.g., teachers and parents) [51].
- The Diagnostic Interview for Social and Communication Disorders (DISCO) is a schedule for the diagnosis of autistic spectrum and related disorders and assessment of individual needs. It enables information to be recorded systematically for a wide range of behaviors and developmental skills and is suitable for use with all ages and levels of ability. In addition to helping the clinician to obtain a profile of each individual's pattern of development and behavior, the DISCO also enables identification of specific features found in autistic spectrum disorders that are relevant for use with established diagnostic systems [52].

4. After diagnosis of ASD, a functional assessment should be completed using for example Vineland II [53], VB-MAPP [54], TTAP [55], or in ASD with severe intellectual disability the Essential for Living assessment [56], too.
5. A neuropsychological assessment is useful to detect specific cognitive deficit (attention, memory, executive functioning, praxia, and gnosia) or for legal purpose, as for evaluation for driving license [57].
6. A psychopathological evaluation is useful to better define the profile of the person. Clinical interviews such as SCID are useful in ASD; otherwise clinicians must be careful in using self-report test as MMPI because the ASD patient could read literally the question and so answer in a wrong way leading to misdiagnosis of psychosis. The Rorschach test could support clinical evaluation with information concerning with psychopathological functioning [58].

1.6 Medical Assessment

The assessment has to take into account and detect possible differential diagnoses and coexisting disorders or conditions. Biological or genetic tests or neuroimaging for diagnostic purposes should not routinely be part of the assessment of ASD in adolescence and adulthood [8, 59]. However, they may be applied if needed to rule out certain disorders or conditions that may mimic ASD, such as severe hearing impairments. An example of this disorders is summarized in the following. We must remember that medical condition could be the trigger of behavioral disorder especially in severe intellectual disability and in language disorder, when the patient is unable to indicate the origin of the pain: so in challenging behavior, a complete medical assessment must be done before considering it as a functional or psychological symptom and before using drugs as antipsychotics that could worsen the medical condition (e.g., slowing gastrointestinal functioning).

Blood examination could be useful, related especially to a diet dysregulation in ASD and the use of psychotropic drug (glycemia, cholesterol, triglycerides, lipase, hepatic markers, and homocysteine).

In ASD, eating difficulties or limited variety of food intake could lead to vitamin or iron deficits (folate, B_{12}, iron, ferritin, and vitamin D); also, endocrinological disorders could worsen the cognitive level of functioning and trigger challenging behavior (TSH reflex, PRL, and cortisol).

Metabolic and genetic disorder could lead to an ASD especially with ID phenotype (organic acid, plasmatic amino acids, ammonia, ferritin, copper, and porphyria): even if this screening should be done in childhood, some late-onset metabolic disorders allow prescribing the screening also in adolescence or early adulthood [60].

Mitochondria play a key role in different cellular functions, especially those related to energy metabolism: ASD patients are more likely to show mitochondrial dysfunctions than neurotypical people [61]. Clinical signs could be weakness in arms and legs, cardiomyopathy, ataxia, epileptic-like episodes and laboratory markers as high level of lactic acid, ammonium, AST, pyruvate, creatine-kinase, and low carnitine. Some authors suggest a mitochondrial subtype of ASD that includes a history of regression and multiorgan system involvement (heart, skeletal muscle, gut, and endocrine system), hypotonia, epilepsy, fatigued with activity.

We also have to consider the possibility of a metabolic disorder causing ASD and/or ID especially in patients coming from nations where the metabolic screening at the moment of birth is not a routine guideline and if there is a neurological disorder in comorbidity, as epilepsy [60, 62]. For example, phenylketonuria may cause neurologic and psychiatric disorders, including intellectual disability, anxiety, depressive disorder, psychosis, epilepsy, neurocognitive dysfunction, Tourette, eating disorders, and autism [63].

An immune dysregulation could be involved in tic symptoms in ASD, as in PANDA's syndrome (VES, PCR, antiDNAse B, Ab anti-mycoplasma).

Genetic syndromes may be associated with behaviors that mimic ASD and are in comorbidity with ASD, too.

In tuberous sclerosis, especially type 2, interaction and communication as well as attention and impulse control are impaired, while ritualized and stereotypic behaviors can be observed less frequently. Epilepsy is common in tuberous sclerosis.

Fragile X syndrome (FXS) is the most common monogenetic cause of intellectual disability. Many of its sufferers, who are predominantly male, show hyperactivity, deficits in attention and self-regulation, and repetitive behaviors. Moreover, social anxiety and shyness in eye-contact may resemble ASD at first glance, while interest in social relations is unaffected. Some authors indicate differences in the profile of social and communicative symptomatology of FXS compared to idiopathic autism and support different and targeted interventions for individuals with FXS [64]. Other than in full syndrome (more than 200 triplets), neuropsychiatric disorder could be observed in pre-mutation, too (50–200 triplets). The mother of the patient has a high risk of thyroid disease and mood disorder and also a higher risk of multiple sclerosis than in general population, and in grandfather a dementia with ataxia could be observed.

Rett syndrome is a unique neurodevelopmental disorder with clear genetic basis that affects mainly girls often misdiagnosed as idiopathic autism or cerebral palsy or nonspecific developmental delay. It has been stressed that children with Rett syndrome appear to be normal in the initial 6–18 months, but the most show delay in rolling over and some in head control. An analysis of home video from birth to 12 months reveals sign of potential difficulty in appearance, posture, movement and contact, and abnormalities in generalized and fine finger movements.

Late infancy to early childhood is the period believed to be associated with the onset of the classic form of Rett syndrome. This is the regression period, and the babies show autistic tendency: delay in motor milestones, speech delay, loosing purposeful hand use (12–18 months) followed by hand stereotypies (washing-hands); toward early childhood muscle hypertonus starting from legs become apparent.

In the period spanning from childhood to adulthood, symptoms become stabilized and autistic features begin to disappear and the child begins to associate with the environment, even if intellectual ability is affected. Dystonic muscle hypertonus increases, scoliosis slowly progresses, breathing abnormalities become evident, and epileptic seizures may occur. The severity score rises until 15 years of age and flatten at 25 years. In adulthood, the condition stabilizes. If dementia progresses, muscle tone shows plastic rigidity and Parkinsonism but without tremor. Knowledge about the underlying genetic syndrome and the associated behavioral phenotypes is supportive to prevent psychiatric misdiagnoses [65, 66].

In Down syndrome, a higher rate of ASD is observed rather than general population. Approximately 10–18% of persons with Down syndrome meet diagnostic criteria for ASD as compared to 1% in the typical population [66]. Dementia is very common in Down syndrome: a complete neuropsychological assessment should be done in Down syndrome in adulthood for screening dementia [67].

Patients with 15q11.2 BP1-BP2 microdeletion (Burnside-Butler syndrome) can present with developmental and language delay, neurobehavioral disturbance, psychiatric problems, and autism with motor delay and microcephaly.

Prader-Willi syndrome and Angelman syndrome are typically caused by a deletion involving the distal breakpoint BP3 and proximally placed breakpoints BP1 or

BP2 (typical 15q11-q13 deletions) and exhibit an interesting model to link genes to glutamate–GABA imbalance.

Phelan Mc Dermid syndrome or 22q13.3 deletion syndrome is a rare neurodevelopmental disorder characterized by generalized developmental delay, intellectual disability, absent or delayed speech, seizures, ASD, neonatal hypotonia, dysmorphic features, and recurrent medical comorbidities. In most cases, it involves SHANK3, a gene encoding a structural component of excitatory synapses indispensable for proper synaptogenesis and neuronal physiology. This syndrome is a model to study targeted therapy as mGluR5 antagonist or IGF1 to treat ASD [68].

Sanfilippo B is a rare autosomal recessive mucopolysaccharidosis (MPS III B) caused by deficiency of N acetyl-alpha-D-glucosaminidase. Accumulation of the substrate leads to neurological degeneration and mental decline. The gene is located on chromosome 17q21.1. Somatic features are relatively mild. Affected individuals may reach late adulthood or even old age. Patients may show autistic-like features, ideomotor apraxia, and weakness in verbal comprehension. Metabolic screening reveals an enhanced concentration of heparin sulfate in urine. Screening for metabolic disorders, as MPS III B, should be considered in patients with the history of intellectual disability and progressive decline [69].

Several genetic syndromes could lead to ASD and psychosis (as del22q11 or Di George syndrome) or to different clinical phenotype in the same family (psychotic or ASD or personality disorder or mood disorders).

By array-CGH analysis, we identified a novel familial 3q29 deletion (1.36 Mb), centromeric to the 3q29 deletion region, which manifests with variable expressivity. The deletion was first identified in a 3-year-old girl diagnosed with ID/DD and autism and segregated in six family members, all affected by severe psychiatric disorders including schizophrenia, major depression, anxiety disorder, and personality disorder. All individuals carrying the deletion were overweight or obese, and anomalies compatible with optic atrophy were observed in three out of four cases examined. Among the ten genes encompassed by the deletion, the haploinsufficiency of optic atrophy 1 (OPA1), associated with autosomal dominant optic atrophy, is likely responsible for the ophthalmological anomalies [14].

We hypothesize that the haploinsufficiency of ATPase type 13A4 (ATP13A4) and/or Hairy/Enhancer of Split Drosophila homolog 1 (HES1) contributes to the neuropsychiatric phenotype, while HES1 deletion might underlie the overweight/obesity. In conclusion, we proposed a novel contiguous gene syndrome due to a proximal 3q29 deletion variably associated with autism, ID/DD, psychiatric traits, and overweight/obesity.

We have to consider a genetic evaluation, starting with FRAXA and CGH array also in adolescence and adulthood, especially when brother or sister of the patients are in fertile age or the high functioning, as in AS, leads to the possibility to become father/mother.

Neurodevelopmental disorders share a common genetic basis: approximately 50–70% of the contributing genetic factors in ASD and ADHD show overlap [70]. A shared genetic and neurobiological underpinnings form an explanation why also psychopathological disorders as psychosis, obsessive-compulsive spectrum disorders, and mood disorder (especially bipolar disorder) occur so frequently within the same patient and family. Schizophrenia spectrum disorder (SCZD), autism spectrum disorder (ASD), and obsessive-compulsive spectrum disorder (OCSD) are considered as three separate psychiatric conditions with, supposedly, different brain alteration patterns. From a neuroimaging perspective, we described a meta-analytic study aimed to address whether this nosographical differentiation is actually supported by different brain patterns of gray matter (GM) or white matter (WM) morphological alterations. We explored two possibilities: a) SCZD, ASD, and OCSD could show distinctive patterns of alterations; b) SCZD, ASD, and OCSD could share common patterns of alterations. Our analysis reveals that these psychiatric spectra do not present clear distinctive patterns of alterations; rather, they all tend to be distributed in two alteration clusters. Cluster 1, that is more specific for SCZD, includes the anterior insular, anterior cingulate cortex, ventromedial prefrontal cortex, and frontopolar areas, which form a network that resembles the *salience detection network*. Cluster 2, more specific for OCDS, presents occipital, temporal, and parietal alteration patterns with the involvement of sensorimotor, premotor, visual, and lingual areas, thus forming a network that is more associated with the auditory-visual, auditory, and premotor visual somatic functions. ASD is shared in the two clusters. The three spectra share a significant set of alterations. This observation support the hypotheses of a large range of genetic vulnerability to neurodevelopmental disorders and common neurobiological damage, possibly related to neuroinflammation during brain development [71].

Both environmental factors and genetic factors are involved in the pathogenesis of ASD. Epigenetics, an essential mechanism for gene regulation based on chemical modifications of DNA and histone proteins is also involved in ASD. Up to 40–50% of variance in ASD liability might be determined by environmental factors, as prenatal exposure to particulate matters or pesticides or high exposure to inorganic mercury in the environment (but not in vaccination) in early life; PCB-95, a polychlorinated could lead to the deletion or duplication of 15q11-q13, a genetic cause of ASD [72–74].

Even if the ASD pathogenetic role of cytomegalovirus and rubeola in pregnancy are well known, otherwise neuropsychiatric Lyme borreliosis is generally misdiagnosed in clinical practice, but there is an increasing evidence that it causes mental symptoms mediated by immune and metabolic effects that result in a gradually developing spectrum of neuropsychiatric symptoms. This may include symptoms such as ASD-like, psychosis, mood disorder, and cognitive disorders. It is caused by *Borrelia burgdorferi* and other Borrelia species. Up to 40% of patients develop neurological involvement (in peripheral or central nervous system). Congenital infections can contribute to developmental disorders and neuropsychiatric impairments; infections can lead to ASD-like syndrome, ADHD, and a broad spectrum of psychiatric and multisystem symptoms, especially irritability or mood swings, anger rage, developmental delays, tic, seizure, photophobia, auditory hyperacuity or sensory hypersensitivity, and cognitive impairment. A clinical screening assessment should include:

- Areas or activities that may expose to ticks
- Family members or dog been infected
- History of tick bite with flu-like illness, bull's eye, or other rash
- A point in the patient history in which the health declined, followed by a fluctuating progression and development of multi-systemic symptoms (cognitive, psychiatric, neurological, and somatic) with functional impairment (school, social life, and work)
- Antibiotics cause a sudden worsening followed by improvement of symptoms
- Relapsing progressive multisystemic symptoms [75]

Epilepsy and ASD commonly co-occur with ASD. The co-occurrence of epilepsy is well documented, and there is also evidence of a higher prevalence of EEG abnormalities with 4–86% of individuals with ASD presenting epileptiform or not epileptiform EEG abnormalities. The presence of epilepsy in people with ASD may be determined by several structural alterations, genetic conditions, or metabolic dysfunctions, known to play a role in the emergence of both epilepsy and autism. The frequent comorbidity between ASD and epilepsy suggests that they are the results of shared underlying neurobiological mechanisms. This could be related to genetic mutations discovered in autism and epilepsy which highlight the presence of abnormalities in both synapse formation and function causing altered balance between neuronal excitation and inhibition that is widely recognized as a cause of seizures and epilepsy and also the basis for new targeted treatment of ASD. The increased excitation has been linked to dysfunctional ion channels that trigger membrane depolarization (e.g., sodium or calcium channelopathy) or to an enhanced excitatory neurotransmission determined, for example, by a greater glutamate release or more glutamatergic synapses; the decreased inhibitory function (potassium channelopathy) or alterations in GABAergic neurotransmission leads to greater susceptibility to seizures. Several genetic mutations that have been found to be linked to the development of ASD and/or epilepsy exert their influence on various aspects of neuronal function and are not limited to ion channels and synaptic physiology. Such mutations affect proteins implicated in neuronal excitability: anchoring synaptic machinery, managing synaptic vesicle release, the control of subcellular signaling pathways, and the regulation of migration of neurons as well the organization of network connections. All seizure types can be associated with ASD, although some studies report partial, atypical absence, myoclonic, and tonic–clonic seizures as the most prevalent types, whereas others indicate generalized tonic–clonic and atypical absence seizures as the most common ones. There are two peaks in the age of onset of epilepsy in ASD: the first in early childhood and the second in (perhaps late) adolescence. In ASD there is a higher prevalence of EEG abnormalities, with estimates varying widely from 4% to 86% of individuals with autism presenting epileptiform EEG abnormalities (spikes, spike waves, and slow waves) or nonspecific changes (asymmetry or slowing). Treatment of epilepsy is always indicated; however, there is insufficient evidence to recommend the use of anticonvulsant medications in children with ASD and EEG abnormalities without seizures, as well as no indication that treatment used to normalize the EEG may have a therapeutic effect on the behavior; on the contrary, some evidences show that anticonvulsant treatment, in the presence of epilepsy, improves autistic symptoms in human beings and in animal models but in some patients with ASD, anticonvulsant drugs may worse challenging behavior [76]. Otherwise, higher rates of psychopathology are observed in people with epilepsy relative to the general population, to other neurologic control groups, and to people with chronic non-neurologic disorders. In particular, increased psychopathology is more common in temporal lobe epilepsy than in generalized epilepsy. The link between epilepsy and psychosis has been discussed during the past century, suggesting the concepts of antagonism, i.e., a protection by seizures vs. psychotic disorders, or agonism, i.e., epileptic facilitation vs. the appearance of psychosis (in the chapter Psychosis and ASD the link between psychosis and epilepsy is described) [62, 76].

In adolescence and adulthood, EEG and neuroimaging are indicated only in worsening of cognitive functioning, or in the onset of psychosis or in presence of neurological symptoms, but they are not routinely indicated in all ASD and especially not in Asperger disorders.

Sleep problems are commonly reported in ASD and include difficulties with sleep onset, settling, and night walking. It has been suggested that abnormalities in melatonin production and circadian timing may contribute to insomnia and circadian sleep disturbance in ASD, and melatonin may be effective in treating insomnia in ASD.

Gastrointestinal problems are one of the most commonly reported health concerns in ASD and a trigger of challenging behavior. Gastrointestinal complaints, constipation, diarrhea, feeding and eating problem, and gastric reflux are common. Sometimes this disorders must be detected by unusual stereotypies (hit the abdomen), especially in intellectual disability and language impairment. Food selectivity may be associated with poor nutrition, altered gut motility, and constipation. Celiac disease and lactose intolerance must be detected. In some patients, gluten- and casein-free diet may improve behavior. A gastroenterologist or dietician specialized should direct a diet because an incorrect food selectivity may worsen cognitive functioning and behavior, too.

1.7 Define a Personalized Project of Treatment

This assessment is the basis to build a personalized project of treatment. Collecting data from family and PWA information, clinical examination, cognitive assessment, psychopathological assessment, and medical-genetic condition gives the clinician the information to define the project. A network with family, teacher, social worker, employing center, and the knowledge of the context of living lead to planning a personalized treatment and habilitative program [77].

References

1. Steinhausen H, Mohr Jensen C, Lauritsen M. A systematic review and meta-analysis of the long-term overall outcome of autism spectrum disorders in adolescence and adulthood. Acta Psychiatr Scand. 2016;133(6):445–52.
2. Hirvikoski T, Mittendorfer-Rutz E, Boman M, Larsson H, Lichtenstein P, Bölte S. Premature mortality in autism spectrum disorder. Br J Psychiatry. 2016;208(3):232–8.
3. Bari S, Tisci R, Burlando R, Keller R. Caring for autistic adults. A qualitative analysis under the lens of capability approach. Ital Sociol Rev. 2018;8(2):243–64.
4. Sappok T, Gaul I, Bergmann T, Dziobek I, Bölte S, Diefenbacher A, et al. The diagnostic behavioral assessment for autism spectrum disorder—revised: a screening instrument for adults with intellectual disability suspected of autism spectrum disorders. Res Autism Spectr Disord. 2014;8(4):362–75.
5. Bergmann T, Sappok T, Diefenbacher A, Dames S, Heinrich M, Ziegler M, et al. Music-based autism diagnostics (MUSAD)—a newly developed diagnostic measure for adults with intellectual developmental disabilities suspected of autism. Res Dev Disabil. 2015;43–44: 123–35.
6. Sappok T, Bergmann T, Keller R. In: Bertelli MO, Deb S, Munir K, Hassiotis A, Salvador-Carulla L, editors. Textbook of psychiatry for intellectual disability and autism spectrum disorder. World Psychiatric Association Series. 1st ed. Springer; 2019. In press.
7. Keller R, Bari S, Aresi A, Notaro L, Bianco F, Pirfo E. Valutazione diagnostica dei disturbi dello spettro autistico in età adulta [Diagnosing autism spectrum disorders in adulthood]. J Psychopathol. 2015;21:13–18.
8. Ziegler A, Rudolph-Rothfeld W, Vonthein R. Genetic testing for autism spectrum disorder is lacking evidence of cost-effectiveness. Method Inform Med. 2017;56(3):268–73.
9. Keller R, et al. Disturbi dello spettro autistico in adolescenza e età adulta. Aspetti diagnostici e proposte di intervento. Trento: Edizioni Erickson; 2016.
10. American Psychiatric Association (APA). Diagnostic and statistical manual of mental disorders: DSM-5. 5th ed. Washington, DC: American Psychiatric Association; 2013.
11. World Health Organization (WHO). The ICD-10 classification of mental and behavioural disorders: clinical descriptions and diagnostic guidelines. Geneva: World Health Organization; 1992.
12. Maenner MJ, Rice CE, Arneson CL, Cunniff C, Schieve LA, Carpenter LA, Van Naarden Braun K, Kirby RS, Bakian AV, Durkin MS. Potential impact of DSM-5 criteria on autism spectrum disorder prevalence estimates. JAMA Psychiatry. 2014;71(3):292–300. https://doi.org/10.1001/jamapsychiatry.2013.3893.
13. Krystal JH, State MW. Psychiatric disorders: diagnosis to therapy. Cell. 2014;157:201–14. https://doi.org/10.1016/j.cell.2014.02.042.
14. Biamino E, Di Gregorio E, Belligni EF, Keller R, Riberi E, Gandione M, Calcia A, Mancini C, Giorgio E, Cavalieri S, Pappi P, Talarico F, Fea AM, De Rubeis S, Cirillo Silengo M, Ferrero GB, Brusco A. A novel 3q29 deletion associated with autism, intellectual disability, psychiatric disorders, and obesity. Am J Med Genet B Neuropsychiatr Genet. 2016;171(2): 290–9.
15. Di Gregorio E, Riberi E, Belligni EF, Biamino E, Spielmann M, Ala U, Calcia A, Bagnasco I, Carli D, Gai G, Giordano M, Guala A, Keller R, Mandrile G, Arduino C, Maffè A, Naretto VG, Sirchia F, Sorasio L, Ungari S, Zonta A, Zacchetti G, Talarico F, Pappi P, Cavalieri S, Giorgio E, Mancini C, Ferrero M, Brussino A, Savin E, Gandione M, Pelle A, Giachino DF, De Marchi M, Restagno G, Provero P, Silengo MC, Grosso E, Buxbaum JD, Pasini B, De Rubeis S, Brusco A, Ferrero GB. CNVs analysis in a cohort of isolated and syndromic DD/ID reveals novel genomic disorders, position effects and candidate disease genes. Clin Genet. 2017;92(4):415–22. https://doi.org/10.1111/cge.13009.
16. Luciano CC, Keller R, Politi P, Aguglia E, Magnano F, et al. Misdiagnosis of high function autism spectrum disorders in adults: an Italian case series. Autism. 2014;4:131. https://doi.org/10.4172/2165-7890.1000131.

17. Roy PP, Pal U, Llados J, Delalandre M. Multi-oriented and multi-sized touching character segmentation using dynamic programming. In: Document analysis and recognition. ICDAR'09. 10th International Conference on (pp. 11–15). IEEE; 2009.
18. Brown-Lavoie SM, Viecili MA, Weiss JA. Sexual knowledge and victimization in adults with autism spectrum disorders. J Autism Dev Disord. 2014;44(9):2185–96. https://doi.org/10.1007/s10803-014-2093-y.
19. Rynkiewicz A, Łucka I. Autism spectrum disorder (ASD) in girls. Co-occurring psychopathology. Sex differences in clinical manifestation. Psychiatr Pol. 2018;52(4):629–39. https://doi.org/10.12740/PP/OnlineFirst/58837.
20. Bargiela S, Steward R, Mandy W. The experiences of late-diagnosed women with autism spectrum conditions: an investigation of the female autism phenotype. J Autism Dev Disord. 2016;46(10):3281.
21. Barahona-Corrêa JB, Filipe CN. A concise history of Asperger syndrome: the short reign of a troublesome diagnosis. Front Psychol. 2016;6:2024.
22. Sappok T, Diefenbacher A, Budczies J, Schade C, Grubich C, Bergmann T, et al. Diagnosing autism in a clinical sample of adults with intellectual disabilities: how useful are the ADOS and the ADI-R? Res Dev Disabil. 2013;34(5):1642–55.
23. Matson J, Dempsey T, LoVullo S, Wilkins J. The effects of intellectual functioning on the range of core symptoms of autism spectrum disorders. Res Dev Disabil. 2008;29(4):341–50.
24. Bettelheim B. Empty fortress. New York: Simon and Schuster; 1972.
25. National Institute for Health and Clinical Excellence (NICE). Autism spectrum disorder in adults: diagnosis and management. 2012. https://www.nice.org.uk/guidance/cg142/chapter/1-guidance.
26. Latino V, Bari S, Keller R. La valutazione dei disturbi specifici dell'apprendimento in presenza di disturbi dello spettro autistico in età adulta e in adolescenza. Giornale Italiano dei disturbi del neurosviluppo. 2018;3(1).
27. Westwood H, Tchanturia K. Autism spectrum disorder in anorexia nervosa: an updated literature review. Curr Psychiatry Rep. 2017;19(7):41.
28. Piedimonte A, Nobile E, Keller R. Motor imagery and motor coordination in autism spectrum disorders: similarities and differences. Int J Neurorehabil. 2018;5:310. https://doi.org/10.4172/2376-0281.1000310.
29. Piedimonte A, Conson M, Frolli A, Bari S, Della Gatta F, Rabuffetti M, Keller R, Berti A, Garbarini F. Dissociation between executed and imagined bimanual movements in autism spectrum conditions. Autism Res. 2018;11(2):376–84. https://doi.org/10.1002/aur.1902. Epub 2017 Dec 1. PMID: 29197168.
30. Freeman N, Perry A. Outcomes of intensive behavioural intervention in the Toronto preschool autism service. J Dev Disabil. 2010;16(2):17.
31. Muthugovindan D, Singer H. Motor stereotypy disorders. Curr Opin Neurol. 2009;22(2):131–6. https://doi.org/10.1097/WCO.0b013e328326f6c8.
32. Keller R, Torta R, Lagget M, Crasto S, Bergamasco B. Psychiatric symptoms as late onset of Wilson's disease: neuroradiological findings, clinical features and treatment. Ital J Neurol Sci. 1999;20:49–54.
33. Wechsler D. WISC-III: Wechsler intelligence scale for children. New York: The Psychological Corporation;1991.
34. Wechsler D. Wechsler adult intelligence scale-revised. New York: The Psychological Corporation; 1981.
35. Leiter RG. The Leiter international performance scale. Santa Barbara: Santa Barbara State College Press; 1940.
36. Raven JC. Standard progressive matrices. Firenze: Giunti OS; 1984.
37. Baron-Cohen S, Wheelwright S. The empathy quotient: an investigation of adults with Asperger syndrome or high functioning autism, and normal sex differences. J Autism Dev Disord. 2004;34:163–75.
38. Baron-Cohen S, Wheelwright S, Skinner R, et al. The autism spectrum quotient (AQ): evidence from Asperger syndrome/high-functioning autism, males and females, scientists and mathematicians. J Autism Dev Disord. 2001;31:5–17.

39. Matson J, Boisjoli J, González M, Smith K, Wilkins J. Norms and cut off scores for the autism spectrum disorders diagnosis for adults (ASD-DA) with intellectual disability. Res Autism Spectr Dis. 2007;1(4):330–8.
40. Rutter M, Bailey A, Berument S, Lord C, Pickles A. Social communication questionnaire (SCQ). Los Angeles: Western Psychological Services; 2001.
41. Sappok T, Brooks W, Heinrich M, McCarthy J, Underwood L. Cross-cultural validity of the social communication questionnaire for adults with intellectual developmental disorder. J Autism Dev Disord. 2016;47(2):393–404.
42. Derks O, Heinrich M, Brooks W, Sterkenburg P, McCarthy J, Underwood L, et al. The social communication questionnaire for adults with intellectual disability: SCQ-AID. Autism Res. 2017;10(9):1481–90.
43. Sappok T, Diefenbacher A, Bergmann T, Bölte S, Gaul I, Heinrich M, Dziobek I. Der Diagnostische Beobachtungsbogen für Autismus-Spektrum-Störungen-Revidiert (DiBAS-R). Ein Screening-Instrument für Erwachsene mit Intelligenzminderung. [The diagnostic behavioral assessment for autism spectrum disorder-revised (DIBAS-R). A screening instrument for adults with intellectual disability]. Bern: Huber; 2015.
44. Bertelli M, Scuticchio D, Ferrandi A, Lassi S, Mango F, Ciavatta C, et al. Reliability and validity of the SPAID-G checklist for detecting psychiatric disorders in adults with intellectual disability. Res Dev Disabil. 2012;33(2):382–90.
45. Kraijer DW, La Malfa G, Lassi S. STA-DI. Scala di valutazione dei tratti autistici nelle persone con disabilità intellettiva. Trento: Erickson; 2006.
46. Lord C, Rutter M, LeCouteur A. Autism diagnostic interview-revised (ADI-R). Los Angeles: Western Psychological Services; 2003.
47. Lord C, Rutter M, DiLavore PC, et al. Autism diagnostic observation schedule: ADOS. Los Angeles: Western Psychological Services; 2002.
48. Gilliam JE. Gilliam autism rating scale (GARS). Austin: Pro-Ed; 1995.
49. Ritvo RA, Ritvo ER, Guthrie D, et al. The Ritvo autism Asperger diagnostic scale-revised (RAADS-R): a scale to assist the diagnosis of autism SPECTRUM disorder in adults: an international validation study. J Autism Dev Disord. 2011;41:1076–89.
50. Baron-Cohen S, Wheelwright S, Robinson J, Woodbury-Smith M. The Adult Asperger Assessment (AAA): a diagnostic method. J Autism Dev Disord. 2005;35(6):807–19.
51. Constantino JN. SRS-2 social responsiveness scale. 2nd ed. Los Angeles: Western Psychological Services; 2012.
52. Wing L, Leekam SR, Libby SJ, Gould J, Larcombe M. The diagnostic interview for social and communication disorders: background, inter-rater reliability and clinical use. J Child Psychol Psychiatry. 2002;43(3):307–25.
53. Sparrow SS, Balla DA, Cicchetti DV. The Vineland adaptive behavior scales. Circle Pines: American Guidance Service; 1984.
54. Sundberg M. Vb-mapp. Verbal behavior milestones assessment and placement program. Firenze: Giunti OS; 2008.
55. Mesibov GB, Thomas JB, Chapman SM, et al. TTAP: TEACHH transition assessment profile. Austin: Pro-Ed; 2007.
56. McGreevy P, Fry T, Cornwall C. The essential for living. 2012.
57. Brighenti S, Schintu S, Liloia D, Keller R. Neuropsychological aspects of Asperger syndrome in adults: a review. Neuropsychol Trends. 2018.
58. Keller R, Bari S, Fratianni B, Piedimonte A, Freilone F. Response to Rorschach test in autism spectrum disorders in adulthood: a pilot study. J Psychopathol. 2018;24:224–9.
59. National Institute for Health and Clinical Excellence (NICE). Evidence update 59—autism in adults; 2014. https://arms.evidence.nhs.uk/resources/hub/1035112/attachment.
60. Sedel F, Baumann N, Turpin JC, Lyon-Caen O, Saudubray JM, Cohen D. Psychiatric manifestations revealing inborn errors of metabolism in adolescents and adults. J Inherit Metab Dis. 2007;30(5):631–41.
61. Marazziti D, Baroni S, Picchetti M, Landi P, Silvestri S, Vatteroni E, Catena Dell'Osso M. Psychiatric disorders and mitochondrial dysfunctions. Eur Rev Med Pharmacol Sci. 2012;16(2):270–5.

62. Keller R, Basta R, Salerno L, Elia M. Autism, epilepsy, and synaptopathies: a not rare association. Neurol Sci. 2017;38(8):1353–61. https://doi.org/10.1007/s10072-017-2974-x. Epub 2017 Apr 28.
63. Bilder DA, Burton BK, Coon H, Leviton L, Ashworth J, Lundy BD, Longo N. Psychiatric symptoms in adults with phenylketonuria. Mol Genet Metab. 2013;108(3):155–60.
64. Hall SS, Lightbody AA, Hirt M, Rezvani A, Reiss AL. Autism in fragile X syndrome: a category mistake? J Am Acad Child Adolesc Psychiatry. 2010;49(9):921–33.
65. Moss J, Howlin P. Autism spectrum disorders in genetic syndromes: implications for diagnosis, intervention and understanding the wider autism spectrum disorder population. J Intellect Disabil Res. 2009;53(10):852–73. https://doi.org/10.1111/j.1365-2788.2009.01197.x.
66. Nomura Y. Early behavior characteristics and sleep disturbance in Rett syndrome. Brain Dev. 2005;27:S35–42.
67. Rachubinski AL, Hepburn S, Elias ER, Gardiner K, Shaikh TH. The co-occurrence of Down syndrome and autism spectrum disorder: is it because of additional genetic variations? Prenat Diagn. 2017;37(1):31–6.
68. Harony-Nicolas H, De Rubeis S, Buxabaum JD. Phelan Mc Dermid syndrome: from genetic discoveries to animal models and treatments. J Child Neurol. 2015;30(14):1861–70.
69. Verhoeven WM, Csepan R, Marcelis CL, Lefeber DJ, Egger JI, Tuinier S. Sanfilippo B in an elderly female psychiatric patient: a rare but relevant diagnosis in presenile dementia. Acta Psychiatr Scand. 2010;122(2):162–5.
70. Craig F, Margari F, Legrottaglie AR, Palumbi R, De Giambattista C, Margari L. A review of executive function deficits in autism spectrum disorder and attention-deficit/hyperactivity disorder. Neuropsychiatr Dis Treat. 2016;12:1191.
71. Cauda F, Costa T, Nani A, Fava L, Palermo S, Bianco F, Duca S, Tatu K, Keller R. Are schizophrenia, autistic, and obsessive spectrum disorders dissociable on the basis of neuroimaging morphological findings? A voxel-based meta-analysis. Autism Res. 2017;10(6):1079–95. https://doi.org/10.1002/aur.1759. Epub 2017 Mar 24.
72. Modabbernia A, Velthorst E, Reichenberg A. Environmental risk factors for autism: an evidence-based review of systematic reviews and meta-analyses. Mol Autism. 2017;8:13.
73. Kubota T, Mochizuki K. Epigenetic effect of environmental factors on autism Spectrum disorders. Int J Environ Res Public Health. 2016;13(5):504. https://doi.org/10.3390/ijerph13050504.
74. Matelski L, Van de Water J. Risk factors in autism: thinking outside the brain. J Autoimmun. 2016;67:1–7.
75. Bransfield RC. Aggressiveness, violence, homicidality, homicide, and Lyme disease. Neuropsychiatr Dis Treat. 2018;14:693–713.
76. Keller R, Torta R. Behavioral, psychotic and anxiety disorders in epilepsy: etiology, clinical features and therapeutic indications. Epilepsia. 1999;40(Suppl 10):S2–S20.
77. Murphy CM, Wilson CE, Robertson DM, Ecker C, Daly EM, Hammond N, McAlonan GM. Autism spectrum disorder in adults: diagnosis, management, and health services development. Neuropsychiatr Dis Treat. 2016;12:1669.

Genomic Architecture of ASD

2

Alfredo Brusco and Giovanni Battista Ferrero

2.1 Introduction

Autism Spectrum Disorders (ASDs) are neurodevelopmental disabilities with a large heritable component. Concordance rate in monozygotic twins is 30–99% depending on the study, whereas concordance rates in dizygotic twins and siblings are 0–65% and 3–30%, with an estimated overall heritability of 0.7–0.8 [1]. ASD is clinically heterogeneous with respect to behavior, intellectual function, anthropometric traits (e.g., head size; BMI), and comorbid conditions [2]. The extreme clinical variability parallels the genetic heterogeneity, which is far to be completely identified. Indeed, even if epidemiological evidence from family and twin studies has convincingly demonstrated a strong genetic component to ASD, identifying the responsible genetic variants has been impaired by the lack of appropriate technical genomic tools. Only in recent years, we have rapidly developed novel and sensitive methods such as microarray analyses and next generation sequencing (NGS), which have allowed identifying several novel ASD-associated genetic and genomic lesions.

Several Mendelian diseases have been linked to ASD and genetic evidence suggests that up to 1500 genes are involved in ASD susceptibility [3]. Copy Number Variants (CNVs) explain 5–15% of ASD cases and pathogenic variants in single Mendelian genes likely account for a further 15–20%. Finally, oligogenic or polygenic inheritance may account for a still undetermined, but surely relevant group of patients.

A. Brusco (✉)
Department of Medical Sciences, University of Torino and Medical Genetics Unit, Città della Salute e della Scienza University Hospital, Torino, Italy
e-mail: alfredo.brusco@unito.it

G. B. Ferrero
Department of Public Health and Pediatrics, University of Torino, Regina Margherita Childrens' Hospital, Torino, Italy
e-mail: giovannibattista.ferrero@unito.it

R. Keller (ed.), *Psychopathology in Adolescents and Adults with Autism Spectrum Disorders*, https://doi.org/10.1007/978-3-030-26276-1_2

On the other hand, it is now clear that the same genetic determinant associated with ASD can also cause other neurodevelopmental anomalies, including isolated intellectual disability, or psychiatric disorders. The reason of this variable clinical expressivity is unknown and may be attributed to the genetic background, epigenetic or environmental factors.

The breakthrough of new genetic technologies has evidenced a determinant contribution of *de novo* genomic and genetic variants in ASD, which account for the rarity of familial cases of ASD. This means that these mutations arise in the parental germ cells or in somatic cells of the developing embryo. As for intellectual disability, the strong impact on phenotype associated with a reduced reproductive fitness of the severe ASD forms indicated *a priori* that *de novo* variants play an important role in ASD [4].

2.2 CNVs Associated with Increased Risk for ASD

More than a decade ago, karyotyping and fluorescence in situ hybridization (FISH) have shown the role of rare genomic alterations in ASD [5], including the 7q11.23, 15q11–13, and 22q11.2 regions, already associated with micro-deletion and micro-duplication syndromes, characterized by autistic symptoms as a component [6, 7]. A breakthrough in the discovery of ASD genetic elements was determined by the development of microarray analyses, such as comparative genomic hybridization (CGH), which allowed a higher resolution—as low as 100 kb—compared with karyotype in the detection of CNVs [8]. The first analyses showed that individuals with ASD had 10–20 times the number of CNVs compared to healthy controls [9, 10]. Since then, a number of studies have consistently confirmed that individuals with ASD have more CNVs than non-related controls. In particular, the study of trios (parents and child) has revealed that part of ASD cases are caused by highly penetrant *de novo* CNVs [11, 12] (Table 2.1). The importance of CNVs in ASD is underlined by the fact that microarray methods to search for genomic deletions and duplications are now recommended as first-line genetic tests in ASD [13–16].

Part of the pathogenic CNVs are recurrent, i.e., involve the same genetic region in different affected subjects with *de novo* CNV. These are mediated by unequal crossing-over events due to a peculiar structure of the genomic region involved. On the other hand, many non-recurrent CNVs have been described, and are generated by different and more complex molecular mechanisms [17].

In both cases, a pathogenic CNV involves one or more dose-sensitive gene(s). This term indicates genes whose product amount is critical for the cell function. Its unbalance is thus associated with a genetic disease, both if decreased, such as in deletions, and increased, such as in duplications [18].

Some of the pathogenic CNVs can result in nearly opposite or mirror phenotypes depending on whether they are duplicated or deleted. This reciprocal impact of deletions/duplications is well-known for the 16p11.2 copy number variant. Severe obesity (deletion) and leanness (duplication) have mirror

Table 2.1 CNVs frequently associated with ASD, and their counterparts

Alternative titles/related syndromes	Locus	CNV	Clinical features	OMIM number
Chromosome 1q21.1 deletion syndrome	1q21.1	Loss	Developmental delay, bone and cardiac anomalies	612474
Chromosome 1q21.1 duplication syndrome	1q21.1	Gain	ASD, schizophrenia	612475
Chromosome 2q37 deletion syndrome	2q37.2-q37.3	Loss	ASD	600430
	2q24.2	Loss	ASD	605556
Chromosome 2p16.3 deletion syndrome	2p16.3	Loss	ASD, MR, schizophrenia	614332
Chromosome 3q29 deletion syndrome	3q29	Loss	MR, ASD, schizophrenia, BD	609425
	3p14.2	Loss	ASD	
	3p14.2	Gain	ASD	
	6p23	Loss	ASD	600511
Williams–Beuren region duplication syndrome	7q11.23	Gain	ASD, speech delay, craniofacial anomalies	609757
	7q36.3	Gain	ID, schizophrenia	613959
	7q31.1	Loss		602081
Saethre–Chrotzen syndrome	7p21.1	Loss	ASD	101400
	10q11.23-q21.2	Gain	ASD	610987
	11q13.3-q13.4	Loss	ASD, ID	603290
	13q14.12-q14.13	Loss	ASD	615609
Chromosome 15q13.3 micro-deletion syndrome	15q13.3	Loss	ID, seizures, schizophrenia, ASD, BPD	612001
Duplication 15q11-q13 syndrome	15q11-q13.33	Gain	ASD	608636
Chromosome 15q11.2 deletion syndrome	15q11.2	Loss	ID, ADHD, schizophrenia, ASD	615656
Chromosome 16p13.3 deletion syndrome (Rubinstein–Taybi)	16p13.3	Loss	ASD	610543
Chromosome 16p13.3 duplication syndrome	16p13.3	Gain	ID, speech problems, mild skeletal anomalies	613458
	16p13.1	Gain	ASD, ID, schizophrenia	
Chromosome 16p11.2 deletion syndrome, 220 kb	16p11.2	Loss	Obesity, obesity with developmental delay	613444
Chromosome 16p11.2 deletion syndrome, 593 kb	16p11.2	Loss	ASD	611913
Chromosome 16p11.2 duplication syndrome	16p11.2	Gain	ASD, schizophrenia, ADHD, microcephaly	614671
Chromosome 16p12.1 deletion syndrome, 520-kb	16p12.1	Loss	Developmental delay and learning disability	136570

(continued)

Table 2.1 (continued)

Alternative titles/related syndromes	Locus	CNV	Clinical features	OMIM number
Smith–Magenis syndrome	17p11.2	Loss	ASD	182290
Potocki–Lupski syndrome	17p11.2	Gain	ASD	610883
Chromosome 17q12 deletion syndrome	17q12	Loss	ID, ASD, schizophrenia	614527
Chromosome 17q12 duplication syndrome	17q12	Gain	ID, behavioral abnormalities, psychomotor delay	614526
	22q13.33	Loss	ASD	606230
Chromosome 22q13 duplication syndrome	22q13.33	Gain	ASD, ID	615538
	20p13	Loss	ASD	
Chromosome 22q11.2 deletion syndrome	22q11.2	Loss	ID, schizophrenia, ADHD, other psychiatric disturbances	188400
Chromosome 22q11.2 duplication syndrome	22q11.2	Gain	ASD	608363
	Xp22.11	Loss	ASD, ADHD	300830
	Xq13.1	Loss	ASD, ID	300336

ADHD attention deficit hyperactivity disorder, *ID* intellectual disability

etiologies, possibly through contrasting effects on metabolism regulating energy balance [19]. A similar mirror phenotype is associated with the 7q11.23 deletion/duplication, both leading to multisystem neurodevelopmental disorders. The former is associated with the Williams–Beuren syndrome characterized by extreme friendliness and sociable traits lying at opposite ends of the same behavioral spectrum in duplication 7q11.23 which has language impairment, and autistic like features [20].

In other CNVs, two pathogenic different models have been proposed: (1) in the dominant model, gene expression changes in one direction only (decrease or increase) may contribute to a specific phenotype, with no effect (on the same trait) for a change in the other direction. An example is the immunodeficiency associated with the 22q11.2 deletion, but not observed in the corresponding duplication. (2) In the U-shaped model, genotype–phenotype correlations in reciprocal CNVs have allowed to demonstrate that a reduced or increased number in the number of copies of causal genes can lead to the same phenotype. Among many examples, the 15q13.3 deletion and duplication syndromes are overlapping (i.e., ID, DD, ASD, schizophrenia, ADHD) except for aggressive/impulsive behavior which are reported in deletion, but not duplication, carriers (up to 35%) [20].

Most recurrent CNVs are large (>400 kb), involving dozens of genes, and are individually rare (<0.1%). There are now several well-characterized rare CNVs, clearly associated with a high risk of ASD (Table 2.1). Very large CNVs seem to be further enriched in individuals who have comorbidity with intellectual disability.

Recurrent CNVs can be distinguished in "syndromic," where they are associated to a highly reproducible set of congenital anomalies, or "variable expressive CNVs," resulting in a broad spectrum of disease phenotypes [21].

One emerging aspect of CNVs associated with ASD is that most manifest a wide range of clinical phenotypes. As an example, the 15q13.3 deletion and duplication are now clearly associated with ASD [22], ID [23], epilepsy [24], and schizophrenia [25].

Some CNVs are not only associated with a variable expressivity, but also with an incomplete penetrance. This is clear in families where the transmitting parent is apparently "unaffected" suggesting these CNVs are not sufficient to determine the disease. Indeed, recent works provide evidence for an oligogenic CNV model, where in addition to the primary CNV, a second CNV (inherited or *de novo*) is required at a different locus for a child to develop ASD. This phenomenon is exemplified by the 520-kb deletion on chromosome 16p12.1 (MIM# 136570), which is associated with developmental delay and extensive phenotypic variability [26]. Interestingly, in most cases, this deletion was inherited from a parent who also manifested mild neuropsychiatric features, and the severely affected children were more likely to carry another large (>500 kb) rare CNV.

These results suggest a contribution of rare variants in the genetic background toward neurodevelopmental disorders, depending upon the extent to which the primary variant sensitizes an individual toward a specific pathological phenotypic trajectory [26].

2.3 Rare Highly Penetrant ASD Genes

CNVs are causative in only 5–15% of individuals with ASD, suggesting that other types of mutations must be operant in ASD as well. Rare Mendelian syndromes have been associated with ASD, showing that at least in part ASD is a monogenic disorder [27, 28]. Among these, fragile X syndrome (*FMR1* gene), Rett syndrome (*MECP2* gene), tuberous sclerosis (*TSC1* and *TSC2* genes), Timothy syndrome (*CACNA1C* gene), all display partial comorbidity with ASD [18].

The recent widespread availability of next generation sequencing (NGS) allowed a further increase in the resolution to detect genetic alteration in ASD. Starting from 2008, NGS has allowed to sequence the coding genes of an entire human genome, the so-called whole exome sequencing (WES) strategy, at affordable prices and without the need of an *a priori* hypothesis on the disease gene. A number of large WES studies have been completed in ASD, now encompassing several thousands of individuals [29–35]. Rare autosomal recessive disorders were identified in consanguineous families, affecting for instance the *AMT, BCKDK, C3ORF58, CNTNAP2, NHE9, PCDH10, PEX7, SYNE1, VPS13B, PAH, POMGNT1,* and *SLC9A9* genes [36–38]. These are associated with highly variable clinical presentation, and ASD can be isolated in patients lacking the diagnostic criteria and features of the associated Mendelian disorders. A limited number of X-linked genes have also identified to contribute to ASD, among these, the already cited *FMR1* and *MECP2*, and neuroligins *NLGN3* and *NLGN4* [39, 40]. However, recently new important X-linked genes are emerging such as the X-linked dominant *DDX3X* gene, affecting females only [41].

The list of these genes is still limited and will surely expand in the next years thanks to the new sequencing methods.

2.4 Novel Highly Penetrant ASD Genes

As for CNVs, also single-nucleotide pathogenic variations so far discovered are mainly *de novo* in highly penetrant ASD. These genes behave as autosomal dominant and are rarely found segregating in families (e.g., *SHANK1, SHANK2,* and *SHANK3*) often because their strong effect on reproductive fitness reduction. WES studies identified a number of high-confidence ASD candidate genes that likely may represent up to 20% of cases [42, 43]. Some of them are recurrently hit among families, such as *CHD8, DYRK1A, KATNAL2, GRIN2B, POGZNTNG1*, and *SCN2A* [44]. However, the general notion is that many genes associated with ASD phenotype are likely to be very rare or even "private," unlikely to be found in many individuals. This suggests that rare variants have a larger than originally expected impact on ASD risk, although large cohorts of patients are needed to deepen the knowledge on this issue.

The list of candidate genes involved in ASD is continuously increasing as the complexity of data supporting their pathogenicity. Several groups have tried to develop criteria to rank and assess the strength of evidence associated with candidate genes. Among these one of the most complete databases is SFARI gene (https://gene.sfari.org/), built on information extracted from peer-reviewed scientific and clinical studies on the molecular genetics and biology of ASD [45]. SFARI gene integrates genetic, neurobiological, and clinical information about genes associated with ASD, reporting a total of 956 genes (version 3.0). The annotation criteria used allow dividing genes into seven categories: syndromic genes predisposing to autism in the context of a syndromic disorder (e.g., fragile X syndrome); categories 1 and 2 (high and strong confidence) contain genes with a genome-wide statistical significance, with independent replication; categories 3 and 4 (suggestive and minimal evidence) list genes reported in relatively small studies, whose evidence is still incomplete. Finally, in category 5 (hypothesized but untested) are reported genes that have been implicated solely by evidence in model organisms or other evidence of a marginal nature, and category 6 (evidence does not support a role) is for those genes that have been tested in a human cohort, but the weight of the evidence argues against a role in ASD (Table 2.2).

Table 2.2 ASD genes reported in SFARI database (November 2018)

Category	Definition	N. of genes
Syndromic	Genes with a substantial degree of increased risk for ASD, and consistently linked to additional characteristics not required for an ASD diagnosis	79
Category 1, high confidence	Genes with evidence of recurrent and convincing mutations (functional or large pedigree segregation) accompanied by a rigorous statistical comparison with the mutation frequency in controls. This category also includes single genes that reached genome-wide significance in association studies independently replicated, or which reached genome-wide significance via meta-analysis of all current association studies	25
Category 2, strong candidate	Rare mutations that are recurrent and convincing (see above), accompanied by a rigorous statistical comparison with the mutation frequency in controls. Rare *de novo* variants, likely to be disruptive, in three or more unrelated cases. Results from association studies must reach genome-wide significance, uniquely implicating a single gene, but with no independent replication. Alternatively, consistently replicated association of the same allele, falling short of genome-wide significance, that must be accompanied by evidence that the risk variant has a relevant functional effect in humans	61
Category 3, suggestive evidence	Genes with consistently replicated association of the same allele, without functional support. Rare *de novo* variants, likely to be disruptive, in two or more unrelated cases. Genes within a CNV, or near a GWAS peak close to significance, with additional accessory evidence	184
Category 4, minimal evidence	Genes in an ASD-associated multi-genic CNV, proximal to genome-wide significant intergenic variants for which there is no other independent evidence. Any significant, convincing, but unreplicated association study data, along with any instances of multiple but inconsistent reports of association that are not overall significant by meta-analysis Genes with a series of two or more putative mutations identified (e.g., non-synonymous substitutions, single-gene deletion, duplication, disruption by translocation) for which there is not rigorous statistical comparison with controls Single rare de novo variants, likely to be disruptive	437
Category 5, hypothesized	Genes for which the only evidence comes from studies of model organisms. Genes in a region of linkage with no unique evidence for that gene versus others. Genes shown to functionally interact with category ASD strong candidates. Genes with a single rare variant observed in a single ASD case/family are placed here	170

This table reports a summary whose full text is available at https://gene.sfari.org/about-gene-scoring/

2.5 Common Variants Risk to ASD

High-throughput genotyping of single-nucleotide polymorphisms (SNP) allowed a large number of genome-wide association studies (GWAS) to identify common variants to ASD risk [46]. The potential number of genes likely able to confer moderately-sized risk for ASD is large. In fact, statistical modeling based on published results of both rare and common variation has predicted that up to 1000–1500 genes may ultimately be found to be associated with ASD [35, 47]. The comprehension of how such a large and varied number of genes can all be associated with one common clinical phenotype will be the major challenge to the field. The challenge of understanding how combinations of susceptibility genes interact during human brain development to cause disease (epistasis) has only begun to be explored.

Common variation throughout the genome exerts substantial additive genetic effects on ASD liability, with simplex/multiplex family status having an impact on the identified composition of that risk. As a fraction of the total variation in liability, the estimated narrow-sense heritability exceeds 60% for ASD individuals from multiplex families and is approximately 40% for simplex families. Genome-wide association studies demonstrate that a myriad of common variants of very small effect impacts ASD liability. The identification of such variants needs huge cohorts of patients to be analyzed and represents the challenge of ASD genetics for the next decades [48].

2.6 Biological Insights into ASD

The genetic architecture of ASD has been proved to be complex and the large majority of cases still have no identifiable genetic cause [3, 49]. Despite these limitations, ASD-causing genes have started providing clues on functional pathways involved in the pathogenesis. WES studies have demonstrated grouping of protein–protein interaction networks, enriched for involvement in beta-catenin, p53 signaling, chromatin remodeling, ubiquitination, and neuronal function [29, 34, 43, 47, 50]. The analyses of convergent pathways integrated with experimental findings based on transcriptomic, and cellular and mouse models are now pointing toward three major cellular pathways interconnected through neuronal activity [44, 51].

1. Synapse development and function. The development and/or maintenance of synaptic function seem a critical factor in development of ASD [52]. Among the important genes are those encoding the presynaptic cell-adhesion molecules (CAMs) neurexins (*NRXN1*) and their postsynaptic partners, neuroligins (*NLGN3* and *NLGN4*). Other molecules involved in pre-post synaptic anchoring are the SHANK family (*SHANK3*) and other molecules connected with the actin cytoskeleton (*CNTNAP2*). The most common electrophysiological and neuroanatomical findings evidenced by mouse models of these genes are altered glutamatergic synaptic transmission, loss of inhibitory GABA interneurons, and impairment in synaptic plasticity attributable to dysfunction of NMDA and

AMPA receptors. Similar findings have been reported in the duplication 15q syndrome mouse models (*UBE3A* gene) which recapitulates the three core ASD features [53]. Glutamatergic transmission might represent a targetable pathway in ASD. Indeed, *Fmr1* knockout mice show a hyperactive mGluR5 signaling, leading to excessive protein synthesis at the synapse and increased trafficking of AMPA receptors [54, 55].

2. Growth, transcription regulation, and protein synthesis. Many ASD risk genes (e.g., *TSC1, TSC2,* and *PTEN*) lie downstream the signaling pathway containing mTOR, a key regulator of cell growth, proliferation, and survival. These genes are predicted to alter protein synthesis within synaptic spines, which is necessary for neuronal plasticity and thus proper cognitive function. Among the recently introduced genes in this list, *CDKL5* (Rett-like syndrome) has recently been shown to affect the mTOR pathway [56]. WNT pathway signaling is also considered to have a key role in the etiology of ASD [57, 58]. Defective synaptogenesis (or synaptic function), altered WNT signaling during brain development, and altered transcription and/or translation in neurons can influence neuronal circuit formation and activity [51].
3. Serotonin signaling and neuropeptides. Alterations in the serotoninergic system were among the earliest evidence of abnormal brain function in ASD [59]. Serotonin mediates neurogenesis, cell migration and survival, synaptogenesis and plasticity [60]. Several variants in the serotonin system have been linked to ASD (*SERT/SLC6A4, MAOA*) [61].

A complementary approach to identify biological relationships among identified genes is to analyze the specific expression time window or molecular process. Two independent works showed that ASD genes are likely expressed in the mid-fetal brain (10–12 weeks of gestation), spatially corresponding to superficial glutamatergic neurons [62, 63]. Interestingly, ASD genes encode messenger RNAs interacting with FMRP, encoded by the *FMR1* gene, suggesting that convergence at common pathways of synaptic plasticity associated with gene regulation is mediated by this protein [47, 64].

Overall, a key role for fetal glutamatergic neuron development has been established for ASD, with a growing evidence for converging pathways in ASD-causing genes, with spatiotemporal specific expression pathways [44].

2.7 Conclusion

In recent years, major progress in understanding the genetic architecture of ASD has been made. We now know that both rare and common variants contribute to ASD, with a number of genes and loci implicated. Much remains unknown: the penetrance and expressivity of many ASD genes is still to be determined, as well as the contribution of low penetrance genes in oligogenic forms. Several large-scale projects have just begun to understand both the genetic architecture and the pathophysiological mechanism of these heterogeneous disorders.

Acknowledgements This research received funding specifically appointed to Department of Medical Sciences from the Italian Ministry for Education, University and Research (Ministero dell'Istruzione, dell'Università e della Ricerca—MIUR) under the program "Dipartimenti di Eccellenza 2018–2022" project D15D18000410001, Associazione "Enrico e Ilaria sono con noi" ONLUS, and Fondazione FORMA.

References

1. Ramaswami G, Geschwind DH. Genetics of autism spectrum disorder. Handb Clin Neurol. 2018;147:321–9.
2. American Psychiatric Association. 5th ed. Washington, DC: American Psychiatric Association; 2013.
3. Berg JM, Geschwind DH. Autism genetics: searching for specificity and convergence. Genome Biol. 2012;13(7):247.
4. Vissers LE, de Ligt J, Gilissen C, Janssen I, Steehouwer M, de Vries P, et al. A de novo paradigm for mental retardation. Nat Genet. 2010;42(12):1109–12.
5. Vorstman JA, Staal WG, van Daalen E, van Engeland H, Hochstenbach PF, Franke L. Identification of novel autism candidate regions through analysis of reported cytogenetic abnormalities associated with autism. Mol Psychiatry. 2006;11(1):1, 18–28
6. Somerville MJ, Mervis CB, Young EJ, Seo EJ, del Campo M, Bamforth S, et al. Severe expressive-language delay related to duplication of the Williams-Beuren locus. N Engl J Med. 2005;353(16):1694–701.
7. Mabb AM, Judson MC, Zylka MJ, Philpot BD. Angelman syndrome: insights into genomic imprinting and neurodevelopmental phenotypes. Trends Neurosci. 2011;34(6):293–303.
8. Alkan C, Coe BP, Eichler EE. Genome structural variation discovery and genotyping. Nat Rev Genet. 2011;12(5):363–76.
9. Jacquemont ML, Sanlaville D, Redon R, Raoul O, Cormier-Daire V, Lyonnet S, et al. Array-based comparative genomic hybridisation identifies high frequency of cryptic chromosomal rearrangements in patients with syndromic autism spectrum disorders. J Med Genet. 2006;43(11):843–9.
10. Sebat J, Lakshmi B, Malhotra D, Troge J, Lese-Martin C, Walsh T, et al. Strong association of de novo copy number mutations with autism. Science. 2007;316(5823):445–9.
11. Pinto D, Delaby E, Merico D, Barbosa M, Merikangas A, Klei L, et al. Convergence of genes and cellular pathways dysregulated in autism spectrum disorders. Am J Hum Genet. 2014;94(5):677–94.
12. Pinto D, Pagnamenta AT, Klei L, Anney R, Merico D, Regan R, et al. Functional impact of global rare copy number variation in autism spectrum disorders. Nature. 2010;466(7304):368–72.
13. Miller DT, Adam MP, Aradhya S, Biesecker LG, Brothman AR, Carter NP, et al. Consensus statement: chromosomal microarray is a first-tier clinical diagnostic test for individuals with developmental disabilities or congenital anomalies. Am J Hum Genet. 2010;86(5):749–64.
14. Manning M, Hudgins L, Professional P, Guidelines C. Array-based technology and recommendations for utilization in medical genetics practice for detection of chromosomal abnormalities. Genet Med. 2010;12(11):742–5.
15. Committee on Bioethics; Committee on Genetics, and; American College of Medical Genetics and; Genomics Social; Ethical; Legal Issues Committee. Ethical and policy issues in genetic testing and screening of children. Pediatrics. 2013;131(3):620–2.
16. Volkmar F, Siegel M, Woodbury-Smith M, King B, McCracken J, State M, et al. Practice parameter for the assessment and treatment of children and adolescents with autism spectrum disorder. J Am Acad Child Adolesc Psychiatry. 2014;53(2):237–57.
17. Zhang F, Gu W, Hurles ME, Lupski JR. Copy number variation in human health, disease, and evolution. Annu Rev Genomics Hum Genet. 2009;10:451–81.
18. Sztainberg Y, Zoghbi HY. Lessons learned from studying syndromic autism spectrum disorders. Nat Neurosci. 2016;19(11):1408–17.

19. Jacquemont S, Reymond A, Zufferey F, Harewood L, Walters RG, Kutalik Z, et al. Mirror extreme BMI phenotypes associated with gene dosage at the chromosome 16p11.2 locus. Nature. 2011;478(7367):97–102.
20. Deshpande A, Weiss LA. Recurrent reciprocal copy number variants: roles and rules in neurodevelopmental disorders. Dev Neurobiol. 2018;78(5):519–30.
21. Girirajan S, Rosenfeld JA, Coe BP, Parikh S, Friedman N, Goldstein A, et al. Phenotypic heterogeneity of genomic disorders and rare copy-number variants. N Engl J Med. 2012;367(14):1321–31.
22. Pagnamenta AT, Wing K, Sadighi Akha E, Knight SJ, Bolte S, Schmotzer G, et al. A 15q13.3 microdeletion segregating with autism. Eur J Hum Genet. 2009;17(5):687–92.
23. Sharp AJ, Mefford HC, Li K, Baker C, Skinner C, Stevenson RE, et al. A recurrent 15q13.3 microdeletion syndrome associated with mental retardation and seizures. Nat Genet. 2008;40(3):322–8.
24. Helbig I, Mefford HC, Sharp AJ, Guipponi M, Fichera M, Franke A, et al. 15q13.3 microdeletions increase risk of idiopathic generalized epilepsy. Nat Genet. 2009;41(2):160–2.
25. Stefansson H, Rujescu D, Cichon S, Pietilainen OP, Ingason A, Steinberg S, et al. Large recurrent microdeletions associated with schizophrenia. Nature. 2008;455(7210):232–6.
26. Pizzo L, Jensen M, Polyak A, Rosenfeld JA, Mannik K, Krishnan A, et al. Rare variants in the genetic background modulate cognitive and developmental phenotypes in individuals carrying disease-associated variants. Genet Med. 2019;21(4):816–25.
27. Abrahams BS, Geschwind DH. Advances in autism genetics: on the threshold of a new neurobiology. Nat Rev Genet. 2008;9(5):341–55.
28. Betancur C. Etiological heterogeneity in autism spectrum disorders: more than 100 genetic and genomic disorders and still counting. Brain Res. 2011;1380:42–77.
29. O'Roak BJ, Vives L, Girirajan S, Karakoc E, Krumm N, Coe BP, et al. Sporadic autism exomes reveal a highly interconnected protein network of de novo mutations. Nature. 2012;485(7397):246–50.
30. O'Roak BJ, Deriziotis P, Lee C, Vives L, Schwartz JJ, Girirajan S, et al. Exome sequencing in sporadic autism spectrum disorders identifies severe de novo mutations. Nat Genet. 2011;43(6):585–9.
31. O'Roak BJ, State MW. Autism genetics: strategies, challenges, and opportunities. Autism Res. 2008;1(1):4–17.
32. O'Roak BJ, Stessman HA, Boyle EA, Witherspoon KT, Martin B, Lee C, et al. Recurrent de novo mutations implicate novel genes underlying simplex autism risk. Nat Commun. 2014;5:5595.
33. O'Roak BJ, Vives L, Fu W, Egertson JD, Stanaway IB, Phelps IG, et al. Multiplex targeted sequencing identifies recurrently mutated genes in autism spectrum disorders. Science. 2012;338(6114):1619–22.
34. Neale BM, Kou Y, Liu L, Ma'ayan A, Samocha KE, Sabo A, et al. Patterns and rates of exonic de novo mutations in autism spectrum disorders. Nature. 2012;485(7397):242–5.
35. Sanders SJ, Murtha MT, Gupta AR, Murdoch JD, Raubeson MJ, Willsey AJ, et al. De novo mutations revealed by whole-exome sequencing are strongly associated with autism. Nature. 2012;485(7397):237–41.
36. Musante L, Ropers HH. Genetics of recessive cognitive disorders. Trends Genet. 2014;30(1):32–9.
37. Yu TW, Chahrour MH, Coulter ME, Jiralerspong S, Okamura-Ikeda K, Ataman B, et al. Using whole-exome sequencing to identify inherited causes of autism. Neuron. 2013;77(2):259–73.
38. Morrow EM, Yoo SY, Flavell SW, Kim TK, Lin Y, Hill RS, et al. Identifying autism loci and genes by tracing recent shared ancestry. Science. 2008;321(5886):218–23.
39. Jamain S, Quach H, Betancur C, Rastam M, Colineaux C, Gillberg IC, et al. Mutations of the X-linked genes encoding neuroligins NLGN3 and NLGN4 are associated with autism. Nat Genet. 2003;34(1):27–9.
40. Nava C, Lamari F, Heron D, Mignot C, Rastetter A, Keren B, et al. Analysis of the chromosome X exome in patients with autism spectrum disorders identified novel candidate genes, including TMLHE. Transl Psychiatry. 2012;2:e179.

41. Wang X, Posey JE, Rosenfeld JA, Bacino CA, Scaglia F, Immken L, et al. Phenotypic expansion in DDX3X—a common cause of intellectual disability in females. Ann Clin Transl Neurol. 2018;5(10):1277–85.
42. Iossifov I, O'Roak BJ, Sanders SJ, Ronemus M, Krumm N, Levy D, et al. The contribution of de novo coding mutations to autism spectrum disorder. Nature. 2014;515(7526):216–21.
43. De Rubeis S, He X, Goldberg AP, Poultney CS, Samocha K, Cicek AE, et al. Synaptic, transcriptional and chromatin genes disrupted in autism. Nature. 2014;515(7526):209–15.
44. Chen JA, Penagarikano O, Belgard TG, Swarup V, Geschwind DH. The emerging picture of autism spectrum disorder: genetics and pathology. Annu Rev Pathol. 2015;10:111–44.
45. Abrahams BS, Arking DE, Campbell DB, Mefford HC, Morrow EM, Weiss LA, et al. SFARI gene 2.0: a community-driven knowledgebase for the autism spectrum disorders (ASDs). Mol Autism. 2013;4(1):36.
46. Gaugler T, Klei L, Sanders SJ, Bodea CA, Goldberg AP, Lee AB, et al. Most genetic risk for autism resides with common variation. Nat Genet. 2014;46(8):881–5.
47. Iossifov I, Ronemus M, Levy D, Wang Z, Hakker I, Rosenbaum J, et al. De novo gene disruptions in children on the autistic spectrum. Neuron. 2012;74(2):285–99.
48. Klei L, Sanders SJ, Murtha MT, Hus V, Lowe JK, Willsey AJ, et al. Common genetic variants, acting additively, are a major source of risk for autism. Mol Autism. 2012;3(1):9.
49. Stein JL, Parikshak NN, Geschwind DH. Rare inherited variation in autism: beginning to see the forest and a few trees. Neuron. 2013;77(2):209–11.
50. Michaelson JJ, Shi Y, Gujral M, Zheng H, Malhotra D, Jin X, et al. Whole-genome sequencing in autism identifies hot spots for de novo germline mutation. Cell. 2012;151(7):1431–42.
51. Quesnel-Vallieres M, Weatheritt RJ, Cordes SP, Blencowe BJ. Autism spectrum disorder: insights into convergent mechanisms from transcriptomics. Nat Rev Genet. 2019;20(1):51–63.
52. Zoghbi HY. Postnatal neurodevelopmental disorders: meeting at the synapse? Science. 2003;302(5646):826–30.
53. Smith SE, Zhou YD, Zhang G, Jin Z, Stoppel DC, Anderson MP. Increased gene dosage of Ube3a results in autism traits and decreased glutamate synaptic transmission in mice. Sci Transl Med. 2011;3(103):103ra97.
54. Bear MF, Huber KM, Warren ST. The mGluR theory of fragile X mental retardation. Trends Neurosci. 2004;27(7):370–7.
55. Huber KM, Gallagher SM, Warren ST, Bear MF. Altered synaptic plasticity in a mouse model of fragile X mental retardation. Proc Natl Acad Sci U S A. 2002;99(11):7746–50.
56. Wang IT, Allen M, Goffin D, Zhu X, Fairless AH, Brodkin ES, et al. Loss of CDKL5 disrupts kinome profile and event-related potentials leading to autistic-like phenotypes in mice. Proc Natl Acad Sci U S A. 2012;109(52):21516–21.
57. Kwan V, Unda BK, Singh KK. Wnt signaling networks in autism spectrum disorder and intellectual disability. J Neurodev Disord. 2016;8:45.
58. Hormozdiari F, Penn O, Borenstein E, Eichler EE. The discovery of integrated gene networks for autism and related disorders. Genome Res. 2015;25(1):142–54.
59. Cook EH, Leventhal BL. The serotonin system in autism. Curr Opin Pediatr. 1996;8(4):348–54.
60. Azmitia EC. Serotonin and brain: evolution, neuroplasticity, and homeostasis. Int Rev Neurobiol. 2007;77:31–56.
61. Veenstra-VanderWeele J, Muller CL, Iwamoto H, Sauer JE, Owens WA, Shah CR, et al. Autism gene variant causes hyperserotonemia, serotonin receptor hypersensitivity, social impairment and repetitive behavior. Proc Natl Acad Sci U S A. 2012;109(14):5469–74.
62. Willsey AJ, Sanders SJ, Li M, Dong S, Tebbenkamp AT, Muhle RA, et al. Coexpression networks implicate human midfetal deep cortical projection neurons in the pathogenesis of autism. Cell. 2013;155(5):997–1007.
63. Parikshak NN, Luo R, Zhang A, Won H, Lowe JK, Chandran V, et al. Integrative functional genomic analyses implicate specific molecular pathways and circuits in autism. Cell. 2013;155(5):1008–21.
64. Steinberg J, Webber C. The roles of FMRP-regulated genes in autism spectrum disorder: single- and multiple-hit genetic etiologies. Am J Hum Genet. 2013;93(5):825–39.

3 Neuropsychology of ASD

Stefania Brighenti and Roberto Keller

Autism spectrum disorder (ASD) is a cluster of neurodevelopmental conditions characterized by persistent deficits in social communication and interaction manifested by difficulties in social-emotional reciprocity and in nonverbal communicative behaviors used for social interaction and relationships [1].

In ASD, restricted, repetitive patterns of behavior, interests, or activities are also present (e.g., stereotyped or repetitive speech, excessive adherence to routines, ritualized patterns of verbal or nonverbal behavior, excessive resistance to change or highly restricted, and fixated interests).

All these symptoms are present in early childhood but may not become fully manifest until social demands impair everyday functioning [1].

ASD broad spectrum can be useful as a general conceptualization of autism, but it includes subtypes of disorders with large differences in functioning, even with different neurobiological bases [1–3].

As mentioned above, it is not so easy to analyze ASD as an unitary clinical condition: the definition of "*spectrum*" is intrinsically characterized by an extreme variability, and in clinical practice, many differences emerge among ASD people, for example, Asperger syndrome (AS) or high-functioning autism (HFA) individuals are substantially different from ASD patients who have intellectual disability and therefore require different treatments.

Here, we synthesize results from recent literature about neuropsychological characteristics of ASD focusing our work on differences and similarities among the "*spectrum*."

After a brief theoretical introduction, we provide an analysis about neuropsychological aspects of autism spectrum disorders in adulthood.

A neuropsychological approach of ASD is useful to better explain overlap between brain and behavior [4]. Actually, in recent years, many studies have pointed

S. Brighenti (✉) · R. Keller
Adult Autism Centre, Mental Health Department, Local Health Unit ASL Città di Torino, Turin, Italy

R. Keller (ed.), *Psychopathology in Adolescents and Adults with Autism Spectrum Disorders*, https://doi.org/10.1007/978-3-030-26276-1_3

out different pattern of brain connectivity in ASD, as recently reviewed [5] findings of both cortical underconnectivity and overconnectivity in ASD have occurred. These alternate patterns of brain connectivity are strictly linked with cognitive functioning and—as a consequence—with behavior.

3.1 A Theoretical Introduction

Many theories tried to explain the core symptoms of autism spectrum disorders focusing their attention on different aspects [1].

For example, ASD deficits in mentalizing, understanding other's intentions, believes, emotions, and feelings have been explained as a manifestation of deficits in "Theory of Mind" [6–13].

Second, difficulties in imitation, understanding other's actions, embodying other's emotions and feelings present in autism spectrum disorders can even be due to an ipo-activation of mirror neuron system as described by "Broken Mirror Neurons Theory" [14–16]; this theory explains peculiar behaviors in social interactions in ASD, communicative deficits, and difficulties in understanding other's intentions and the functional meaning of other's actions [1].

Moreover, deficits in mentalizing (e.g., social skills, communication, and imagination) and strength in systemizing (islets of abilities and restricted interest, preference for recurrences and systems, and repetitive behaviors) can be considered as an expression of an "Extreme Systematizing Brain" or an "Extreme Male Brain" [17, 18] accounting for systemizing tendencies and the restricted interests present in autism spectrum disorders.

In recent years, some theory tried to understand autistic symptoms focusing their analysis on neurocognitive characteristics of ASD. Autistic people show strength in capturing details and deficits in synthetizing stimuli in a global representation ("Weak Central Coherence Theory") [19, 20], but enhanced perceptual abilities may be the result of an "Enhanced Perceptual Functioning" [21, 22].

Instead, other theories tried to explain restricted and repetitive behavior and interests, necessity of predictability, and deficits in social cognition, as a manifestation of an "Executive Dysfunctions" [23–26].

3.2 Intelligence

"Intelligence" is a complex concept that "*may be approximately described, but cannot be fully defined.*"[1] Synthetizing different conceptualizations [27], "intelligence" can been defined as the ability to use, to manipulate information in order to solve problems, to make decisions, to judge, and, generally, to act behavior.

"Intelligence" is strictly connected with other cognitive domains like attention, memory, executive functioning and emotional, perceptual, and sensory processing.

[1] Legg S, Hutter M. A collection of definitions of intelligence. AGI; 2006. p. 1.

In clinical practice, the main utilized scales to evaluate IQ are Wechsler Adult Intelligence Scales [28–30].

Until 2008, IQ scores have been calculated with two sub-scores: the Performance IQ (PIQ) and the Verbal IQ (VIQ). The first one allowed to obtain a quantification of verbal abilities, verbal and logic reasoning while the second one could be used to quantify visual and nonverbal reasoning.

After the publication of WAIS-IV [31], the Full Scale IQ is now accompanied by four indices: the Verbal Comprehension Index (similar to VIQ), the Perceptive Reasoning Index (similar to PIQ); the Working Memory Index (working memory and short-term auditory and verbal memory), and Processing Speed Index (selective attention, visual-spatial exploration, and executive speed).

ASD level of intelligence varied from cases with intellectual disability to cases with extremely high IQ: considering this variability and that IQ score seems to remain stable lifetime [32], IQ score can be a considered as a predictor of capabilities outcomes [32, 33].

Our research group recently conduct a preliminary study [34] on 110 ASD (level 1 and 2) adults (mean age 28.16 ± 10.7; 17–58) in order to define their intelligence profiles. On WAIS-IV, 57% of our participants reached a Full Scale IQ score below the average, 36% of the participants achieved a FSIQ in the normative range, and, finally, the 7% obtained a Full Scale IQ score above the average.

Considering the whole sample, the worse index was the Working Memory Index followed by the Processing Speed Index and the Verbal Comprehension Index, whereas the participants obtained better scores on Perceptual Reasoning Index.

Finally, the percentage of normative range scores was similarly distributed between indices.

Numbers of studies have underlined the cognitive variance among ASD spectrum [35, 36] especially between AS and HF.

For example, AS obtain better scores on Full Scale IQ than other individuals with ASD [37].

Comparing HF, AS, and controls, other authors [38] find that HF group showed lower scores than controls regarding Verbal Comprehension and Processing Speed Indices.

Contrarily, no difference have been found between AS and controls on Verbal Comprehension Index, Perceptual Reasoning Index, and Working Memory Index. Comparing HF to AS, AS performance on Processing Speed Index subtests is better than HF. Finally, ASD (both HFA and AS) obtain lower Processing Speed Index score than the control group [38].

Moreover, it seems that those with Asperger syndrome show superior verbal intelligence compared with nonverbal intelligence [39] and obtain verbal IQ scores generally higher than their nonverbal scores even if there is no agreement between authors [37, 38, 40–44].

In this regard, some authors notice an overlap between AS and nonverbal learning disabilities [45].

Contrarily, HF shows the opposite pattern; in high-functioning individuals' PIQ is higher than VIQ [46].

However, other authors shed lights on the fact that both HF and AS individuals showed good performance in visual reasoning tasks and that can be considered as a manifestation of the enhanced perceptual abilities distinctive of the whole autistic spectrum [22]; this hypothesis can be preliminarily confirmed by our previously exposed results too [34].

In summary, the evaluation of general intelligence level could be helpful to understand the cognitive functioning of ASD people in order to better understand how a person may benefit from rehabilitative activities. Furthermore, considering the variability between people IQ and indices scores cloud help to understand how those rehabilitative activities should be designed and tailored. This evaluation should be done for all ASD people adopting adequate tools for each individuals; it is important to examine the intellectual abilities of nonverbal individuals through neuropsychological instruments that allow the assessment by nonverbal stimuli too (for example, Raven Matrices) [21, 22, 47]. The risk is that the level and the nature of intelligence of nonverbal autistic could be underestimated.

3.3 Attentional and Perceptual Abilities

In recent years, many authors provide different models of attentional functions, but there is a certain agreement on a multi-componential definition of "attention" [48].

"Alertness" allows to facilitate the cognitive performance and to maintain a state of general activation working with information processing, whereas "sustained attention" and "vigilance" are necessary to retain an adequate level of responsivity.

"Divided attention" allows to execute two (or more) tasks simultaneously and independently.

"Selective Attention," instead, helps to discriminate the relevant stimuli ignoring the irrelevant ones, focusing the cognitive resources to reach a goal.

There are many neuropsychological instrument to assess attentional abilities [1].

One of those is Trail Making Test (TMT) [49]. This test is employed to evaluate attentive functions, visual scanning, and cognitive speed [50]. TMT is composed of two parts [50]: TMT-A provides a measure of visual-spatial exploration and scanning abilities while TMT-B provides a measure of cognitive and attentional shifting and visual-spatial exploration.

There is an evidence of slower processing speeds in adults with ASD [51] and, regarding Asperger syndrome, using TMT and concerning with attentional abilities, seems to be difficulties in executive speed, visual-spatial exploration, and attentional shifting [1, 24, 52, 53].

To evaluate selective attention, generally visual searching tasks are used.

ASD people show strength in visual searching tasks both when the target item shares many attributes with the distractors and when the target shares less attributes with non-target stimuli. Even when the number of the stimuli is very high, ASD individuals show faster performances than controls [54].

People with ASD seem to have some advantages in visual processing and in visual search tasks as well as in divided-attention tasks, as recently reported [55].

In addition, some authors underlined the presence of intact or superior attention abilities in ASD [56].

Considering the peculiar capacities shown by ASD in visual perception (very good abilities in copy ambiguous figures and less susceptibility of optical illusions [54]), some studies [19, 20] have investigated the perceptual shifting in ASD.

To assess perceptual shifting and local versus global visual perceptual predominance, the Navon task [57] is commonly used.

Individuals with AS have difficulties in shifting from the local to the global elaboration of the stimuli, whereas the control group shows the opposite pattern [58].

The preference for a local elaboration has been recently supported [59]; however, other authors [40] failed to find differences between AS and controls.

The Embedded Figures Test (EFT) [60] is a perceptual task generally used to evaluate the ability to distinguish and discriminate simple shapes from a complex figure [61].

On EFT, there were no differences between AS, HF, and controls in terms of accuracy, but both AS and HF groups were significantly faster than controls [62].

These results are in contrast with recent finding [63] that did not evidence strengths in AS or HF compared to controls on the same test and did not find significant differences between AS, HF, and controls [64].

Finally, as recently reported [65], many studies underling the co-occurrence of attention deficit and hyperactivity disorder (ADHD) in ASD.

In a recent study [66], the effect of the combination of ASD with ADHD was studied: these dysfunctions seem to not be a simple summary of the dysfunctions found in the ASD and in ADHD.

Also, adults with ASD and ADHD showed comparable performance on selective attention tasks, but significant differences emerged in attentional switching: ASD adults are slower and more accurate, whereas ADHD adults were significantly faster and more inaccurate [67].

In any case, in clinical practice, this overlap needs to be deepen.

3.4 Memory

Memory abilities are a range of different cognitive functions [48].

"Memory" can be distinguished primarily relatively to time duration of information in the system in "short-term memory" (brief time) and "long-term memory" (long time of duration).

Depending on the type of the stimuli, long-term memory can be distinct in "episodic" ("autobiographic") and "semantic" memory: the first one operates information about ourselves while the second one allows to memorize and recall events, knowledges, and facts concerning world. These two types of memory are comprised in the "explicit memory" in contrast to "implicit memory": the distinction is based on the possibility consciously and verbally explains the memories: "implicit memory," for example, allows us to go by bike and to drive.

Long-term memory processes are divided into different phases: "learning" and "coding" contribute to elaborate the stimuli, "consolidation" to generate a representation of the information into the system, "storing" allows to record the information whereas "recall" to retrieve the information.

Based on the quality of the stimuli, memory can also been divided into "verbal" and "visual" memory ("visuospatial" as well as "visual" in the strictest sense of the word) [48].

The Rey Auditory Verbal Learning test (RAVLT) [68] is commonly used to evaluate the short-term and long-term verbal memory and verbal learning through a 15-word repetition tasks [69].

Nonverbal memory deficits were found in adults with AS on learning and delayed recall tasks as measured by the RAVLT [52], and on Warrington Recognition Memory Test [70], no significant differences were found between AS individuals and controls in verbal memory tasks [40].

Other authors [71] did not find any impairment in Asperger syndrome on verbal index from Doors and People Battery [72]. The same authors did not find impairment on Wechsler Memory Scale–Revised [73]. These results have been replicated employing Doors and People Battery [53].

No differences in verbal memory between AS individuals and controls as well as between Asperger and high-functioning individuals have been recently found [64] contrasting with the previously findings that underlined deficits in verbal memory in high-functioning autism but not in Asperger syndrome [74].

Concerning verbal memory, as recently summarize [75], ASD used atypical strategies in memory tasks as reduced/absent primacy effect (in contrast to intact recency effect) and show difficulties in using strategies to support episodic memory [76].

Finally, in Asperger syndrome, there seems to be a dissociation between long-term versus short-term verbal memory: despite, as summarized before, some studies [40, 53, 71] reported no impairments in long-term verbal memory, other authors [52] found a significant difference in short-term verbal memory between AS and controls as measured by the Digit Span Forward [73].

In addition, regarding "episodic memory," some authors [77] analyzed "autobiographic memory" in Asperger individuals hypothesizing a possible relationship between autobiographic memory and social problem-solving: in this sense, the "autobiographic memory" would be useful to provide a corpus of experiences and situations from which the individuals would extract information useful to solve social problems. The results of their study showed that AS individuals, compared to the control group, were slower in recalling specific autobiographic episodes.

Lastly, considering differences between types of memory, some authors shed lights on the difficulties in explicit memory but not implicit memory in autism [78].

To quantified long-term visual-spatial memory, the Rey Complex Figure Test (RCFT) [68, 79] is typically used [80].

Measured by RCFT, long-term visual memory of AS did not differ from that of controls [40, 52].

Conversely, other studies [40, 53, 71] found that AS performance is impaired using other visual neuropsychological tools.

Summarizing, there is not agreement concerning visual-spatial memory abilities in Asperger syndrome, and it may be due to the different neuropsychological tools employed [1].

Finally, considering the whole autistic spectrum, visual recognition memory for unknown faces seems to be poorer than controls [81].

3.5 Executive Functions

"Executive Functions" (EF) is a term used to describe human abilities, primarily represented in prefrontal cerebral circuits, to manipulate information in order to direct behavior.

The term comprises a set of high-level cognitive capacity like [65, 82]:

- Flexibly switching between tasks [5, 83] adapting behavior to changes ("flexibility" and "shifting")
- The ability to recall words ("fluency") and to generate different pattern according to executive speed and memory ("generativity")
- The capacity to temporarily maintain and use information during a task ("working memory")
- The abilities to use information from the context in order to plan, to monitor, and to update and consequently to make decision and to act behaviors ("planning," "problem-solving," "judgment," and "reasoning")
- The capacity to inhibit unappropriated response according to different contexts ("inhibitory control").

In any case, executive functions act with all cognitive abilities, linking with attention, memory, language, perceptual capacities.

In clinical practice, there is a variety of neuropsychological tools used to evaluate the executive functions.

For example, planning abilities are assessed employing the Tower of London task [84] or the Hanoi Tower Task [85].

To measure the inhibitory control and the ability to resist to interference, in clinical practice, the Stroop task [86] and Go-no-go tasks [23] are used whereas to assess cognitive flexibility the commonly used test is The Wisconsin Card Sorting Test [87].

The most extensive analysis of cognitive profiles in ASD has been developed within the "Executive Dysfunction Theory" [23, 24].

ASD show impairments in cognitive and conceptual flexibility tasks, in switching and set-shifting [4] planning, mental flexibility, and generativity (verbal and design fluency), but no inhibition or self-monitoring deficits are shown [23].

There are some evidence of a dissociation between verbal and spatial working memory in ASD: verbal working memory seems to be intact while spatial working memory seems to be impaired [88].

In a recent meta-analysis, some evidences of a general impairments in working memory in ASD emerged; this impairment seems to be more consistent in spatial tasks than in verbal tasks [89].

As we recently described [1] regarding Asperger syndrome results are divergent.

On the one hand, there is no agreement if cognitive flexibility is impaired [24, 43, 52, 53, 71] even if there are evidence to support difficulties in set-shifting in individuals with AS [90].

On the other hand, inhibitory control is shown to be a strength [23, 24, 43, 53, 64].

Contrarily, individuals with AS show impairment in planning and problem-solving [23, 24, 41].

Concerning generativity, there is disagreement regarding the presence of deficits in verbal fluency tasks [24, 43, 52, 64, 71, 91].

Lastly, decision-making seems to be in the normal range [52] for Asperger individuals; however, despite comparable performance, AS and controls used different strategies to make decisions.

3.6 Male/Female Differences in Cognition

The "female ASD phenotype" is generally associated with attenuated symptomatology, better language abilities, less repetitive, and stereotyped behavior [92]. In a recent literature review [93], some characteristic often present in ASD female have been reported as, for example, more desire to relate and interact with other people, to camouflage social difficulties, to develop more compensatory strategies, better imagination and fantasy, less bizarre restricted interests.

Considering that evidences, in recent years, beside the previously cited "Extreme Male Brain Theory" and "Female Protectiveness" have been hypothesized [94].

In women, "camouflaging" (to mask autistic traits by imitating others in social interactions and to find compensatory strategies to act like other people) tangles clinical diagnosis of AS, and it also plays a role in the observed male preponderance in ASD [92, 93].

Recent studies underlined the difference between female and male with ASD in terms of cognitive profiles [65].

Comparing ASD female to male, equal mean score on Full Scale IQ have been found [94]. Anyway, the authors found out a more homogeneous cognitive profile in females. Nevertheless, females show higher verbal abilities while males show better executive functions and processing speed.

We recently [34] conduct a preliminary study on a sample of 110 ASD (level 1 and 2) adults (mean age 28.16 ± 10.7; range 17–58). Participants were both ASD men and women (female = 25, 23%; male = 85, 77%); female:male ratio = 1.34.

For each one of the participants, we calculated Full Scale IQ, Verbal Comprehension Index, Visuo-Perceptual Index, Working Memory Index, and Processing Speed Index.

According to the gender, some differences have been found in Full Scale IQ: 56% of female and 57.65% of male show an FSIQ below the normal range; 40% of female and 34.11% of male obtained an FSIQ in the normal range, whereas 4% of female and 8.24% of male showed an FSIQ above the normal range.

Considering Verbal Comprehension Index, no difference has been found; a larger number of male obtained a Perceptive Reasoning Index score above average; a larger number of female obtained a Working Memory Index score below the average, and no female showed Working Memory Index above average. Finally, considering the Processing Speed Index, a larger number of male achieve below average scores; conversely, the number of female who reached a Processing Speed Index score above the range is three times higher than male.

3.7 Cognition Across Life Span

Considering the observed brain connectivity changes across life span in autism spectrum disorders (overconnectivity has been find in children while underconnectivity in adolescents and adults) [5] and the increasing population of adults diagnosed with ASD, recent studies in neuropsychology investigated the cognitive changes across life span in ASD in order to underline cognitive changes and to discover the correspondence between ASD and typical development elderly.

Typical cognitive changes due to age seem to be characterized by worsening of executive functions (working memory and flexibility), memory (episodic memory) and processing speed [95].

Some authors [96] shed light on poorer performance of ASD in respect to elderly with typical development in attentional and executive functioning tasks (working memory and fluency), whereas it seems that ASD show similar performance on processing speed, cognitive flexibility, and working memory tasks.

Other authors underlined the fact that age is related to a poorer cognitive performance in ASD compared to controls, specifically in relation to a decline in executive functioning [95].

ASD elderly and age-matched controls performed likewise on verbal memory task (RAVLT) and visual searching test but (EFT) differences have been found between the two groups on cognitive flexibility (WCST) [97].

Moreover, ASD elderly reported more subjective complaints of cognitive decline of executive functions even when no differences have been found in neuropsychological evaluation [98].

These findings suggest that aging in ASD may affect some cognitive domains while leaving others relatively intact or affected to the same for typical aging [95].

Furthermore, other authors suggest that ASD maybe protective against age-relate cognitive changes [99].

Finally, as previously described, we recently [34] conducted a preliminary study on 110 ASD adults (mean age 28.16 ± 10.7; 17–58) calculating for each one of the participants Full Scale IQ and related indices on WAIS-IV. We stratified results based on age creating four subgroups (age 17–28 = 70, age 29–38 = 23, age 39–48 = 6, age 49–58 = 11).

According to age, we find that, increasing age, the percentage of Full Scale IQ scores below the average diminished; moreover, the percentage of younger participants who showed Full Scale IQ below the average is three times higher while the difference between younger and older participants who achieved Full Scale IQ above the average is 8.5 times higher.

In the younger group (age 17–28), the majority of participants obtained a Full Scale IQ score below the average; in the young adults group (age 29–38), no one reached Full Scale IQ above the average.

We found that the Verbal Comprehension Index score was worse in younger participants (age 17–28) and better for the older group (age 49–58).

Perceptive Reasoning Index score was worse for younger (age 17–28) group and higher for the middle age group (age 39–48).

Regarding Working Memory Index, it was worse for the young adults group (age 29–38), and it was better for elderly (age 49–58); no one of younger participants obtained a Working Memory Index score above the average.

Finally, considering Processing Speed Index, elderly (age 49–58) obtained better cores, whereas younger ASD participants (age 17–28) showed worse scores.

Considering overexposed results, a deepening neuropsychological evaluation in clinical and research context should be done for autistic elderly in order to discriminate and better characterize cognitive "physiological" decline from specific cognitive changes due to age in ASD. Lastly, this assessment will help to define the developmental trajectory of autism spectrum disorders as far as old-age.

3.8 Conclusions

Given the above, neuropsychological difficulties could be present in daily living context and limit the autonomy of ASD people.

Considering the variability of ASD and the impact of neuropsychological deficits in everyday life, a neuropsychological assessment in ASD could be very informative because it provides an overview of strengths and weaknesses for each individual. These information could be precious to support diagnosis as well as to tailor the rehabilitative treatments.

All cognitive functions could be deepened to define activities carried in rehabilitative contexts, in workplaces, and schooling.

References

1. Brighenti S, Schintu S, Liloia D, Keller R. Neuropsychological aspects of Asperger syndrome in adults: a review. Neuropsychol Trends. 2018;24:63–95. https://doi.org/10.7358/neur-2018-024-brig.
2. Biamino E, Di Gregorio E, Belligni EF, Keller R, Riberi E, Gandione M, Calcia A, Mancini C, Giorgio E, Cavalieri S, Pappi P, Talarico F, Fea AM, De Rubeis S, Cirillo Silengo M, Ferrero GB, Brusco A. A novel 3q29 deletion associated with autism, intellectual disability, psychiatric disorders, and obesity. Am J Med Genet B Neuropsychiatr Genet. 2016;171(2):290–9.

3. Di Gregorio E, Riberi E, Belligni EF, Biamino E, Spielmann M, Ala U, Calcia A, Bagnasco I, Carli D, Gai G, Giordano M, Guala A, Keller R, Mandrile G, Arduino C, Maffè A, Naretto VG, Sirchia F, Sorasio L, Ungari S, Zonta A, Zacchetti G, Talarico F, Pappi P, Cavalieri S, Giorgio E, Mancini C, Ferrero M, Brussino A, Savin E, Gandione M, Pelle A, Giachino DF, De Marchi M, Restagno G, Provero P, Cirillo Silengo M, Grosso E, Buxbaum JD, Pasini B, De Rubeis S, Brusco A, Ferrero GB. Copy number variants analysis in a cohort of isolated and syndromic developmental delay/intellectual disability reveals novel genomic disorders, position effects and candidate disease genes. Clin Genet. 2017;92(4):415–22.
4. Joseph RM. Neuropsychological frameworks for understanding autism. Int Rev Psychiatry. 1999;11(4):309–24.
5. Maximo JO, Cadena EJ, Kana RK. The implications of brain connectivity in the neuropsychology of autism. Neuropsychol Rev. 2014;24(1):16–31. https://doi.org/10.1007/s11065-014-9250-0.
6. Pino MC, Mazza M, Mariano M, Peretti S, Dimitriou D, Masedu F, Valenti M, Franco F. Simple mindreading abilities predict complex theory of mind: developmental delay in autism spectrum disorders. J Autism Dev Disord. 2017;47(9):2743–56. https://doi.org/10.1007/s10803-017-3194-1.
7. Baron-Cohen S, Ring H, Moriarty J, Schmitz B, Costa D, Ell P. Recognition of mental state terms. Clinical findings in children with autism and a functional neuroimaging study of normal adults. Br J Psychiatry. 1994;165(5):640–9.
8. Baron-Cohen S, Leslie AM, Frith U. Does the autistic child have a "theory of mind"? Cognition. 1985;21(1):37–46.
9. Fonagy P, Target M. Attachment and reflective function: their role in self-organization. Dev Psychopathol. 1997;9(4):679–700.
10. Frith CD, Frith U. Interacting minds—a biological basis. Science. 1999;286(5445):1692–5.
11. Hadwin J, Baron-Cohen S, Howlin P, Hill K. Does teaching theory of mind have an effect on the ability to develop conversation in children with autism? J Autism Dev Disord. 1997;27(5):519–37.
12. Holroyd S, Baron-Cohen S. Brief report: how far can people with autism go in developing a theory of mind? J Autism Dev Disord. 1993;23(2):379–85.
13. Premack D, Woodruff G. Does the chimpanzee have a theory of mind? Behav Brain Sci. 1978;1(4):515–26.
14. Keller R, Bugiani S, Fantin P, Pirfo E. Mirror neurons and autism. J Psychopathol. 2011;17:404–12.
15. Rizzolatti G, Fabbri-Destro M. Mirror neurons: from discovery to autism. Exp Brain Res. 2010;200(3–4):223–37.
16. Saffin JM, Tohid H. Walk like me, talk like me. The connection between mirror neurons and autism spectrum disorder. Neurosciences (Riyadh). 2016;21(2):108–19.
17. Baron-Cohen S. The extreme male brain theory of autism. Trends Cogn Sci. 2002;6(6):248–54.
18. Baron-Cohen S. The cognitive neuroscience of autism. J Neurol Neurosurg Psychiatry. 2004;75:945–8.
19. Frith U. Autism: explaining the enigma, vol. 1989. Hoboken: Wiley Online Library; 1989.
20. Happé F. Autism: cognitive deficit or cognitive style? Trends Cogn Sci. 1999;3(6):216–22.
21. Mottron L, Dawson M, Soulieres I, Hubert B, Burack J. Enhanced perceptual functioning in autism: an update, and eight principles of autistic perception. J Autism Dev Disord. 2006;36(1):27–43.
22. Mottron L, Bouvet L, Bonnel A, Samson F, Burack JA, Dawson M, Heaton P. Veridical mapping in the development of exceptional autistic abilities. Neurosci Biobehav Rev. 2013;37(2):209–28.
23. Hill EL. Evaluating the theory of executive dysfunction in autism. Dev Rev. 2004;24(2):189–233.
24. Hill EL, Bird CM. Executive processes in Asperger syndrome: patterns of performance in a multiple case series. Neuropsychologia. 2006;44(14):2822–35.
25. Ozonoff S, Jensen J. Brief report: specific executive function profiles in three neurodevelopmental disorders. J Autism Dev Disord. 1999;29(2):171–7.

26. Russell JE. Autism as an executive disorder. New York: Oxford University Press; 1997.
27. Legg S, Hutter M. A collection of definitions of intelligence: AGI; 2006.
28. Wechsler D. Manual for the Wechsler adult intelligence scale-revised. New York: Psychological Corporation; 1981.
29. Wechsler D. WAIS-III: Wechsler adult intelligence scale. San Antonio: Psychological Corporation; 1997.
30. Wechsler D. Wechsler abbreviated scale of intelligence. San Antonio: Psychological Corporation; 1999.
31. Wechsler D. Wechsler adult intelligence scale–fourth edition (WAIS–IV). San Antonio: NCS Pearson; 2008.
32. Magiati I, Tay XW, Howlin P. Cognitive, language, social and behavioural outcomes in adults with autism spectrum disorders: a systematic review of longitudinal follow-up studies in adulthood. Clin Psychol Rev. 2014;34(1):73–86. https://doi.org/10.1016/j.cpr.2013.11.002. Epub 2013 Dec 4.
33. Rutter M. Language disorder and infantile autism. In: Rutter M, Schopler E, editors. Autism: a reappraisal of concepts and treatment. New York: Plenum; 1978.
34. Brighenti S, Bari S, Borroz E, Monti C, Tonella E, Castaldo R, Keller R. Caratterizzazione del profilo intellettivo in pazienti adulti con disturbo dello spettro autistico: analisi descrittive preliminari VII Congresso della Società Italiana di Neuropsicologia, Roma, 23–24 novembre 2018.
35. Morris RG, Rowe A, Fox N, Feigenbaum J, Miotto E, Howlin P. Spatial working memory in Asperger's syndrome and in patients with focal frontal and temporal lobe lesions. Brain Cogn. 1999;41(1):9–26.
36. Noterdaeme M, Wriedt E, Höhne C. Asperger's syndrome and high-functioning autism: language, motor and cognitive profiles. Eur Child Adolesc Psychiatry. 2010;19(6):475–81.
37. Cederlund M, Hagberg B, Gillberg C. Asperger syndrome in adolescent and young adult males. Interview, self-and parent assessment of social, emotional, and cognitive problems. Res Dev Disabil. 2010;31(2):287–98.
38. Holdnack J, Goldstein G, Drozdick L. Social perception and WAIS-IV performance in adolescents and adults diagnosed with Asperger's syndrome and autism. Assessment. 2011;18(2):192–200.
39. Planche P, Lemonnier E. Research in autism spectrum disorders children with high-functioning autism and Asperger's syndrome: can we differentiate their cognitive profiles? Res Autism Spectr Disord. 2012;6(2):939–48.
40. Gunter HL, Ghaziuddin M, Ellis HD. Asperger syndrome: tests of right hemisphere functioning and interhemispheric communication. J Autism Dev Disord. 2002;32(4):263–81.
41. Hagberg BS, Nydén A, Cederlund M, Gillberg C. Asperger syndrome and "non-verbal learning problems" in a longitudinal perspective: neuropsychological and social adaptive outcome in early adult life. Psychiatry Res. 2013;210(2):553–8.
42. Hagberg B, Billstedt E, Nydén A, Gillberg C. Asperger syndrome and nonverbal learning difficulties in adult males: self–and parent–reported autism, attention and executive problems. Eur Child Adolesc Psychiatry. 2015;24(8):969–77.
43. Kleinhans N, Akshoomoff N, Delis DC. Executive functions in autism and Asperger's disorder: flexibility, fluency, and inhibition. Dev Neuropsychol. 2005;27(3):379–401.
44. Soulières I, Dawson M, Gernsbacher MA, Mottron L. The level and nature of autistic intelligence II: what about Asperger syndrome? PLoS One. 2011;6(9):e25372.
45. Klin A, Volkmar FR, Sparrow SS, Cicchetti D, Rourke BP. Validity and neuropsychological characterization of Asperger syndrome: convergence with nonverbal learning disabilities syndrome. J Child Psychol Psychiatry. 1995;36(7):1127–40.
46. Montgomery CB, Allison C, Lai MC, Cassidy S, Langdon PE, Baron-Cohen S. Do adults with high functioning autism or Asperger syndrome differ in empathy and emotion recognition? J Autism Dev Disord. 2016;46(6):1931–40.
47. Raven JC. Standardization of progressive matrices, 1938. Psychol Psychother Theory Res Pract. 1941;19(1):137–50.

48. Vallar G, Papagno C, Manuale di Neuropsicologia. Il Mulino Ed., Bologna; 2007.
49. Reitan RM. Validity of the trail making test as an indicator of organic brain damage. Percept Mot Skills. 1958;8(3):271–6.
50. Tombaugh T. Trail making test A and B: normative data stratified by age and education. Arch Clin Neuropsychol. 2004;19(2):203–14.
51. Haigh SM, Walsh JA, Mazefsky CA, Minshew NJ, Eack SM. Processing speed is impaired in adults with autism spectrum disorder and relates to social communication abilities. J Autism Dev Disord. 2018;48(8):2653–62. https://doi.org/10.1007/s10803-018-3515-z.
52. Torralva T, Gleichgerrcht E, Roca M, Ibanez A, Marenco V, Rattazzi A, Manes F. Impaired theory of mind but intact decision-making in Asperger syndrome: implications for the relationship between these cognitive domains. Psychiatry Res. 2013;205(3):282–4.
53. Towgood KJ, Meuwese JD, Gilbert SJ, Turner MS, Burgess PW. Advantages of the multiple case series approach to the study of cognitive deficits in autism spectrum disorder. Neuropsychologia. 2009;47(13):2981–8.
54. Vivanti G. La mente autistica; le risposte della ricerca scientifica al mistero dell'autismo. Omega Ed. Torino; 2010.
55. Rutherford MD, Richards ED, Moldes V, Sekuler AB. Evidence of a divided-attention advantage in autism. Cogn Neuropsychol. 2007;24(5):505–15. https://doi.org/10.1080/02643290701508224.
56. Minshew N, Goldstein G, Siegel D. Neuropsychologic functioning in autism: profile of a complex information processing disorder. J Int Neuropsychol Soc. 1997;3(4):303–16.
57. Navon D. Forest before trees: the precedence of global features in visual perception. Cogn Psychol. 1977;9(3):353–83.
58. Katagiri M, Kasai T, Kamio Y, Murohashi H. Individuals with Asperger's disorder exhibit difficulty in switching attention from a local level to a global level. J Autism Dev Disord. 2013;43(2):395–403.
59. Carther-Krone TA, Shomstein S, Marotta JJ. Looking without perceiving: impaired preattentive perceptual grouping in autism spectrum disorder. PLoS One. 2016;11(6):e0158566.
60. Witkin HA, Oltman PK, Raskin E, Karp SA. A manual for the embedded figures test. Palo Alto: Consulting Psychologists Press; 1971.
61. Happé F. Embedded figures test (EFT). In: Volkmar FR, editor. Encyclopedia of autism spectrum disorders. New York: Springer; 2013. p. 1077–8.
62. Jolliffe T, Baron-Cohen S. Are people with autism and Asperger syndrome faster than normal on the embedded figures test? J Child Psychol Psychiatry. 1997;38(5):527–34.
63. Spek AA, Scholte EM, van Berckelaer-Onnes IA. Local information processing in adults with high functioning autism and Asperger syndrome: the usefulness of neuropsychological tests and self-reports. J Autism Dev Disord. 2011;41(7):859–69.
64. Wilson CE, Happé F, Wheelwright SJ, Ecker C, Lombardo MV, Johnston P, Daly E, Murphy CM, Spain D, Lai MC, Chakrabarti B, Sauter DA, MRC AIMS Consortium, Baron-Cohen S, Murphy DG. The neuropsychology of male adults with high-functioning autism or Asperger syndrome. Autism Res. 2014;7(5):568–81.
65. Zwick GP. Neuropsychological assessment in autism spectrum disorder and related conditions. Dialogues Clin Neurosci. 2017;19(4):373–9.
66. Nydén A, Niklasson L, Stahlberg O, Anckarsater H, Wentz E, Rastam M, Gillberg C. Adults with autism spectrum disorders and ADHD neuropsychological aspects. Am J Psychiatry. 2006;163:1239–44.
67. Johnston K, Dittner A, Bramham J, Murphy C, Knight A, Russell A. Attention deficit hyperactivity disorder symptoms in adults with autism Spectrum disorders. Autism Res. 2013;6(4):225–36. https://doi.org/10.1002/aur.1283.
68. Rey A. L'examen psychologique dans les cas d'encéphalopathie traumatique. (Les problems). Archives de psychologie. 1941;28:215–85.
69. Baddeley AD, Kopelman MD, Wilson BA. The handbook of memory disorders. New York: Wiley; 2002.

70. Warrington EK. Recognition memory test: Rmt.(words). Test booklet 1. Nashville: NFER-Nelson Publishing Company; 1984.
71. Ambery FZ, Russell AJ, Perry K, Morris R, Murphy DG. Neuropsychological functioning in adults with Asperger syndrome. Autism. 2006;10(6):551–64.
72. Baddeley AD, Emslie H, Nimmo-Smith I. Doors and people: a test of visual and verbal recall and recognition. San Antonio: Harcourt Assessment; 2006.
73. Wechsler D. Wechsler memory scale. San Antonio: Psychological Corporation; 1945.
74. Ozonoff S, Rogers SJ, Pennington BF. Asperger's syndrome: evidence of an empirical distinction from high-functioning autism. J Child Psychol Psychiatry. 1991;32:1107–22. https://doi.org/10.1111/j.1469-7610.1991.tb00352.x.
75. Shalom DB. Memory in autism: review and synthesis. Cortex. 2003;39(4–5):1129–38. https://doi.org/10.1016/S0010-9452(08)70881-5.
76. Williams DL, Minshew NJ, Goldstein G, Mazefsky CA. Long-term memory in older children/adolescents and adults with autism spectrum disorder. Autism Res. 2017;10:1523–32. https://doi.org/10.1002/aur.1801.
77. Goddard L, Howlin P, Dritschel B, Patel T. Autobiographical memory and social problem-solving in Asperger syndrome. J Autism Dev Disord. 2007;37(2):291–300. https://doi.org/10.1007/s10803-006-0168-0.
78. Ring M, Gaigg SB, Bowler DM. Object-location memory in adults with autism spectrum disorder. Autism Res. 2015;8:609–19. https://doi.org/10.1002/aur.1478.
79. Osterrieth P. Test of copying a complex figures: contribution to the study of perception and memory. Arch Psychol. 1944;20:206–356.
80. McKinlay A. Rey complex figure test encyclopedia of child behavior and development. Boston: Springer; 2011. p. 1264–5.
81. Blair RJ, Frith U, Smith N, Abell F, Cipolotti L. Fractionation of visual memory: agency detection and its impairment in autism. Neuropsychologia. 2002;40(1):108–18.
82. Chung HJ, Weyandt LL, Swentosky A. The physiology of executive functioning. In: Goldstein S, editor. Jack A. Naglieri handbook of executive functioning. New York: Springer-Verlag; 2014.
83. Miyake A, Friedman NP, Emerson MJ, Witzki AH, Howerter A. The unity and diversity of executive functions and their contributions to complex "frontal lobe" tasks: a latent variable analysis. Cogn Psychol. 2000;41:49–100.
84. Shallice T. Specific impairments of planning. Philos Trans R Soc Lond B Biol Sci. 1982;298(1089):199–209.
85. Bishop D, Aamodt-Leeper G, Creswell C, McGurk R, Skuse D. Individual differences in cognitive planning on the tower of Hanoi task: neuropsychological maturity or measurement error? J Child Psychol Psychiatry Allied Discip. 2001;42(4):551–6.
86. Stroop JR. Studies of interference in serial verbal reactions. J Exp Psychol. 1935;18(6):643–62.
87. Berg EA. A simple objective technique for measuring flexibility in thinking. J Gen Psychol. 1948;39(1):15–22.
88. Williams DL, Goldstein G, Carpenter PA, Minshew NJ. Verbal and spatial working memory in autism. J Autism Dev Disord. 2017;35(6):747.
89. Wang Y, Zhang YB, Liu LL, Cui JF, Wang J, Shum DH, van Amelsvoort T, Chan RC. A meta-analysis of working memory impairments in autism Spectrum disorders. Neuropsychol Rev. 2017;27(1):46–61. https://doi.org/10.1007/s11065-016-9336-y. Epub 2017 Jan 19.
90. Brady DI, Schwean VL, Saklofske DH, McCrimmon AW, Montgomery JM, Thorne KJ. Conceptual and perceptual set-shifting executive abilities in young adults with Asperger's syndrome. Res Autism Spectr Disord. 2013;7(12):1631–7.
91. Spek AA, Schatorje T, Scholte E, van Berckelaer-Onnes I. Verbal fluency in adults with high functioning autism or Asperger syndrome. Neuropsychologia. 2009;47(3):652–6.
92. Lai M-C, Lombardo MV, Ruigrok AN, Chakrabarti B, Auyeung B, Szatmari P, Happé F, Baron-Cohen S, MRC AIMS Consortium. Quantifying and exploring camouflaging in men and women with autism. Autism. 2017;21(6):690–702.

93. Lai MC, Lombardo MV, Auyeung B, Chakrabarti B, Baron-Cohen S. Sex/gender differences and autism: setting the scene for future research. J Am Acad Child Adolesc Psychiatry. 2015;54(1):11–24.
94. Lehnhardt FG, Falter CM, Gawronski A, Pfeiffer K, Tepest R, Franklin J, Vogeley K. Sex-related cognitive profile in autism spectrum disorders diagnosed late in life: implications for the female autistic phenotype. J Autism Dev Disord. 2016;46(1):139–54. https://doi.org/10.1007/s10803-015-2558-7.
95. Powell PS, Klinger LG, Klinger MR. Patterns of age-related cognitive difference in adults with autism spectrum disorders. J Autism Dev Disord. 2017;47:3204. https://doi.org/10.1007/s10803-017-3238-6.
96. Geurts HM, Vissers ME. Elderly with autism: executive functions and memory. J Autism Dev Disord. 2012;42:665–75.
97. Braden B, Smith CJ, Thompson A, Glaspy TK, Wood E, Vatsa D, et al. Executive function and functional and structural brain differences in middle-age adults with autism spectrum disorder. Autism Res. 2017;10(12):1945–59. https://doi.org/10.1002/aur.1842.
98. Davids RD, Groen Y, Berg IJ, Tucha OM, van Balkom IC. Executive functions in older adults with autism spectrum disorder: objective performance and subjective complaints. J Autism Dev Disord. 2016;46(9):2859–73. https://doi.org/10.1007/s10803-016-2831-4.
99. Lever AG, Geurts HM. Age-related differences in cognition across the adult lifespan in autism spectrum disorder. Autism Res. 2016;9:666–76. https://doi.org/10.1002/aur.1545.

4 Psychosis and ASD

Roberto Keller and Stefania Bari

4.1 Clinical Evaluation

The strict relationship between psychosis and ASD was present since the first definition of "autism" itself.

Kanner, in his description of the first autistic patients, took the term "autism" from Bleuler, who had collocated this characteristic within the core clinical symptom of schizophrenia [1, 2].

Initially and until the *DSM III*, we observed an almost complete overlapping between "childhood schizophrenia" and ASD. This overlapping was followed, later, by a rigid division of these two disorders, without the possibility of comorbidity; now, in the *DSM 5* [3], it is possible to define comorbidity between autism and schizophrenia when both the positive symptoms of schizophrenia (SCZ) and the characteristics of ASD are present in a patient [4].

A considerable number of ASD patients meet the criteria for a psychotic disorder (12–15%) [5–7].

Up to 40% of ASD patients meet formal criteria for a schizotypal personality disorder.

Autistic behavior traits may overlap with the schizotypal and schizoid ones [8].

We described through case series the possible clinical characteristics found in the comorbidity between psychotic disorders and ASD [9].

We observe several different types of relationship between psychosis and ASD.

R. Keller (✉) · S. Bari
Adult Autism Centre, Mental Health Department, Local Health Unit ASL Città di Torino, Turin, Italy

R. Keller (ed.), *Psychopathology in Adolescents and Adults with Autism Spectrum Disorders*, https://doi.org/10.1007/978-3-030-26276-1_4

4.1.1 Misdiagnosis of Psychosis Instead of ASD

It is possible in clinical practice to observe patients diagnosed with schizophrenia or schizotypal personality disorder that are non-recognized ASD. This possibility is more frequent in older patients in Europe and in higher functioning autism, especially Asperger syndrome, because this syndrome was unknown in the past to psychiatrist who considered only Kanner's autism. So, a misdiagnosis of schizophrenia instead of ASD could be related to the historical data that nosographic description of Asperger syndrome, defined in 1944 by Hans Asperger, was not yet diffused in Europe since its translation made by Lorna Wing. Thus, persons with Asperger syndrome (now defined as ASD level 1 in *DSM 5*) who received a diagnosis from psychiatrists before this period were frequently considered part of other diagnostic categories instead of ASD and, in primis, schizophrenia.

We observed several cases of ASD misdiagnosis that share common clinical features [10]. All are characterized by normal verbal communication and fluent grammar, and all were brought to the attention of a physician because of relational problems, perceived not by the patient but by his/her family members or school teachers. Behaviors concerning interpersonal communication difficulties and patterns of repetitive behavior are less commonly perceived by the patient and his/her environment as a good reason to visit a doctor. The correct diagnosis could be made only after considering all the clinical features and especially a detailed developmental history of their early childhood that is the clinical key for distinguishing SCZ from ASD. Otherwise, if only a single cluster of symptoms is taken into account without neurodevelopmental patient data, cases can easily suggest other psychiatric or personality disorders, which are more familiar to the psychiatrist. Thus, aberration in language and apparently bizarre behavior can induce a misdiagnosis of schizophrenia, and chronic social withdrawal and difficulty in relationship with others can induce a misdiagnosis of schizoid/schizotypal personality disorder and so on.

The negative and catatonic manifestations of SCZD are similar to the social withdrawal and communicative difficulty in ASD that even specific tests, such as the Autism Diagnostic Observation Schedule (ADOS) [11], sometimes fail and produce false ASD positives if performed on adolescent patients with SCZD [12].

Also the RAADS—*Ritvo Autism and Asperger's Diagnostic Scale-Revised* [13]—evaluation must be related to patient neurodevelopmental history and not used as unique test to differential diagnosis between ASD and SCZ. The same is for Minnesota Multiphasic Personality Inventory (MMPI), if used as self-reported test, because persons with autism (PWA) may answer to question literally, and this may lead to misdiagnosis of psychosis. Rorschach test could be useful in ASD to detect psychotic functioning [14]. ADI-r interview could help clinician to a correct analysis of first years of patient's life, but in Asperger syndrome we can also observe false negative in ADI-r because symptoms are detected only when the child go to school, where higher social skills are requested [15].

One of the distinguishing features of schizoid personality disorder is a marked narrowing of effect with an impaired capacity for emotional experience and expression. Differently from ASD, schizoid personality disorder does not show pleasure in sexual and affective relationship and does not really want others; on the contrary, PWA generally lack the social skill to easily get a sexual or affective relationship or to have a family, but they like it.

Schizotypal personality disorder is typified by seemingly eccentric social contact behavior with apparently paranoid perceptual distortion and bizarre convictions (magical thinking), but differently from schizophrenia, there aren't delusions or hallucinations.

Persons with ASD are hypomentalizers and fail to recognize social cues such as verbal hints, body language, and gesticulations, but persons with schizophrenia-like personality disorders tend to be hypermentalizers, overinterpreting such cues in a generally suspicious way. Most people with schizophrenia and schizophrenia-like personality disorders displayed well-adapted social behavior in childhood, along with apparently normal emotional function. Autistic signs are common in adolescents with schizotypal personality disorder, but autistic features are not linked with conversion to psychosis [16].

4.1.2 Autistic Pseudopsychosis

Persons with autism (PWA) may consider the reality from a literal point of view. So they can misread a joke as a serious event. They may also react to a change of their rigid routine or to a hypersensoriality stimulus (visual, noise, etc.) with tantrum or irritability, or psychomotor agitation apparently without significance. So they may be driven to Emergency Psychiatric Ward and diagnosed as acute psychosis.

A challenge behavior may also be related to physical pain that the persons with autism (PWA) are unable to describe.

Also a typical autistic meltdown, with psychomotor agitation, or an acute shutdown, with acute social withdrawal, linked for example to a sensory or activity overload, could be misdiagnosed as an acute psychotic episode.

So, visiting a PWA with psychomotor agitation, we have to first check some of the following items:

1. Is there pain? Is there an organic cause of the agitation? Is it possible to use a drug for pain such as paracetamol to detect this possibility? The PWA must be examined from an organic point of view.
2. Has the PWA routine changed and was he not prepared to change? We have to collect information from parents, social workers, etc.
3. Is there a sensorial stimulus as a trigger of agitation? We must know the characteristic of PWA, and his reaction to specific sensorial stimulus.
4. Does the PWA have difficulty to understand the environment? We must know that PWA may have difficulty in prosody or may detect external situations from a single detail and that if we change a single detail, it is a "world change" for the PWA, and that he prefers visual communication, so we have to explain how to read the reality correctly.

4.1.3 Transitory Reactive Paranoid Psychosis

In patients affected by ASD, and in particular in the Asperger syndrome, the scholastic or work discrimination is a frequent event and represents a stressful trigger that in turn elicits anxiety, depressive, and transient psychotic episodes. This happens in particular when a patient does not know to be affected by ASD (especially by Asperger), and thus, he does not know how to adequately relate or comprehend the hostility of the external environment, considering that often this hostility is caused accidentally by the patient behavior itself: he does not understand the world and the world does not understand him.

Clinicians must be careful because an acute paranoid psychosis could cover a misdiagnosed ASD.

4.1.4 Comorbidity of ASD and Paranoid Personality Disorder and/or Narcissistic Personality Disorder

Personality disorders may be observed in comorbidity with ASD. In these patients, we observe two distinct aspects: The classical "vengeance" thirst proper of a paranoid personality, associated with a narcissistic aspect (e.g., reflected in their need to write to the maxim authority) and also the ingenuity of the Asperger syndrome, (the patient could describe to unknown people his private life in public Facebook profile).

The presence of these comorbidities renders complex the treatment of Asperger syndrome because the narcissistic paranoid aspects are amplified when they are under the stress of a relationship and when they have to work with other people, and difficulties in relationship are also strictly related to Asperger syndrome, so it became a circuit that could lead to acute psychotic paranoid episodes.

4.1.5 Schizophrenic Evolution of an ASD

Some patients, diagnosed with ASD in their childhood, show a schizophrenic development in adolescence or adulthood, accompanied by neurodegenerative aspects and cognitive impairment [9].

As we know, we cannot wait for positive symptoms of psychosis (as requested in *DSM 5*) to diagnose this "comorbidity" (or, better, this psychotic evolution).

We must take care to a decline in cognitive functioning and in academical results that could be a symptom of the ASD neurodegenerative evolution toward schizophrenia [17–24]. School performance is a point of strength in high functioning ASD and especially in Asperger syndrome, so a decline is not usual in ASD without comorbidity. Visuospatial processing impairment and some memory deficits are apparent before the full expression of psychotic illness, and ultra-high risk patients who develop psychosis have impairment in the visual reproduction subtest and verbal memory index owing to low logical memory scores of the Wechsler Memory Scale [23]. In schizophrenia, negative symptoms are related to a pervasive pattern of worsening performance across a broad range of neuropsychological function as verbal memory, abstraction and executive function, perceptual and motor speed, attentional function, and vigilance. Sustained attention and working memory deficit are trait markers of schizophrenia not consequent to delusions or side effects of drugs. Also a selective impairment in the attentional ability to inhibit prepotent response during attentional task (as detected by Stroop index color-word) is related to psychosis. Crystallized verbal skill is related to impairment in neurocognitive function and performance-based skills in everyday life function [25]. A neuropsychological evaluation of ASD patients may help to detect cognitive worsening, that if related to patient functioning impairment could be a marker of psychosis; in this situation, we can help patients before that full-blown positive symptoms (delusion and hallucinations) occur, as requested in *DSM 5*. Useful tests for clinical practice are Wechsler Intelligence Scale, Repeatable Battery for the Assessment of Neuropsychological Status—RBANS, the MATRICS Evaluation, the Brief Assessment of Cognition in Schizophrenia, the Brief Cognitive Assessment, and the Social Cognition Assessment [26, 27]. A neurocognitive rehabilitation treatment could be useful in this situation and also in detecting of trigger events to avoid them [28].

4.1.6 Affective Psychosis, Especially in Bipolar Disorder

In adolescence, an acute psychotic episode may represent the onset of a bipolar disorder, especially after the use of antidepressant drugs.

As described in the chapter of bipolar disorder, this comorbidity is higher in ASD compared to general population.

The first acute psychotic episode, also with delusion or hallucination, must not lead directly to a diagnosis of schizophrenia, because a psychotic mania is very similar in clinical presentation to schizophrenia, also with paranoid delusion that could also be present in mania.

4.2 Neurobiological Basis

There are numerous clinical and neurobiological links between SCZ and ASD that lead to hypothesize a deficit of a transdiagnostic cognitive circuitry linked to genetic–environmental pathogenesis of a unique neurodevelopmental disorder [17, 29–31].

Individuals with ASD and those with schizophrenia (SCZ) are characterized by marked social deficits, with impoverished social networks. Both groups are impaired in basic emotion perception. SCZ and ASD perform similarly to one another on social cognitive tasks and in social perceptual theory of mind [32].

ASD shows impaired performance on most domain of executive function (mental flexibility, sustained attention, and fluency), and early psychosis shows impairment on sustained attention and attentional shifting [29].

A substantial proportion of adults with schizophrenia (and bipolar disorder) show high autistic-like traits and symptoms, suggesting a shared pathophysiology among ASD and SCZ.

In schizophrenia, the distributed nature of brain region abnormalities suggests that multiple brain circuits are impaired, a neural feature that may be better addressed with network level analyses [33].

SCZ is related to neuropathological brain changes which are believed to disrupt connectivity between brain processes. In the first psychotic episode, SCZ patients show evidence of GM loss in cortical areas and in limbic structure as hippocampus, thalamus, striatum, and cerebellum. Consistent with disturbed neural connectivity, WM alterations have been observed in limbic structures, corpus callosum, and many subgyral and sublobar regions in the parietal, temporal, and frontal lobes [34]. Poor performance on the WCST in early psychosis subjects identifies those who have more marked cognitive impairment [35].

Even if schizophrenia spectrum disorder (SCZD), autism spectrum disorder (ASD), and obsessive compulsive spectrum disorder (OCSD) are considered in *DSM 5* as clinically separate psychiatric conditions with, supposedly, different brain alteration patterns, we described a meta-analytic study from a neuroimaging perspective aimed to address whether this nosographical differentiation is actually supported by different brain patterns of gray matter (GM) or white matter (WM) morphological alterations. Our analysis reveals that these psychiatric spectra do not present clear distinctive patterns of alterations; rather, they all tend to be distributed in two alteration clusters:

- Cluster 1, which is more specific for SCZD, includes the anterior insular, anterior cingulate cortex, ventromedial prefrontal cortex, and frontopolar areas, which are parts of the cognitive control system.
- Cluster 2, which is more specific for OCSD, presents occipital, temporal, and parietal alteration patterns with the involvement of sensorimotor, premotor, visual, and lingual areas, thus forming a network that is more associated with the auditory-visual, auditory, and premotor visual somatic functions. In turn, ASD appears to be uniformly distributed in the two clusters [36].

Studying the patterns of co-alteration distribution from voxel-based morphological data, we analyzed the patterns of brain alterations of SCZD, ASD, and OCSD. The analysis of the co-atrophy network of schizophrenia spectrum disorder (SCZD), ASD, and obsessive compulsive spectrum disorder (OCSD) reveals that alterations in certain GM sites appear to be statistically related to alterations of other GM regions. Although this finding has already been proven to be the case in neurodegenerative diseases, it has never been found before in psychiatric conditions [37].

The clusters of co-altered areas form a net of alterations that can be defined as morphometric co-alteration network (MCN) or co-atrophy network (in the case of gray matter decreases). Within this network, specific cerebral areas can be identified as pathoconnectivity hubs, the alteration of which is supposed to enhance the development of neuronal abnormalities. Within the morphometric co-atrophy network of SCZD, ASD, and OCSD, a subnetwork composed of 11 highly connected nodes can be distinguished. This subnetwork encompasses the anterior insula, inferior frontal areas, left superior temporal areas, left parahippocampal regions, left thalamus, and right precentral gyri. The co-altered areas also exhibit a normal structural covariance pattern which overlaps, for some of these areas (like the insula), the co-alteration pattern. These findings reveal that, similarly to neurodegenerative diseases, psychiatric disorders are characterized by anatomical alterations that distribute according to connectivity constraints so as to form identifiable morphometric co-atrophy patterns.

In particular, our results indicate that a small number of brain areas show a high degree of pathoconnectivity and only a few cerebral areas appear to be particularly co-altered with several other regions; so, regions that play an important role in the formation and development of the MCN can be thought of as pathoconnectivity hubs. Brain sites with the highest network degree were found to be the insula and the prefrontal cortices, which are also strictly connected with each other. These regions are therefore pathoconnectivity hubs and can be considered as primary altered areas, whereas the other brain regions, which have a lower network degree and appear to be connected only with specific pathoconnectivity hubs, can be considered as secondary altered areas. We identify within the MCN a "core" subnetwork composed of 11 nodes located in the insula, inferior frontal gyrus, superior temporal gyrus, thalamus, and right precentral gyrus. Some of these regions are involved in supporting the salience network, an essential part of the frontoparietal control system. The disruption of the functional integrity of this network would account for the executive deficits that are frequently observed across schizophrenia and ASD. Alteration of the areas forming the MCN may lead to a disruption of social cognition, which is frequently associated with ASD and SCZD [38]. Social cognition refers to our abilities to recognize, manipulate, and behave with respect to socially relevant information, including the ability to construct representation flexibly to guide social behavior. Amygdala is part of the structures that form the basis of social cognition, and bilateral damage to the human amygdala has been found to impair social judgments of trustworthiness and approachability of people based on their faces. There is a clear relationship between the aspects of functional outcome and social cognition in schizophrenia and autism.

The insula has a role in the integration of external sensory stimuli with emotions, the conscious perception of error, the generation and maintenance of a state of awareness associated with the body's condition [39–43]. The anterior insula is involved in interoceptive, affective, and empathic processes and is a part of the salience network integrating external sensory stimuli with internal states as a hub mediating interactions between large-scale networks involved in externally and internally oriented cognitive processing: dysfunctional anterior insula connectivity plays an important role in autism [44].

Our analysis reveals that particularly the anterior part of the insular cortex seems to be mostly involved in the formation of the MCN associated with SCZD and ASD.

The STG multimodal areas are involved in cortical integration of both sensory and limbic information implicated in the social perceptual skills. STG is thought to process the biological motion [45, 46] and has been associated with some verbal and nonverbal communication impairments observed in patients with ASD [47].

Precentral and inferior frontal gyri are involved in the mirror neuron system; GM thinning in regions associated with the mirror neuron system has been correlated with social and communication deficits in patients with ASD [48–51].

The disruption of the thalamus has been variously associated with SCZD and ASD, and a reduced GM density in the thalamus, right cerebellum hemisphere, and left temporoparietal cortex is related to intellectual disabilities in ASD [52]. Other findings suggest a relationship between hypoconnectivity disturbances in the thalamofrontal system and ASD [53]. The thalamus is also supposed to play an important role in the inflammatory processes.

In both ASD and SCZD, disruption of the loop system of the basal ganglia is thought to explain impaired sensorimotor access, which reflects the ability of an organism to filter out irrelevant stimuli; hippocampal disruption has been associated with both ASD and SCZD [54]. Hippocampal deficits are an established feature of schizophrenia and are complementary with evidences of marked allocentric processing deficits of psychosis; hippocampal could be viewed as a cognitive map, with spatial maps built in right hippocampus and semantic maps in left hippocampus.

The fact that neuronal abnormalities caused by SCZD and ASD converge on a set of core areas that are associated with cognitive control functions [55, 56] is also consistent with previous evidence showing that in brain disorders GM alterations and WM alterations tend to exhibit concordant patterns of distribution, which are influenced by brain connectivity [57–60].

Proteins such as astrotactin have been suggested as a common genetic link among these different spectra, because they are fundamental in guiding neuron migration during brain development [61].

Oxytocin, a hormone related to the regulation of social behavior and the formation of pair bonds, has been found to be involved in psychiatric disorders, including ASD and SCZD. In patients with ASD, oxytocin appears to be related to social recognition, attachment, and stereotyped behaviors, whereas in patients with SCZD it has been associated with a potential antipsychotic effect [62–66].

The relative symptomatic similarity between ASD and SCZD is consistent with a neurobiological model that suggests a common basis for SCZD and ASD, with a number of genetic alterations (SHANK 3 variations, DISC 1, dysregulation of CYFIP1, SCN2A, NRXN1 neurexin gene, or RELN), cytoarchitectural abnormalities (about proliferation, migration, and lamination defects), neuropsychological deficit, neuroimaging investigations (about GM/WM abnormalities and structural/functional connectivity alterations), and clinical observations [31, 67–74].

It is possible that there are genes that can be linked to the social cognitive defects, such as Disrupted in Schizophrenia 1 (DISC 1) gene, choroidal neurovascularization disruption of the neurexin-1 (NRXN1) gene, in both SCZ and ASD.

Autistic-like traits, detected also with Social Responsiveness Scale for Adults, are higher in subjects with schizophrenia and bipolar disorder than in general population, suggesting a shared pathophysiology among ASD and SCZ and bipolar disorder [75]. The high "comorbidity" between ASD, ADHD, intellectual disability, SCZ, and bipolar disorder challenge the etiological basis of current diagnostic categories and suggest that we should consider neurodevelopmental disorders as a unique group of related and overlapping syndromes that result in part as a combination of genetic and environmental effects on brain development [76]. All the clinical data might be accounted for by finding out the common genetic roots at the basis of neurodevelopment disorders, which bring about phenotypic expressions with different timings and modalities, due to epigenetic factors affecting the production of proteins with regulatory function over the brain organization and development [77]. This hypothesis is consistent with the clinical examination of families of patients with ASD, in which phenotypic expressions bear psychiatric disorders different from ASD and SCZD [78]. The relationship between genes, epigenetic, and environmental factors could emerge from the specific patterns of structural alterations, and brain hubs are likely to be the areas in which this relationship appears to be stronger. Both schizophrenia and ASD are highly heritable, with 25–33% genetic contribution to schizophrenia and 49% to ASD.

A genetic model of the link between SCZ and ASD could be the 22q11.2 deletion syndrome (Di George syndrome), a neurogenetic disorder affecting 1 in 2000–4000 live births. This syndrome in 90% of cases arises from de novo mutation and is associated with high rates of psychosis (41%) and ASD (14–50%); also ADHD is frequent in this syndrome (37%) overrepresented in males, and anxiety disorders and mood disorders, too [79]. Up to 30% of adolescents and adults develop a schizophrenia-like psychosis [80]. ASD and SCZ represent two unrelated phenotypic manifestations consistent with a neuropsychiatry pleiotropy model. This genetic lesion provides a unique model for the discovery of specific genome risk and potentially protective factors for neuropsychiatric disease. The rate of psychosis and mood disorders increases dramatically in adolescence and young adulthood, and a cognitive deterioration in adolescence is a dynamic phenotype that may be a potent predictor of psychosis in the 22q11 deletion syndrome. In this syndrome, we could also observe an early onset Parkinson's disease that suggests a role of a dopaminergic system disruption in older patients [80, 81]. Other than velocardiofacial signs, in these patients seizures could be observed, which are typically related to hypocalcemia, an easily identifiable specific factor [82–84].

The neurobiological substrate of common alterations in ASD and SCZS may involve a neurochemical unbalance, especially an alteration in the ratios of GABA–glutamate on the one hand and oxytocin–vasopressin on the other, which could be the targets of specific pharmacological therapies for ASD [85, 86], as balovaptan. In syndromic ASD, metabotropic glutamate receptor 5 (mGLUr5) CNVs are more prevalent; the dysregulation of the mGLUr network is a possible permissive factor that increases propensity to develop an ASD [87]. Deficits of synchronous firing of neurons required for higher order cognitive functioning have been observed in SCZ and have been attributed to deficits of GABA signaling-related mRNAs and proteins; also GABAergic neurons in the subcortical white matter are affected in psychosis [88]. ASD and SCZ have an overlap linked to social disorganization, and the high expression of the SD phenotype may be associated with increased glutamate/GABA ratio in the right auditory regions, which may affect prosody processing [85].

Several studies have supported a role of neuroinflammation in the etiology of ASD, SCZD, and other brain disorders [89, 90]. In fact, an increased inflammatory response in the central nervous system is supposed to activate microglial cells, the activity of which leads to the release of pro-inflammatory cytokines, including interleukin (IL)-1b, IL-6, and tumor necrosis factor-a. In turn, pro-inflammatory cytokines aggravate and propagate neuroinflammation, thus degenerating healthy neurons and impairing brain functions. The activated microglia may contribute to the generation of GM abnormalities and, consequently, to the pathogenesis of psychiatric disorders [91]. Microglia is supposed to regulate excitatory and inhibitory input to pyramidal neurons [92]. Differences in neuroinflammatory response in individual immune response and environmental factors may explain different age of clinical onset of ASD and SCZ. The development of ASD, differently from SCZD, appears to be more related to cerebellar dysfunction and subsequent thalamic hyperactivation in early childhood. In contrast, SCZD seems to be triggered by thalamic hyperactivation in late adolescence, whereas hippocampal aberration can possibly originate in childhood. The possible culprits could be found in the metal homeostasis disturbances, which can induce dysfunction of blood–cerebrospinal fluid barrier. Thalamic hyperactivation is thought to be produced by microglia-mediated neuroinflammation as well as by abnormalities of the intracerebral environment. Consequently, it is likely that thalamic hyperactivation leads to the dysregulation of the circuit formed by dorsolateral prefrontal cortex and lower brain regions related to social cognition [37, 89].

Evidence support the role of neuroinflammation in the link between ASD and SCZ that involve microglia (the inflammatory brain-resident myeloid cells) and biomarkers (cytokines, oxidative stress markers, and microRNA players) that influence cellular processes at brain and immune levels.

Approaches of functional connectivity reveal that specific parameters of connectivity networks present heritability and are associated with familial risk for psychopathology, suggesting a genetic role not only with regard to single psychiatric categories but with regard to the brain inter-regional synchronization, thus confirming liability to broad dimensions of symptomatically related disorders [55, 93]. Mental illness is generally characterized by polygenic inheritance, which constantly causes genetic liability. This defies the validity of rigid categorical models of psychiatric disorder and risk, as it implies also that brain disorders can be viewed as the extreme manifestations of distributed quantitative traits; so the presence of ASD and SCZ in a patient could be viewed as a unique neurodevelopmental disorder, with early onset in ASD and late onset in SCZ. So it is not correct to describe the association ASD–SCZ in a patient as a "comorbidity," but we have to think better as a "schizophrenic evolution of ASD" or a late onset of a unique neurodevelopmental disorder, linked to common genetic basis, too [94].

4.3 Treatment

Otherwise, we must remember that ASD and SCZ need specific and distinct treatment and that if we observe a schizophrenic evolution of an ASD, we have to consider both the treatment, for psychosis and for ASD. ASD is not a psychosis, indeed.

Using antipsychotic drugs in ASD could be related to:

- Treating symptoms not related to ASD core symptoms, as irritability, and in this case risperidone and aripiprazole are FDA-approved drugs [95, 96].
- Treating true psychotic symptoms in ASD. This is related to the same treatment of psychosis than in general population.

We have to take care that ASD population may have very individually specific response to the drugs; so, the response to the specific drug and side effects are less predictable than in general population, and so the dose of the drug must be strictly personalized with a "tailor" technique, with frequent controls of the patient especially in the first period of treatment itself.

A role in pathogenesis and in the treatment of biological condition linked to ASD and psychosis could be related to microbiome. The extinction of key "heirloom" taxa can deprive individuals of metabolic pathways that have been present in their ancestors for millennia. Some of these pathways support essential synthesis and toxin clearance processes. So clinicians must pay attention to a microbiome equilibrium that could be one of the pieces of the complexity of the treatment [97].

References

1. Bolte S, Rudolf L, Poustka F. The cognitive structure of higher functioning autism and schizophrenia: a comparative study. Compr Psychiatry. 2002;43(4):325–30.
2. Tarazi FI, Sahli ZT, Pleskow J, Mousa SA. Asperger's syndrome: diagnosis, comorbidity and therapy. Expert Rev Neurother. 2015;15(3):281–93.
3. American Psychiatric Association (APA). Diagnostic and statistical manual of mental disorders: DSM-5. 5th ed. Washington, DC: American Psychiatric Association; 2013.
4. Carpenter WT, Tandon R. Psychotic disorders in DSM-5: summary of changes. Asian J Psychiatr. 2013;6(3):266–8.
5. Hofvander B, Delorme R, Chaste P, Nyden A, Wentz E, Stahlberg O, Hebrecht E, Stopin A, Anckarsater H, Gillberg C, Rastam M, Leboyer M. Psychiatric and psychosocial problems in adults with normal—intelligence autism spectrum disorders. BMC Psychiatry. 2009;9:35.
6. Lugnegard T, Hallerback MU, Gillberg C. Psychiatric comorbidity in young adults with a clinical diagnosis of Asperger syndrome. Res Dev Disabil. 2011;32(5):1910–7.
7. Larson FV, Wagner AP, Jones PB, Tantam D, Lai M-C, Baron-Cohen S, Holland A. Psychosis in autism: comparison of the features of both conditions in a dually affected cohort. Br J Psychiatry. 2017;210(4):269–75.
8. Lehnhardt F, Gawronski A, Pfeiffer K, Kockler H, Schilbach L, Vogeley K. The investigation and differential diagnosis of Asperger syndrome in adults. Dtsch Arztebl Int. 2013;110(45):755–63.
9. Keller R, Piedimonte A, Bianco F, Bari S, Cauda F. Diagnostic characteristics of psychosis and autism spectrum disorder in adolescence and adulthood. A case series. Autism Open Access. 2015;6:159.
10. Luciano CC, Keller R, Politi P, Aguglia E, Magnano F, et al. Misdiagnosis of high function autism spectrum disorders in adults: an Italian case series. Autism. 2014;4:131.
11. Lord C, Rutter M, Di Lavore PC, et al. Autism diagnostic observation schedule: ADOS. Los Angeles: Western Psychological Services; 2002.
12. Bertelli MO, Rossi M, Scuticchio S, Bianco A. Diagnosing psychiatric disorders in people with intellectual disabilities: issues and achievements. Adv Ment Health Intellect Disabil. 2015;9(5):230–42.

13. Ritvo RA, Ritvo ER, Guthrie D, et al. The Ritvo Autism Asperger Diagnostic Scale-Revised (RAADS-R): a scale to assist the diagnosis of Autism Spectrum Disorder in adults: an international validation study. J Autism Dev Disord. 2011;41:1076–89.
14. Keller R, Bari S, Fratianni B, Piedimonte A, Freilone F. Response to Rorschach test in autism spectrum disorders in adulthood: a pilot study. J Psychopathol. 2018;24:224–9.
15. Lord C, Rutter M, LeCouteur A. Autism Diagnostic Interview-Revised (ADI-R). Los Angeles: Western Psychological Services; 2003.
16. Esterberg ML, Trotman HD, Brasfield JL, Compton MT, Walker EF. Childhood and current autistic features in adolescents with schizotypal personality disorder. Schizophr Res. 2008;104:265–73.
17. Mayoral M, Merchan-Naranjo J, Rapado M, Leiva M, Moreno C, Giraldez M, Arango C, Parellda M. Neurological soft signs in juvenile patients with Asperger syndrome, early onset psychosis, and healthy controls. Early Interv Psychiatry. 2010;4:283–90.
18. Kern RS, Neuchterlein KH, Green MF, Baade LE, Fenton WS, Gold JM, Keefe RSE, Mesholam-gately R, Mintz J, Seidman LJ, Stover E, Marder S. The MATRICS consensus cognitive battery, part 2: co-norming and standardization. Am J Psychiatr. 2008;165: 214–20.
19. Fitzgerald D, Lucas S, Redoblado MA, Winter V, Brennan J, Anderson J, et al. Cognitive functioning in young people with first episode psychosis: relationship to diagnosis and clinical characteristics. Aust N Z J Psychiatry. 2004;38:501–10.
20. Howes OD, Fusar-Poli P, Bloomfield M, Selvaraj S, McGuire P. From the prodrome to chronic schizophrenia: the neurobiology underlying psychotic symptoms and cognitive impairments. Curr Pharm Des. 2012;18(4):459–65.
21. Harvey PD, Green MF, Keefe RS, Velligan DI. Cognitive functioning in schizophrenia: a consensus statement on its role in definition and evaluation of effective treatments for the illness. J Clin Psychiatry. 2004;65(3):361–72.
22. Rund BR, Melle I, Friis S, Larsen TK, Midbøe LJ, Opjordsmoen S, Simonsen E, Vaglum P, McGlashan T. Neurocognitive dysfunction in first-episode psychosis: correlates with symptoms, premorbid adjustment, and duration of untreated psychosis. Am J Psychiatry. 2004;161(3):466–72.
23. Brewer WJ, Francey SM, Wood SJ, Jackson H, Pantelis C, Philiès LJ, Yung AR, Anderson VA, McGorry PD. Memory impairments identified in people at ultra-high risk of psychosis who later develop first-episode psychosis. Am J Psychiatr. 2005;162(1):71–8.
24. Casacchia M, Mazza M, Roncone R. Theory of mind, social development and psychosis. Curr Psychiatry Rep. 2004;6:183–9.
25. Kurtz MM, Donato J, Rose J. Crystallized verbal skills in schizophrenia: relationship to neurocognition symptoms, and functional status. Neuropsychology. 2011;25(6):784–91.
26. Rocca P, Castagna F, Marchiaro L, Rasetti R, Rivoira E, Bogetto F. Neuropsychological correlates of reality distortion in schizophrenic patients. Psychiatry Res. 2006;145:49–60.
27. Montemagni C, Rocca P. Assessing cognition and real-world functioning in schizophrenia. J Psychopathol. 2018;24:49–59.
28. Cavallaro R, Bechi M, Spangaro M. Targeting social cognition to improve functional outcome of patients with schizophrenia: clinical evidence. Journal of Psychopathol. 2018;24:88–92.
29. Demetriou EA, Song CY, Park SH, Pepper KL, Naismith SL, Hermens DF, Hickie IB, Thomas EE, Norton A, White D, Guastella AJ. Autism, early psychosis, and social anxiety disorder: a transdiagnostic examination of executive function cognitive circuitry and contribution to disability. Transl Psychiatry. 2018;8(1):200. https://doi.org/10.1038/s41398-018-0193-8.
30. Uher R, Zwicker A. Etiology in psychiatry: embracing the reality of poly-gene-environmental causation of mental illness. World Psychiatry. 2017;16:121–9.
31. De Lacy N, King BH. Revisiting the relationship between autism and schizophrenia: toward an integrated neurobiology. Annu Rev Clin Psychol. 2013;9:555–87.
32. Couture SM, Penn DL, Losh M, Adolphs R, Hurley R, Piven J. Comparison of social cognitive functioning in schizophrenia and high functioning autism: more convergence than divergence. Psychol Med. 2010;40(4):569–79.

33. Wheeler AL, Voineskos AN. A review of structural neuroimaging in schizophrenia: from connectivity to connectomics. Front Hum Neurosci. 2014;8:653.
34. Watson DR, Anderson JME, Bai F, Barrett SL, McGinnity TM, Mulholland CC, Rushe TM, Cooper SJ. A voxel based morphometry study investigating brain structural changes in first episode psychosis. Behav Brain Res. 2012;227(1):91–9.
35. Addington J, Saeedi H, Addington D. The course of cognitive functioning in first episode psychosis: changes over time and impact on outcome. Schizophr Res. 2005;78:35–43.
36. Cauda F, Costa T, Nani A, Fava L, Palermo S, Bianco F, Duca S, Tatu K, Keller R. Are schizophrenia, autistic, and obsessive spectrum disorders dissociable on the basis of neuroimaging morphological findings?: a voxel-based meta-analysis. Autism Res. 2017;10(6):1079–95.
37. Cauda F, Nani A, Costa T, Palermo S, Tatu K, Manuello J, Duca S, Fox PT, Keller R. The morphometric co-atrophy networking of schizophrenia, autistic and obsessive spectrum disorders. Hum Brain Mapp. 2018;39(5):1898–928.
38. Bicks LK, Koike H, Akbarian S, Morishita H. Prefrontal cortex and social cognition in mouse and man. Front Psychol. 2015;6:1805.
39. Cauda F, Costa T, Torta DM, Sacco K, D'agata F, Duca S, Vercelli A. Meta-analytic clustering of the insular cortex: characterizing the meta-analytic connectivity of the insula when involved in active tasks. Neuroimage. 2012;62:343–55.
40. Cauda F, Geda E, Sacco K, D'agata F, Duca S, Geminiani G, Keller R. Grey matter abnormality in autism spectrum disorder: an activation likelihood estimation metaanalysis study. J Neurol Neurosurg Psychiatry. 2011;82:1304–13.
41. Klein TA, Ullsperger M, Danielmeier C. Error awareness and the insula: links to neurological and psychiatric diseases. Front Hum Neurosci. 2013;7:14.
42. Vercelli U, Diano M, Costa T, Nani A, Duca S, Geminiani G, Cauda F. Node detection using high-dimensional fuzzy parcellation applied to the insular cortex. Neural Plast. 2016;2016:1938292.
43. Wylie KP, Tregellas JR. The role of the insula in schizophrenia. Schizophr Res. 2010;123:93.
44. Uddin QL, Menon V. The anterior insula in autism: under-connected and under-examined. Neurosci Biobehav Rev. 2009;33:1198–203.
45. Jou RJ, Jackowski AP, Papademetris X, Rajeevan N, Staib LH, Volkmar FR. Diffusion tensor imaging in autism spectrum disorders: preliminary evidence of abnormal neural connectivity. Aust N Z J Psychiatry. 2011;45:153–62.
46. Jou RJ, Mateljevic N, Kaiser MD, Sugrue DR, Volkmar FR, Pelphrey KA. Structural neural phenotype of autism: preliminary evidence from a diffusion tensor imaging study using tract-based spatial statistics. AJNR Am J Neuroradiol. 2011;32:1607–13.
47. Radua J, Via E, Catani M, Mataix-Cols D. Voxel-based meta-analysis of regional white-matter volume differences in autism spectrum disorder versus healthy controls. Psychol Med. 2011;41:1539–50.
48. Cattaneo L, Rizzolatti G. The mirror neuron system. Arch Neurol. 2009;66:557–60.
49. Keller R, Bugiani S, Fantin P, Pirfo E. Mirror neurons and autism. Giornale Italiano Psicopatologia. 2011;17:404–12.
50. Kilner JM, Friston KJ, Frith CD. The mirror-neuron system: a Bayesian perspective. Neuroreport. 2007;18:619–23.
51. Rizzolatti G, Craighero L. The mirror-neuron system. Annu Rev Neurosci. 2004;27:169–92.
52. Spencer MD, Moorhead TW, Lymer GK, Job DE, Muir WJ, Hoare P, Johnstone EC. Structural correlates of intellectual impairment and autistic features in adolescents. NeuroImage. 2006;33:1136–44.
53. Cheon KA, Kim YS, Oh SH, Park SY, Yoon HW, Herrington J, Schultz RT. Involvement of the anterior thalamic radiation in boys with high functioning autism spectrum disorders: a diffusion tensor imaging study. Brain Res. 2011;1417:77–86.
54. Wible CG. Hippocampal temporal-parietal junction interaction in the production of psychotic symptoms: a framework for understanding the schizophrenic syndrome. Front Hum Neurosci. 2012;6:180.

55. Buckholtz JW, Meyer-Lindenberg A. Psychopathology and the human connectome: toward a transdiagnostic model of risk for mental illness. Neuron. 2012;74:990–1004.
56. McTeague LM, Goodkind MS, Etkin A. Transdiagnostic impairment of cognitive control in mental illness. J Psychiatr Res. 2016;83:37–46.
57. Iturria-Medina Y, Evans AC. On the central role of brain connectivity in neurodegenerative disease progression. Front Aging Neurosci. 2015;7:90.
58. Raj A, Kuceyeski A, Weiner M. A network diffusion model of disease progression in dementia. Neuron. 2012;73:1204–15.
59. Voytek B, Knight RT. Dynamic network communication as a unifying neural basis for cognition, development, aging, and disease. Biol Psychiatry. 2015;77:1089–97.
60. Zhou J, Gennatas ED, Kramer JH, Miller BL, Seeley WW. Predicting regional neurodegeneration from the healthy brain functional connectome. Neuron. 2012;73:1216–27.
61. Lionel AC, Tammimies K, Vaags AK, Rosenfeld JA, Ahn JW, Scherer SW. Disruption of the ASTN2/TRIM32 locus at 9q33.1 is a risk factor in males for autism spectrum disorders, ADHD and other neurodevelopmental phenotypes. Hum Mol Genet. 2014;23:2752–68.
62. Cochran DM, Fallon D, Hill M, Frazier JA. The role of oxytocin in psychiatric disorders: a review of biological and therapeutic research findings. Harv Rev Psychiatry. 2013;21:219–47.
63. Humble MB, Uvnas-Moberg K, Engstrom I, Bejerot S. Plasma oxytocin changes and anti-obsessive response during serotonin reuptake inhibitor treatment: a placebo controlled study. BMC Psychiatry. 2013;13:344.
64. Romano A, Tempesta B, Micioni Di Bonaventura MV, Gaetani S. From autism to eating disorders and more: the role of oxytocin in neuropsychiatric disorders. Front Neurosci. 2015;9:497.
65. Shin NY, Park HY, Jung WH, Park JW, Yun JY, Jang JH, Kwon JS. Effects of oxytocin on neural response to facial expressions in patients with schizophrenia. Neuropsychopharmacology. 2015;40(8):1919–27.
66. Strauss GP, Keller WR, Koenig JI, Gold JM, Frost KH, Buchanan RW. Plasma oxytocin levels predict social cue recognition in individuals with schizophrenia. Schizophr Res. 2015;162:47.
67. Baribeau DA, Anagnostou E. A comparison of neuroimaging findings in childhood onset schizophrenia and autism spectrum disorder: a review of the literature. Front Psych. 2013;4:175.
68. Cauda F, Costa T, Nani A, Fava L, Palermo S, Bianco F, Keller R. Are schizophrenia, autistic, and obsessive spectrum disorders dissociable on the basis of neuroimaging morphological findings?: a voxel-based meta-analysis. Autism Res. 2017;10(6):1079–95.
69. Cauda F, Costa T, Palermo S, D'agata F, Diano M, Bianco F, Keller R. Concordance of white matter and gray matter abnormalities in autism spectrum disorders: a voxel-based meta-analysis study. Hum Brain Map. 2014;35:2073–98.
70. Cauda F, Geda E, Sacco K, D'agata F, Duca S, Geminiani G, Keller R. Grey matter abnormality in autism spectrum disorder: an activation likelihood estimation meta-analysis study. J Neurol Neurosurg Psychiatry. 2011;82:1304–13.
71. Cheung C, Yu K, Fung G, Leung M, Wong C, Li Q, McAlonan G. Autistic disorders and schizophrenia: related or remote? An anatomical likelihood estimation. PLoS One. 2010;5:e12233.
72. Chisholm K, Lin A, Abu-Akel A, Wood SJ. The association between autism and schizophrenia spectrum disorders: a review of eight alternate models of co-occurrence. Neurosci Biobehav Rev. 2015;55:173–83.
73. King BH, Lord C. Is schizophrenia on the autism spectrum? Brain Res. 2011;1380:34–41.
74. Pathania M, Davenport EC, Muir J, Sheehan DF, Lopez-Domenech G, Kittler JT. The autism and schizophrenia associated gene CYFIP1 is critical for the maintenance of dendritic complexity and the stabilization of mature spines. Transl Psychiatry. 2014;4:e374.
75. Matsuo J, Kamio Y, Takahaski H, Ota M, Teraishi T, Hori H, Nagashima A, Takej R, Higuchi T, Motohashi N, Kunugi H. Autistic-like traits in adult patients with mood disorders and schizophrenia. PLoS One. 2015;10(4):e0122711.
76. Owen MJ, O'Donovan M, Thapar A, Craddock N. Neurodevelopmental hypothesis of schizophrenia. Br J Psychiatry. 2011;198(3):173–5.
77. Di Gregorio E, Riberi E, Belligni EF, Biamino E, Spielmann M, Ala U, Calcia A, Bagnasco I, Carli D, Gai G, Giordano M, Guala A, Keller R, Mandrile G, Arduino C, Maffè A, Naretto

VG, Sirchia F, Sorasio L, Ungari S, Zonta A, Zacchetti G, Talarico F, Pappi P, Cavalieri S, Giorgio E, Mancini C, Ferrero M, Brussino A, Savin E, Gandione M, Pelle A, Giachino DF, De Marchi M, Restagno G, Provero P, Silengo MC, Grosso E, Buxbaum JD, Pasini B, De Rubeis S, Brusco A, Ferrero GB. CNVs analysis in a cohort of isolated and syndromic DD/ID reveals novel genomic disorders, position effects and candidate disease genes. Clin Genet. 2017;92(4):415–22.
78. Biamino E, Di Gregorio E, Belligni EF, Keller R, Riberi E, Gandione M, Pappi P. A novel 3q29 deletion associated with autism, intellectual disability, psychiatric disorders, and obesity. Am J Med Genet B Neuropsychiatr Genet. 2016;171(2):290–9.
79. Schneider M, et al. Psychiatric disorders from childhood to adulthood in 22q11.2 deletion syndrome: results from the international consortium on brain and behavior in 22q1.2 deletion syndrome. Am J Psychiatr. 2014;171(6):627–39.
80. Jonas RK, Montojo CA, Bearden CE. The 22q11.2 deletion syndrome as a window into complex neuropsychiatric disorders over the lifespan. Biol Psychiatry. 2015;75(5):351–60.
81. Bulent H, Duygu H, Kenan D. 22q11.2 deletion syndrome: current perspective. Appl Clin Genet. 2015;8:123–32.
82. Fung WLA, et al. Practical guidelines for managing adults with 22q11.2 deletion syndrome. Genet Med. 2015;17(8):599–609.
83. Burnside RD. 22q11.21 deletion syndromes: a review of proximal, central and distal deletions and their associated features. Cytogenet Genome Res. 2015;146:89–99.
84. Bertran M, Tagle FP, Irarrazaval YM. Manifestaciones psiquiatricas del sindrome de delecion 22q11.2: una revision de la literatura. Neurologia. 2015;33(2):121–8.
85. Ford TC, Nibbs R, Crewther DP. Glutamate/GABA1 ratio is associated with the psychosocial domain of autistic and schizotypal traits. PLoS One. 2017;12:e0181961.
86. LeBlanc JJ, Fagiolini M. Autism: a "critical period" disorder? Neural Plast. 2011;2011:921680.
87. Wenger TL, et al. The role of mGluR Copy Number Variation in Genetic and environmental forms of syndromic autism spectrum disorder. Sci Rep. 2016;6:19372.
88. Connor MC, Crawford CB, Akbarian S. White matter neuron alterations in schizophrenia and related disorders. Int J Dev Neurosci. 2011;29(3):325–34.
89. Nagakawa Y, Chiba K. Involvement of neuroinflammation during brain developmental in social cognitive deficits in autism spectrum disorder and schizophrenia. J Pharmacol Exp Ther. 2016;358:504–15.
90. Larsen KM, Dzafic I, Siebner RH, Garrido MI. Alteration of functional brain architecture in 22q11.2 deletion syndrome—insights into susceptibility for psychosis. Neuroimage. 2019;190:154–71.
91. Hong H, Kim BS, Im HI. Pathophysiological role of neuroinflammation in neurodegenerative diseases and psychiatric disorders. Int Neurourol J. 2016;20:S2–7.
92. Volk DW. Role of microglia disturbances and immune-related marker abnormalities in cortical circuitry dysfunction in schizophrenia. Neurobiol Dis. 2017;99:58–65.
93. Caspi A, Houts RM, Belsky DW, Goldman-Mellor SJ, Harrington H, Israel S, et al. The p factor: one general psychopathology factor in the structure of psychiatric disorders? Clin Psychol Sci. 2014;2:119–37.
94. Davenport EC, Szulc BR, Drew J, Taylor J, Morgan T, Higgs NF, López-Doménech G, Kittler JT. Autism and schizophrenia-associated CYFIP1 regulates the balance of synaptic excitation and inhibition. Cell Rep. 2019;26(8):2037–2051.e6. https://doi.org/10.1016/j.celrep.2019.01.092.
95. Politte LC, McDougle CJ. Atypical antipsychotics in the treatment of children and adolescents with pervasive developmental disorders. Psychopharmacology (Berl). 2014;231(6):1023–36.
96. Bertelli MO, Rossi M, Keller R, Lassi S. Update on psychopharmacology for autism spectrum disorders. Adv Ment Health Intellect Disabil. 2016;10(1):6–26.
97. Skolnick SD, Greig NH. Microbes and monoamines: potential neuropsychiatric consequences of dysbiosis. Trends Neurosci. 2019;42(3):151–63. https://doi.org/10.1016/j.tins.2018.12.005. Epub 2019 Feb 19.

Adolescents and Adults with ASD and Obsessive Compulsive Disorder

5

Giuseppe Maina, Stefano Bramante, and Sylvia Rigardetto

5.1 Introduction

Autism spectrum disorder (ASD) is a neurodevelopmental disorder with social/communicative dysfunctions, restricted interest, and repetitive behaviours. These symptoms usually appear in the early years of life. ASD is known as a 'spectrum' disorder because there is a wide variation in the type and severity of symptoms people experience. In addition to the core symptoms of autism, comorbid psychiatric illnesses are highly prevalent, aggravating impairment and complicating diagnosis and treatment. Among psychiatric disorder, there is a considerable evidence that patients with ASD frequently present a comorbid obsessive-compulsive disorder (OCD), which might be a result of a common neurological dysfunction located on the basal ganglia [1].

5.2 Epidemiology

Reports on the prevalence of obsessive-compulsive disorder in ASD patients have varied significantly across the years, due to different reasons. Three elements should be considered when it comes to precisely determine the prevalence of ASD/OCD: changes in classification methods, clinical aspects of the two disorders and assessment issues.

- Current prevalence rates using the *DSM-5* (*Diagnostic and Statistical Manual of Mental Disorders-Version 5*) are yet to be established. Most of the data available are derived from studies based on *DSM-IV*: OCD is classified as an anxiety

G. Maina · S. Bramante · S. Rigardetto (✉)
SCDU Psichiatria, AOU San Luigi Gonzaga, Dipartimento di Neuroscienze, Università degli Studi di Torino, Turin, Italy
e-mail: giuseppe.maina@unito.it; stefano.bramante@unito.it

R. Keller (ed.), *Psychopathology in Adolescents and Adults with Autism Spectrum Disorders*, https://doi.org/10.1007/978-3-030-26276-1_5

disorder and there is not a separate categorical diagnosis of 'Hoarding Disorder'. Considering the high prevalence of hoarding behaviours in ASD patients, there is a need of future research with a specific focus on these symptoms to understand if hoarding is a manifestation of a real OCD or of a hoarding disorder, as defined in *DSM-5*.

- Due to the 'spectrum' nature of autism, ASD's manifestations vary depending on age and on the level of development. When this continuum nature is considered, dimensional rather than categorical approach may be more preferable in order to examine the correlation between OCD and ASD. As a result, many authors have come to focus on traits/symptoms and not on disorders as defined on *DSM*, with a resulting risk of overestimating this comorbidity. On the other hand, assessment challenges exist also with individuals who are verbally fluent: despite average language skills, patients may be unable to describe their emotional and internal states or recognise the connection between obsessions and compulsions due to deficits in emotion recognition or insight. Furthermore, overlapping symptoms and the uncommon presentation of comorbid illness in ASD contribute to underestimate the real prevalence of the association of ASD/OCD.
- Many studies use assessment tools not designed for such patients.

Regarding children and adolescents with OCD, the prevalence of autism spectrum disorder varies from 4% to 8%, while diagnosis of obsessive-compulsive disorder has been found in 17% of subjects diagnosed with ASD. In adult OCD patients, up to 35% of the subjects exhibited autistic traits [2]. However, most of the research into the relationship between autism and OCD has been performed in paediatric patients with autism spectrum disorder, with a resulting insufficient awareness of the prevalence rates in adult samples. This might partly due to a lack of knowledge of adult clinicians regarding childhood-onset disorders with the consequence that ASD symptoms are often underestimated [3].

5.3 Psychopathology

As mentioned before, autism spectrum disorder and obsessive-compulsive disorder shared some clinical features. For that reason, it might be difficult to distinguish phenomenological characteristics of these two disorders. Only a precise knowledge of the psychopathology of these conditions, associated with a careful assessment process of differential diagnosis, can help clinicians to recognise such patients. While psychopathology of ASD has been discussed before, we will now focus on OCD.

Obsessive-compulsive disorder is a common, chronic, and long-lasting disorder in which a person has uncontrollable, reoccurring thoughts (obsessions) and behaviours (compulsions). These symptoms can interfere with all aspects of life.

Obsessions are repeated thoughts or mental images that cause high level of anxiety. Common symptoms include fear of contamination, unwanted and forbidden thoughts involving sex, religion and harm; aggressive thoughts; having things symmetrical or in a perfect order. Obsessions are defined by three psychopathological features:

- Persistence: obsessions continue to occur in patient's mind.
- Ego-dystonia: obsessions are in conflict or dissonant with the subject's characteristics and will.
- Incoercibility: patients cannot control their thoughts, even when those thoughts or behaviours are recognised as excessive.

Compulsions are repetitive behaviours that a patient performs to reduce anxiety, generated by the obsessive thought. Common compulsions include excessive cleaning and/or handwashing; ordering and arranging things in a particular and precise way and repeatedly checking on things. Compulsion features are:

- Intent: patients perform compulsions consciously.
- Purpose: the aim of the compulsion is to reduce the distress generated by the obsession.
- Repeatability.

In the last years, a considerable effort has been put into identifying distinct symptom dimensions within obsessive-compulsive disorder. Most of these works have been based on adult samples and factor analysis of the Yale Brown Obsessive Compulsive Scale (Y-BOCS). Five dimensions have been identified as the most frequent: (1) contamination: a fear of contamination due to dirt, germs, viruses and a multitude of other substances or items, including chemicals, radioactivity, greasy or sticky substances, bodily excretions (urine, faeces), bodily secretions (sweat, saliva, mucus, tears, etc.) and blood associated with washing compulsion; (2) harming: fear of harming oneself or others, with compulsion of control; (3) symmetry/ordering: symmetry obsessions are characterised by the need for things to be perfect, exact or 'just right', symmetrical or correctly aligned, and related compulsions include ordering and arranging, evening up or aligning things and touching or tapping; (4) pure obsessions: usually sexual and religious obsession; (5) hoarding: persistent difficulty discarding or parting with possessions, regardless of their actual value [1]. Data of literature are not clear regarding the impact of ASD symptoms and OCD phenomenology in terms of clinical expression and severity. Regarding paediatric samples, patients with ASD and OCD were found to be less likely to have washing/checking symptoms, dimensions and magical thinking [4]; however, adult OCD/ASD samples showed elevated levels of checking and ordering. Other studies reported non-significant differences in obsessive-compulsive dimensions between comorbid ASD/OCD and OCD-only subjects. Furthermore, some authors suggest that patients with obsessive-compulsive disorder and autism are more likely to have hoarding symptom dimensions [5, 6]. Two different hypotheses could be advanced to explain the occurrence of hoarding symptoms in ASD/OCD subjects. First of all, hoarding symptoms are usually common in the secondary form of obsessive-compulsive disorder. As observed in patients affected by bipolar disorder, secondary

OCD shows high rates of hoarding symptoms. In these subjects, obsessive compulsive symptoms should be interpreted as a phenotypic expression of a more severe form of the mood disorder, with specific consequences on management and treatment of these patients. Secondly, ASD subjects without a comorbid OCD often experience intense and restricted interests, which may lead them to acquire and collect items, and have psychosocial characteristics, including attachment to objects, social isolation and impairments. These features may be related to difficulties in discarding items or to a lack of insight regarding problematic aspects of hoarding's behaviour. From this perspective, a comorbid obsessive-compulsive disorder contributes to reveal some clinical features already present in ASD patients [5]. However, more studies and discussions are needed to examine such clinical issues. Furthermore, preliminary data suggest that ASD/OCD subjects show the highest rates of comorbid psychiatric disorder, such as major depressive disorder and anxiety disorder, and medical comorbidities, like tic disorder [5]. All these aspects contribute to complicate the diagnostic assessment and treatment.

5.4 Differential Diagnosis

The similar behavioural profiles of autism spectrum disorder and obsessive-compulsive disorder present the potential for confusion regarding diagnoses and intervention efforts. In particular, restricted and repetitive behaviours (RRBs), defined as frequent behaviours that occur in a manner that is both inappropriate to the situation and context, tend to develop with some similarity in both illness and play an important role in the functional impairments of both patient groups. In ASD, RRBs are stereotyped movements, repetitive use of specific objects, ritualistic habits and restricted interests (abnormal preoccupation with a particular object or topic in terms of specificity and intensity with which it is expressed), with the first ones being linked to compulsions and the last to obsessions in OCD. Restricted interests/obsessions and repetitive behaviours/compulsions are topographically quite similar. Therefore, in order to precisely differentiate subjects with ASD and OCD and to identify the group of patients with a co-occurring ASD/OCD, it is important to focus on some clinical elements: age of onset of the disorders, cognitive and language skills, the ego-syntonic/ego-dystonic nature of the symptoms and phenomenological features of RRBs, such as anxiety and executive functions.

- Age of onset: due to the different nature of these two illness (neurodevelopmental vs. psychiatric disorder), while ASD begins in the first years of life, age of onset of OCD presents distinct peak in childhood and in adulthood, with a typical age of onset of 19 years. Therefore, restricted and repetitive behaviours occurred in the early years should direct clinicians to a possible diagnosis of autism, especially when they are associated with other clinical features such as cognitive and language deficit. However, because ASD patients show a great variation in the type and severity of symptoms, subject without a severe cognitive disability and with mild RRB symptoms might not be recognised until they become adult. At that time, these individuals could be misdiagnosed as affected by obsessive-compulsive disorder.

- Cognitive and language skills: patients with autism spectrum disorder commonly have some difficulties in communication, social interactions, and cognitive functions. These deficits concern both verbal and non-verbal communication and both receptive and expressive skills, with a wide range from patients with normal IQ and normal communications abilities to subjects with severe impairment. In fact, some children with autism show a good grasp on comprehension, but lack expressive skills and vice versa. It is also reported that patients with autism present difficulty with non-verbal communication. Furthermore, subjects with autism often fail to understand words or phrases that are abstract or that have a double meaning and tend to interpret things very literally. Instead, patients with obsessive-compulsive disorder usually present normal cognitive and communication skills, and as a result, the presence of RRBs in a young individual with social and cognitive impairment should direct the diagnoses on ASD. However, because ASD patients show a great variation in the type and severity of symptoms, subjects with autism could not have a severe cognitive disability and, with mild RRBs symptoms, they might not recognise until they become adult and misdiagnosed as affected by OCD.
- Ego-syntonic/ego-dystonic nature of the symptoms: another clinical element that could help psychiatrists to differentiate the two disorders is the ego-syntonic nature of RRBs in ASD compared to those present in OCD. In contrast to the distress experienced with obsessions and compulsions in OCD, subjects with ASD may not struggle against their repetitive behaviours. In many patients with ASD, the RRBs are preferred activities and frustration and protest may occur when the subject is asked to stop the behaviour. However, as mentioned before, because ASD individuals usually have cognitive and communication impairments, they might be unable to differentiate such feelings, especially during childhood, with a resulting more complicated process of differential diagnosis.
- Anxiety: the role of anxiety underlines the distinctions between these two illnesses. As explained before, individuals affected by OCD feel anxiety as a result of obsessive thoughts, images or doubt, while compulsions relieve that anxiety. In ASD patients, the way in which anxiety is related to RRBs is not clearly defined: some authors suggest that RRBs could perpetuate the presence of anxiety, while others interpret RRBs as a form of relief. The going assumption is that insistence behaviours may function as an anxiety-reduction technique performed as a consequence of stressful events. This hypothesis comes from the observation that events that claim anxiety are usually followed by engagement with insistence on sameness behaviours [4].
- Executive functioning: ASD and OCD both experience significant deficit in executive functioning. However, despite both disorders show similar impairments in different cognitive constructs, some elements could be recognising as typical features of different diagnosis. In particular, some authors suggest that deficit in cognitive flexibility and set-shifting (ability to appropriately switch between different concepts or behaviours) are consistently associated with the

presence of RRBs in ASD. Regarding obsessive-compulsive disorder, researchers report that problems with inhibition are more present in such patients. Poor inhibition seems to reflect a function of lowered control which corresponds to the automaticity that accompanies performance of compulsions in OCD. Indeed, despite inhibition is specifically related to total severity scores of the Y-BOCS (Yale Brown Obsessive Compulsive Scale), this correlation is highly related to compulsion scores and only weakly related to obsession scores [4].

5.5 Assessment

Assessment of obsessive-compulsive disorder in autism is a real challenge for clinicians. Some clinical features of ASD, such as cognitive disability, social impairments with deficit in communication, lack of insight and ability to recognise emotions may complicate the evaluation process. Therefore, some recommendations could be made. For individuals with intellectual disability, defined by IQ ≤ 70, with language deficit, the diagnostic process should rely on information obtained by caregivers or teacher. However, even for caregivers it could be hard to recognise anxiety or obsessive-compulsive symptoms in ASD patients: repetitive behaviour, such as arm or hand-flapping, finger-flicking or repetitive use of an object, may appear to be part of OCD. Even in individuals with adequate language skills and cognitive ability, the diagnostic process should be performed with the presence of caregivers. Indeed, deficit in emotion recognition or insight could complicate the use of self-report instruments as well as the ability of clinicians to understand precisely the internal state of the patient. Moreover, there is a lack of assessment tools specifically designed to evaluate obsessive-compulsive symptoms in adult ASD individuals. Regarding youth patients, the modified version of the Children's Yale Brown Obsessive Compulsive Scale for autism (CYBOCS-ASD) has been shown to be a reliable measure to evaluate repetitive behaviours in autistics subjects. The original CYBOCS is a clinician-rated interview designed to rate the severity of obsessive and compulsive symptoms in children and adolescents aged 6–17 years. It can be administered by a clinician or by a trained interviewer in a semi-structured fashion. The ratings depend on the child's and parent's reports, but the final rating is based on the clinical judgement of the interviewer. The evaluation of each item should be done thinking about the prior week up until, and including, the time of the interview. It contains separate checklists for obsessions and compulsions, five severity items for obsessions and five for compulsions. The severity items are scored from 0 (not present) to 4 (extreme), yielding an obsession score of 0 to 20, a compulsion score of 0 to 20 and a total of 0 to 40. As mentioned before, due to the difficulty to evaluate obsessions in individuals with ASD, the modified version (CYBOCS-ASD) is composed only of the five compulsion items (time spent, interference, distress, resistance and control) and has more items in the compulsion checklist. The revised instrument has demonstrated reliability and validity and has also sensitivity to change [7].

5.6 Treatment

International guidelines suggest pharmacological and psychological approach, sometimes in combination, as a first line treatment of Obsessive Compulsive Disorder [8].

Regarding medications, drugs approved by the Food and Drug Administration (FDA) to treat OCD include high doses of SSRI and clomipramine:

- Clomipramine, for adults and children 10 years and older
- Fluoxetine, for adults and children 7 years and older
- Fluvoxamine, for adults and children 8 years and older (not approved in Italy for paediatric population)
- Paroxetine, for adults only
- Sertraline, for adults and children 6 years and older

Treatment response, defined by a reduction of the YBOCS's score ≥ 35% compared to baseline, should be evaluated following 12 weeks at effective dose. In patients with lack of response, this treatment may be associated with low-doses of antipsychotics.

Regarding psychological interventions, cognitive behavioural therapy (CBT) is the only psychotherapy approved for individuals affected by OCD. The most studied and validated type of behavioural technique is the exposure and response prevention (ERP). ERP involves gradually exposing subjects to a feared object or obsession, such as dirt. As a result, individuals learn healthy ways to cope anxiety and learn to manage obsessions and compulsions.

Treatment of patients with a comorbid ASD/OCD is a real challenge for clinicians.

Research on the use of SSRI and clomipramine in such individuals is lacking. Moreover, most of the studies have investigated the use of these drugs in mixed samples of patient with ASD and anxiety disorders, as classified in *DSM-IV*, without considering OCD as a different disease. However, two important considerations could be advanced:

- Prescribing antidepressants to ASD/OCD patients should be approached cautiously. Indeed, some evidences suggest that such patients are particularly vulnerable to the behavioural activation of these drugs, with a resulting increased level of energy, disinhibition and sleep disorders to the point of psychomotor agitation [9].
- Considering a hierarchical approach, as observed in other psychiatric disorders such as bipolar disorder (BD) and major depressive disorder, secondary OCD should be interpreted as a phenotypic expression of a more severe form of the main disorder. As a result, in ASD/OCD individuals, therapeutic interventions should target the principal disease (autism), with a resulting improvement of the comorbid disorder associated.

Regarding CBT, behavioural treatment for individuals with OCD and ASD has received less attention in comparison with CBT in patients with ASD and anxiety disorders. Some research studies suggest that obsessive-compulsive symptoms can improve with such treatment [10]; however, most CBT trials have been conducted with moderate to high functioning patient, with adequate communication skills, and it is unclear if this treatment is appropriate for lower functioning individuals. Regardless CBT in ASD/OCD subjects, authors tend to focus on which components of CBT work best and for whom. Due to the specific features of autistic patients, some clinical issues should be underlined:

- Psychological treatment for patients with ASD should be personalised and individualised to suit the clinical presentation, interests, cognitive and social skills of the patients and may demand longer duration.
- The use of special interests may facilitate therapeutic participation and alliance, especially in paediatric population.
- CBT may require some level of focus on social skills deficit. One of the key differences between the use of standardised CBT and ASD-specific treatment protocols is the addition of social skills training components adapted to the baseline level of communication abilities.
- CBT may include direct intervention to improve independent daily living skills, associated with concomitant psychoeducation strategies addressed to the family members, for the purpose of reducing family accommodation.

In conclusion, pharmacological and psychological interventions for OCD patients can be used in ASD/OCD with a close clinical monitoring and a more personalised approach, in order to develop ASD-specific CBT protocols. However, large-scale double-blind, placebo-controlled trials are needed to establish the real effectiveness of these strategies in such patients.

References

1. Markarian Y, Larson MJ, Aldea MA, et al. Multiple pathways to functional impairment in obsessive-compulsive disorder. Clin Psychol Rev. 2010;30:78–88.
2. Özyurt G, Beşiroğlu L. Autism spectrum symptoms in children and adolescents with obsessive compulsive disorder and their mothers. Noro Psikiyatr Ars. 2018;55(1):40–8.
3. Anholt GE, Cath DC, van Oppen P, et al. Autism and ADHD symptoms in patients with OCD: are they associated with specific OC symptom dimensions or OC symptom severity? J Autism Dev Disord. 2010;40(5):580–9.
4. Jiujias M, Kellery E, Hall L. Restricted, repetitive, behaviors in autism spectrum disorder and obsessive-compulsive disorder: a comparative review. Child Psychiatry Hum Dev. 2017;48:944–59.
5. Mito H, Matsuura N, Mukai K, et al. The impact of elevated autism spectrum disorder traits on clinical and psychosocial features and long-term treatment outcome in adult patients with obsessive-compulsive disorder. Compr Psychiatry. 2014;55:1526–33.
6. La Buissonnière-Ariza V, Wood JJ, Kendall PC, et al. Presentation and correlates of hoarding behaviors in children with autism spectrum disorders and comorbid anxiety or obsessive-compulsive symptoms. J Autism Dev Disord. 2018;48(12):4167–78.

7. Scahill L, Dimitropoulos A, McDougle CJ, et al. Children's Yale-Brown obsessive compulsive scale in autism spectrum disorder: component structure and correlates of symptom checklist. J Am Acad Child Adolesc Psychiatry. 2014;53:97–107.
8. Katzman MA, Bleau P, Blier P, et al. Canadian clinical practice guidelines for the management of anxiety, posttraumatic stress and obsessive-compulsive disorders. BMC Psychiatry. 2014;14(Suppl 1):S1.
9. Postorino V, Kerns CM, Vivanti G, et al. Anxiety Disorders and Obsessive-Compulsive Disorder in Individuals with autism spectrum disorder. Curr Psychiatry Rep. 2017;19:92.
10. Russell AJ, Jassi A, Fullana MA, et al. Cognitive behavior therapy for comorbid obsessive-compulsive disorder in high-functioning autism spectrum disorders: a randomized controlled trial. Depress Anxiety. 2013;30:697–708.

6 Depressive Disorders and ASD

Roberto Keller, Erika Borroz, and Silvia Chieregato

6.1 Introduction

Individuals with ASD have a higher risk of depressive disorders rather than general population, with reported rates in adults that range from 18% to 70%. By age 27 years, 19.8% of individuals diagnosed having ASD has a diagnosis of depression compared with 6% of the general population. In a study of Rai, the risk of depression diagnosis was higher in ASD without intellectual disability [1]. Hedley reports 48.6% rate of depression in ASD [2] and Cassidy 35% [3].

Depression can worse ASD symptomatology and especially social withdrawal but may also lead to suicide or catatonia, unemployment and difficulties in independent living.

Depression is present clinically lifetime and it is related to painful consciousness of their disability and to be different from other people.

Risk factors for depressive disorders in ASD are higher cognitive ability, less social impairment, others psychiatric disorders, rumination and bullying [4].

Awareness of one's own role in failed social situation and assumption of responsibility for negative events contribute to lower self-esteem and discouragement, which may increase the risk for depression in ASD. So higher functioning individuals with ASD could be aware of their social difficulties, and this awareness and the perception of dissimilarity may lead to increase in distress and the development of co-occurrence of psychiatric disorders, as depression. Having the motivation and desire to form social relationship, combined with impairments in the skill necessary to do so, can lead to failed attempts to interact and the inability to form successful relationships. The presence of rituals or compulsions and anxiety may also exacerbate difficulties in adults with ASD [5].

R. Keller (✉) · E. Borroz · S. Chieregato
Adult Autism Centre, Mental Health Department, Local Health Unit ASL Città di Torino, Turin, Italy

R. Keller (ed.), *Psychopathology in Adolescents and Adults with Autism Spectrum Disorders*, https://doi.org/10.1007/978-3-030-26276-1_6

Lack of correct ASD treatment and social support lead to more risk of depressive disorder, too.

A higher intelligence quotient is more related to depression. This factor could be related to a greater capacity of introspection. But we have to consider also that mood disorder is frequently underdiagnosed in intellectual disability and that behaviour equivalent of depressive symptoms is not recognized by clinicians. So, worsening of social withdrawal, reduced repetitive behaviour and aggressive behaviour could be the clinical presentation of depressive disorder in ASD with intellectual disability. And the presence of hallucinations in nonverbal patient could be detected only by behaviour.

6.2 Psychopathology

Self-focused attention (awareness of internally generated information relevant to the self) plays an important role, increasing the salience of perceived parts of the self and so perpetuating depressive cognition. Rumination maintains and worsens mood by increasing negative thought content and reducing problem-solving. Persons with autism (PWA) have a tendency to repetitive thinking that can worsen depressive rumination. Otherwise PWA may have difficulties in awareness of their feelings, mental states, affective conditions and mentalizing. Deficit in non-verbal communication may contribute to difficulty in managing the affective state.

In Asperger syndrome (ASD level 1 in *DSM 5*), the higher level of autism functioning, even if depressed mood is the most frequently cited marker of depression, unfrequently depressed mood is directly reported by the affected individuals, but usually by parents [6].

6.3 Difficulties in Recognizing ASD with Higher Risk for Depression

In ASD, depressive disorder can reduce the repetitive behaviour linked to a special autistic interest. This change could be viewed as an improvement of ASD syndrome and not as a depressive symptom, so masking depression in ASD.

Persons with Asperger syndrome could not be recognized as autistic and so arrive in adolescence and adulthood without psychological support. They live in a world that does not understand them, but they do not understand the world, too. This condition made them vulnerable to psychiatric disorder and especially depressive disorder. They are alone. And frequently bullying is the trigger for psychopathological conditions [7, 8].

In female with Asperger syndrome, the diagnosis of ASD is more difficult. Particularly female with ASD 'camouflage' their social communication difficulties: this behaviour requires considerable cognitive efforts and leads to increase stress, anxiety and depression [9]. Examples of camouflaging include making eye contact during conversation, using learned phrases or prepared jokes in conversation, mimicking other's social behaviours, imitating facial expression or gestures, learning and following social scripts. The constant cognitive effort could be exhausting and may lead to social overload and meltdown/shut down. Camouflage has an important role in increasing ASD underdiagnosed in female.

6.4 Family of ASD and Depressive Disorder

Autism and depression are genetic-related syndrome, and a higher prevalence of affective disorders among parents, particularly mothers, as well as siblings of individuals with ASD, has been reported.

Non-autistic full-siblings and half-siblings have a higher risk of depression than the general population. Compared with their non-autistic full-siblings, individuals with ASD have more than a twofold risk of depression diagnosis in young adulthood [1].

Among siblings, sisters report higher level of depressive disorders and anxiety symptoms than brothers. Having a family history of ASD is associated with depressive but not anxiety symptoms: a diathesis-stress model is only partially supported, primarily through the findings that sibling sub-threshold autism characteristics are associated with depressive and anxiety symptoms in siblings, but only in the presence of a high number of stressful life events [10].

Increased rates of depression in parents of individuals with ASD is so accounted by the stress associated by parenting a child with ASD but also by the presence of the broader autism phenotype (BAP). BAP is a subclinical set of personality and other features that is thought to index genetic liability to ASD. In parents with ASD, it could be observed a higher rate of mood disorder, obsessive compulsive disorder, autism and other psychopathological disorder than in general population [11].

The genetic vulnerability could be linked to a broader neurodevelopmental disorder, including obsessive compulsive disorder, mood disorder and psychosis other than autism and not only strictly to autism. In a circular way, the higher stress to have a child with autism is added to the genetic vulnerability for mood disorder, increasing the frequency of depressive phenotype in parents.

Familial-genetic factors play an important role in the aetiology of depression in children and adults with ASD.

In ASD there is a lack of gender effect, which is present in general population and which could be linked more to a neurobiological basis independently of sex.

Negative life events play a role in precipitating depression. Life events as parents getting divorced, illnesses, death, frequent parental discord, changing residence and especially bullying have been related to depression [12].

6.5 Suicide

Suicide is a global public health crisis: in the United States, 12.93 per 100,000 individuals die by suicide per year, making it the tenth leading cause of death overall, and the second leading cause of death among young people aged 10–34 in general population (CDC, 2016) [13].

But most studies are usually related only to completed suicide, so the real prevalence is unknown and especially in ASD is underestimated. One third of ASD individuals reports suicidal ideation, indeed [2].

Autism diagnosis and autistic traits explain significant additional variance in suicidality beyond a range of known risk factors and are therefore independent risk markers for suicidality: so ASD diagnosis is an independent risk marker for suicide attempts [3].

Non-suicidal self-injury is higher in ASD individuals (63.6%) than in general population (29.8%) and significantly predicts suicidality in ASD individuals [3].

Life-time suicide attempts in ASD individuals (38%) are also higher than in general population (8%) [3].

In the study of Kirby (2019), the cumulative incidence of suicide is 0.17% in ASD individuals (between 2013 and 2017) that is significantly higher than in general population (0.11%): the difference is driven by suicide among females with ASD, that is over three times higher than in females without ASD [13]. Age of death by suicide ranges from 14 to 70 years. Individuals with ASD are less likely to use firearms as a method of suicide [13].

Clinical symptoms of ASD may mask depressive symptoms and especially symptoms related to immediate risk of suicide. Camouflaging is an important barrier to timely ASD diagnosis and has a negative impact on mental health and risk of suicidality. Camouflaging is primarily experienced by autistic females and may at least in part explain why this group has been under-diagnosed [7]. Camouflaging significantly predicts suicidality in ASD [3].

ASD with impaired social communication has a higher risk of self-harm with suicidal intent, suicidal thoughts and suicidal plan (but not self-harm without suicidal intent), compared to those without, at age 16. Is important to assess if self-injurious behaviour occurs in the context of suicidal ideation [14].

Lower levels of social support, in terms of both the number of social supports and satisfaction with the available social support, and increased loneliness are associated with depression and suicidal ideation, as in general population. Greater severity of ASD traits is associated with increased loneliness and lower levels of satisfaction with social support, as well as with higher depression severity. Thus, ASD trait severity may represent a risk factor for the development and maintenance of psychiatric disorders and predict depression, even if in low functioning individuals, psychiatric assessment could be difficult and need specific evaluation. But ASD severity traits are not correlated with suicidal ideation [2].

IQ level is positively associated with the awareness of social limitations. Individuals with ASD who are higher functioning may attempt or commit suicide especially when experiencing frustration even because they are not used to self-report or confide in others when experiencing depressed mood. So, it is imperative that clinicians actively detect depressive symptoms during the evaluation and screen for suicidal thoughts [5].

It may be beneficial for interventions to assist individuals to identify and increase the availability of quality social support networks and to provide opportunity for regular social interaction, to minimize potentially harmful effects of social isolation [2].

The ability to confide in a friend about worries has been associated with a significantly decreased likelihood of lifetime suicide attempt, controlling for psychopathological and demographic variables [15].

Tangible support but not appraisal or belonging may act as an indirect protective factor against suicide in ASD [15].

ASD individuals are lonelier and have poorer quality friendship in terms of companionship, security and help than neuro-typically persons. In ASD, isolation and loneliness have been associated with increased rate of depression and decreased life satisfaction. Deficit in social relationship is a core symptom of ASD. Social skill training is a cognitive-metacognitive treatment that may improve the ability to create new relationship in ASD, teaching the skill to communicate with others in an appropriate manner; this technique could be used in group treatment and so can also improve meeting other people.

Suicide could also be related to auditory hallucinations in psychosis in comorbidity of ASD, especially at the onset of psychosis, and the trigger for psychotic onset could be the bullying, or drug abuse to attempt to reduce social phobia (as THC) [16, 17].

In nations where euthanasia and assisted suicide have been legally possible (as in the Netherlands since 2001), people with intellectual disability and autism have been included in the programme, too [18].

Another important issue concerns with how assessment of suicidality has been made in ASD. Cassidy describes the measurement properties of tools used to assess suicidality in autistic trial and that many studies of suicidality have used clinical settings or existing database or not appropriate testing. So, the lack of standardized assessment is problematic, and many of measures lack evidence of validity; this could explain the wide range of suicidality estimates of suicidal ideation (11–66%) and attempts (1–35%) in ASD. A recommendation for future suicidality research in ASD is to start using suicidality assessment tools with high-quality evidence in support of their measurement properties (COSMIN criteria) [3].

6.6 Brief Focused Psychotherapy for the End-of-Life Understanding in ASD with Intellectual Disability

We propose a psychotherapeutic-educational focused brief treatment for ASD with associated intellectual disability for 'the end-of-life understanding'. This treatment originates from the attempt to structure some (limited duration) psycho-educational paths consisting of variable number of sessions (from six to twelve), with the target to understand the 'concept of death', as an event of human life and to observe the different consequences involving persons involved in this experience.

Before starting the specific treatment with the person with ASD and ID, the programme requires a preliminary phase of preparation, in order to know the person and to structure and adapt the treatment to the specific needs. This first step consists of interviewing the family, or other caregiver, and collecting an accurate history of all the information about the context and life experience.

The focused treatment begins creating a pairing, that is to say a relationship between patient and therapist, focusing also on assessing the attention span, and the ability of understanding verbal, written and image communication of the person involved.

The focused therapy is structured, based on the stability of the setting, the organization of the contents and the duration of the activity. Scripts are used to support the verbal treatment, and images and social stories are used to make the contents more effective.

It is also possible, in case of necessity, to alternate the step of specific treatment with structured leisure activities. This allows to a simultaneous control on both relationship with the therapist and motivation and interest in the activity.

Every aspects of the programme, as the frequency of sessions, the request, the alternation of treatment and leisure time and, in particular, the care in maintaining stability in the sequence of activities presented should be drawn up as clear as possible, even visually.

In order to respect a linearity of thought, the content analysis is based on a deductive method (from the general to the particular). This process starts focusing on the description of life cycle of living beings, then gradually introducing the concept of 'end of life' and then specifically facing the personal mourning experience.

The understanding of human loss also considers the emotional aspects related to this issue. It is therefore important to use some items of cognitive-affective education, for example, trying to work on the link to experience and emotions, between emotions and behaviour, and to the expression of emotions.

Grieving and mourning processes are complex path that takes a long time. Precisely for this reason, it is important to work as much as possible in a network perspective, sharing goals and strategies of the psycho-educational path with the caregivers in the contexts of patient life, in order to facilitate this process and the generalization of learning outside the therapeutic setting.

6.7 Cognitive Therapy of Depression and Autism Spectrum Disorder

According to cognitive psychotherapy, feelings and behaviours are strictly connected to the way how everyone structures their own vision of themselves, of other people and of the world.

Through our previous experiences, we develop basic assumptions hierarchically organized in relatively stable and functional constructs that Beck (1976) called 'schemas' [19]. A schema is a structure, a framework imposed on reality to help individuals explain it and to guide their responses. Schemas can be adaptive or maladaptive, and many of them are formed early in life, continued to be elaborated and then superimposed on later life experiences, even when they are no longer applicable [20].

Guidano (1987), from a constructivist perspective, said that these basic assumptions constitute 'core organizing processes' that constrain the human psychological experience for making sense and that are involved in the development and maintenance of personal identity or 'self': knowledge is selected and organized around 'nuclei of personal meaning' that form a deep structure, a 'personal cognitive organization' [21].

People who develop a depressive disorder often have a psychological organization characterized by an image of themselves and a system of expectations based on a sense of personal inadequacy, failure and loneliness.

Failures and invalidations happen in everyone's life and often lead to an increase of the complexity of self and to a personal growth. In depressive disorders, suffering thoughts remain stable over time without leading to a new equilibrium: intense emotions like anxiety, despair, shame and anger appear, and interpretations of reality and expectations become rigid and self-centred, and they tend to confirm maladaptive models and dysfunctional beliefs.

We can suppose that, in people who have an autism spectrum disorder, all these aspects are intensified.

Many authors describe how individuals with ASD have difficulty processing their own and other people's emotions [22, 23], and how this could relate to ineffective emotion regulation [24–26]. It can therefore be supposed that people with autism could be easily overwhelmed by their intensive negative emotions.

Ineffective emotion regulation could also be explained by core deficits in the theory of mind [23], which make them perceive their own mental states as hazy and make the understanding of the mental states of other people difficult. The world appears confused and unpredictable; therefore, the person might think that, in a situation like this, it becomes hard to detach oneself from rigid models that give security, even if they are dysfunctional. This psychological process is strengthened by cognitive rigidity and self-focused attention, both of which are characteristic in autism, and they are connected to depression in adults with ASD [4].

In the cognitive 'rationalist' psychotherapy, therapeutic techniques are used to let the patients recognize their automatic negative thoughts and their cognitive distortions. The patients are taught to verify and modify dysfunctional beliefs underlying the cognitions: in this way, they can think more realistically and act more adaptively reducing the psychological suffering. The final aim of therapy is the 'cognitive restructuring', namely to be able to change the way in which situations are interpreted and evaluated. The correction of the distorted evaluations regarding oneself, one's life or one's future leads to a gradual change on the emotional and behavioural levels [27].

The cognitive 'constructivist' psychology puts more emphasis on the fact that the suffering and the perception of impotence are not determined by events and by reality, but by our way of interpreting them, of 'narrating' them and reacting to them. According to Guidano (1991), we cannot live without describing to ourselves what we are living and without giving sense to what we are experiencing, because our interpretations are essential to us in order to adapt to our world. We select from the environment the information that confirm our sense of identity and create a path to reading the 'reality' that is consistent with it; therefore, our mental representations always guide how we act in the world in order to confirm what we already know. As a consequence, real mental habits are created; they take the form of priority activation of typical cognitive-emotional-somatic patterns in response to certain situations, and such patterns tend to become automatic and maintain over time [28].

The purpose of cognitive-constructivist psychotherapy is to help the patients to become aware that their narratives do not correspond to reality but rather they are the result of a choice. For this reason, when persons realize that a specific narrative is dysfunctional, they can choose to narrate in a more useful narrative, which allows to contemplate new possibilities, and which establishes action and change in the real life. So, the therapists, through 'emotional perturbation' techniques, help the patients explore new points of view [29].

To get rid of dysfunctional narratives and thoughts, it is necessary to assume a 'meta-observational' position towards them, observing them from a detached point of view and giving attention to processes rather than to the content of thoughts.

Also mindfulness-based cognitive therapy meditation helps people to distance from negative thoughts and ruminations that can cause relapses to depressive disorders.

There are many evidences of effectiveness of CBT interventions (using both cognitive and behavioural techniques) for the treatment of depression in adults with ASD [30–32]. Cognitive therapy using mindfulness-based techniques adapted to autism has also been found effective in reducing depressive symptoms [33].

Although there are no specific studies about the use of cognitive psychotherapy for the treatment of depressive disorders in autism, there are reasons to think it may hold a number of advantages for people with ASD, albeit with adjustments suitable for autistic functioning (like using a more directive approach or avoiding the use of metaphors and abstract concepts) [34]. Cognitive psychotherapy gives a great emphasis on the internal experiences of the individual. The patient is encouraged to understand the connections among thoughts, feelings and behaviours of one's own and of other people, exploring and making mental states explicit, and therefore promoting insight, metacognition and theory of mind functions. This is important because people with ASD often have difficulties with mind reading.

Exploring new narratives and new points of view promotes the ability to move the attention to other people and loosens the cognitive rigidity, which is so peculiar in persons with autism. Training the ability to assume a meta-observational position in relation to one's own mental states also improves cognitive flexibility and stimulates the patients to decentralize themselves from their own negative thoughts and ruminations.

Cognitive psychotherapy also gives great importance to the exploration and recognition of one's emotions and uses techniques to promote emotion regulation. On the other hand, rationalist techniques, guiding the patients in the verification and refutation of their dysfunctional beliefs, can be thought as being logical as the autistic way of thinking.

Moreover, a psychological treatment concerning with the profound processes used in order to construct the own way of maintaining a sense of self and reality improves self-consciousness in a supported context, not leaving the persons with autism alone in exploring how to interpret the world and themselves [4].

6.8 Treating Depressive Disorder in ASD: Consider Not Only the Brain

The treatment of depressive disorder in ASD is not different from treating mood disorder in general population even if we have to take care of some items related to autism.

First, in ASD with ID, we must detect if the psychiatric disorder is an epiphenomenon of an organic disease or not.

In ASD with high functioning, and especially in Asperger disorder, there is an high risk of bipolar disorder; so clinicians must be careful in using an antidepressant drug in a major depression that could be the first episode of a bipolar disorder; if a relative has a bipolar disorder, we should consider this depressive episode with high probability as a bipolar depression, and so prefer, in adulthood, drugs with no tendency to switch to mania, as quetiapine slow-release, or with low tendency to activate bipolarity, as bupropion. Another possibility could be to associate a mood stabilizer, as valproate to the antidepressant drug.

In ASD with intellectual disability, the response to a drug is highly individualized and low predictable, so we should taper the antidepressant drug slower than in general population and with more frequent patient assessment.

In treating depressive disorder in ASD, we should also promote physical activity, especially daily aerobic one (such as walking and swimming) [35].

An interesting role in mood disorder in ASD is related to gut microbiota. The inflammatory state alteration in autism and mood disorder (but also in schizophrenia) strongly recalls the microbiota alteration and the role of gastrointestinal system in neuropsychiatric disorders. The application of therapeutic modulators of gut microbiota to autism and mood disorders has been experienced in experimental settings with promising results. In particular, the dysbiosis and the consequent alteration of intestinal permeability lead to the production of a potent pro-inflammatory endotoxine, namely lipopolysaccaride (LPS). LPS influences the modulation of central nervous system, increasing the amygdale activity, and leads to the production of inflammatory cytokines that alter the brain activity modulating the neuropeptides synthesis. Gut and brain have a bidirectional connection also in the enterochromaffin cells, related to serotonin levels. So the CNS is able to change the composition of microbiota through the activation of the hypothalamus-pituitary-adrenal (HPA) axis. Specific antibiotic treatment that reduces LPS luminal levels lead to attenuate HPA axis stress response, and some studies have tested minocycline in treating depression or vancomycin in improving ASD symptoms. Also probiotics modulate immune and inflammatory response by promoting T cells, regulating Th1 response, inhibiting the production of proinflammatory cytokines (such as IL-12, TNF-alpha and INF-alpha) or increasing anti-inflammatory mediators (such as IL-10 and beta-TFGF). Faecal microbiota transplantation (an injection of filtrate stools from a healthy donor to the patient) has not only been used in treating infection of clostridium difficile but also improved sexual function in Crohn's disease, showing a gut–brain connection and in several cases ameliorate autistic symptoms [36]. Also the use of well-balanced omega-3/6-fatty acid in the diet could ameliorate the stabilization of mood symptoms in ASD.

So in treating mood disorder in ASD, we have to consider a complete body–mind treatment and not only use antidepressant drugs [37].

References

1. Rai D, Heuvelman H, Dalman C, Culpin I, Lundberg M, Carpenter P, et al. Association between autism spectrum disorders with or without intellectual disability and depression in young adulthood. JAMA Netw Open. 2018;1(4):e181465.
2. Hedley D, Uljarević M, Foley K-R, Richdale A, Trollor J. Risk and protective factors underlying depression and suicidal ideation in Autism Spectrum Disorder. Depress Anxiety. 2018;35(7):648–57.
3. Cassidy S, Bradley L, Shaw R, Baron-Cohen S. Risk markers for suicidality in autistic adults. Mol Autism. 2018;9:42.
4. Burns A, Irvine M, Woodcock K. Self-focused attention and depressive symptoms in adults with autistic spectrum disorder (ASD). J Autism Dev Disord. 2019;49(2):692–703.
5. Sterling L, Dawson G, Estes A, Greenson J. Characteristics associated with presence of depressive symptoms in adults with autism spectrum disorder. J Autism Dev Disord. 2008;38(6):1011–8.
6. Stewart ME, Barnard L, Pearson J, Hasan R, O'Brien G. Presentation of depression in autism and Asperger syndrome: a review. Autism. 2006;10(1):103–16.
7. Luciano CC, Keller R, Politi P, Aguglia E, Magnano F, et al. Misdiagnosis of high function autism spectrum disorders in adults: an Italian case series. Autism. 2014;4:131.
8. Rai D, Culpin I, Heuvelman H, Magnusson CMK, Carpenter P, Jones HJ, et al. Association of autistic traits with depression from childhood to age 18 years. JAMA Psychiatry. 2018;75(8):835–43.
9. Lai M-C, Lombardo MV, Ruigrok AN, Chakrabarti B, Auyeung B, Szatmari P, et al. Quantifying and exploring camouflaging in men and women with autism. Autism. 2017;21(6):690–702.
10. Orsmond GI, Seltzer MM. Adolescent siblings of individuals with an autism spectrum disorder: testing a diathesis-stress model of sibling well-being. J Autism Dev Disord. 2009;39(7):1053–65.
11. Ingersoll B, Meyer K, Becker MW. Increased rates of depressed mood in mothers of children with ASD associated with the presence of the broader autism phenotype. Autism Res. 2011;4(2):143–8.
12. De-la-Iglesia M, Olivar J-S. Risk factors for depression in children and adolescents with high functioning autism spectrum disorders. Sci World J. 2015;2015:127853.
13. Kirby AV, Bakian AV, Zhang Y, Bilder DA, Keeshin BR, Coon H. A 20-year study of suicide death in a statewide autism population. Autism Res. 2019;12(4):658–66.
14. Culpin I, Mars B, Pearson RM, Golding J, Heron J, Bubak I, et al. Autistic traits and suicidal thoughts, plans, and self-harm in late adolescence: population-based cohort study. J Am Acad Child Adolesc Psychiatry. 2018;57(5):313–320.e6.
15. Hedley D, Uljarević M, Wilmot M, Richdale A, Dissanayake C. Brief report: social support, depression and suicidal ideation in adults with autism spectrum disorder. J Autism Dev Disord. 2017;47(11):3669–77.
16. Karakoç Demirkaya S, Tutkunkardaş MD, Mukaddes NM. Assessment of suicidality in children and adolescents with diagnosis of high functioning autism spectrum disorder in a Turkish clinical sample. Neuropsychiatr Dis Treat. 2016;12:2921–6.
17. Keller R, Piedimonte A, Bianco F, Bari S, Cauda F. Diagnostic characteristics of psychosis and autism spectrum disorder in adolescence and adulthood. A case series. Autism Open Access. 2015;6:159.
18. Tuffrey-Wijne I, Curfs L, Finlay I, Hollins S. Euthanasia and assisted suicide for people with an intellectual disability and/or autism spectrum disorder: an examination of nine relevant euthanasia cases in the Netherlands (2012-2016). BMC Med Ethics. 2018;19(1):17.

19. Beck AT. Cognitive therapy and the emotional disorders. New York: International Universities Press; 1976. 372 p.
20. Young JE, Klosko JS, Weishaar ME. Schema therapy: a practitioner's guide. 1st ed. New York: Guilford Press; 2006. 436 p.
21. Guidano VF. Complexity of the self: a developmental approach to psychopathology and therapy. New York: Guilford Press; 1987. 270 p.
22. Hill E, Berthoz S, Frith U. Brief report: cognitive processing of own emotions in individuals with autistic spectrum disorder and in their relatives. J Autism Dev Disord. 2004;34(2):229–35.
23. Samson AC, Huber O, Gross JJ. Emotion regulation in Asperger's syndrome and high-functioning autism. Emotion. 2012;12(4):659–65.
24. Barrett FL, Gross J, Christensen TC, Benvenuto M. Knowing what you're feeling and knowing what to do about it: mapping the relation between emotion differentiation and emotion regulation. Cognit Emot. 2001;15(6):713–24.
25. Lambie JA, Marcel AJ. Consciousness and the varieties of emotion experience: a theoretical, framework. Psychol Rev. 2002;109:219–59.
26. Bruggink A, Huisman S, Vuijk R, Kraaij V, Garnefski N. Cognitive emotion regulation, anxiety and depression in adults with autism spectrum disorder. Res Autism Spectr Disord. 2016;22:34–44.
27. Beck AT. Cognitive therapy of depression. New York: Guilford Press; 1979. 442 p.
28. Guidano VF. The self in process: toward a post-rationalist cognitive therapy. New York: Guilford Press; 1991. 256 p.
29. Bara BG. Manuale di Psicoterapia Cognitiva. Torino: Bollati Boringhieri; 1996. 812 p.
30. Spain D, Sin J, Chalder T, Murphy D, Happé F. Cognitive behaviour therapy for adults with autism spectrum disorders and psychiatric co-morbidity: a review. Res Autism Spectr Disord. 2015;9:151–62.
31. Weiss JA, Lunsky Y. Group cognitive behaviour therapy for adults with Asperger syndrome and anxiety or mood disorder: a case series. Clin Psychol Psychother. 2010;17(5):438–46.
32. McGillivray JA, Evert HT. Group cognitive behavioural therapy program shows potential in reducing symptoms of depression and stress among young people with ASD. J Autism Dev Disord. 2014;44(8):2041–51.
33. Spek AA, van Ham NC, Nyklíček I. Mindfulness-based therapy in adults with an autism spectrum disorder: a randomized controlled trial. Res Dev Disabil. 2013;34:246–53.
34. Anderson S, Morris J. Cognitive behaviour therapy for people with Asperger syndrome. Behav Cogn Psychother. 2006;34(3):293–303.
35. Keller R, editors. I Disturbi dello spettro autistico in adolescenza e età adulta. Aspetti diagnostici e proposte di intervento. Edizioni Erickson Trento; 2016.
36. Mangiola F, Ianiro G, Franceschi F, Fagiuoli S, Gasbarrini G, Gasbarrini A. Gut microbiota in autism and mood disorders. World J Gastroenterol. 2016;22(1):361–8.
37. Bertelli MO, Rossi M, Keller R, Lassi S. Update on psychopharmacology for autism spectrum disorders. Adv Ment Health Intellect Disabil. 2016;10(1):6–26.

7 Bipolar Disorder and ASD

Giulia Vannucchi, Giulio Perugi, and Gabriele Masi

7.1 Introduction

Autism spectrum disorder (ASD) is the label given in *DSM-5* to a variety of neurodevelopmental conditions grouped in by impairment in social communication and restricted, repetitive, and stereotyped interests and behavior [1]. This is the so-called umbrella diagnosis including very heterogeneous early onset neurodevelopmental syndromes. Heterogeneity is expressed at genetic, neuroanatomical, neurobiological, and clinical levels. The complexity of individuals with ASD and the "dimensionality" of the diagnosis can be shaped by means of clinical and severity specifiers allowing the distinction of different ASD phenotypes for both clinical and research purposes. From a practical perspective, the distinction between high- and low-functioning ASD is relevant: high functioning autisms (HFA) is defined by "less marked general impairment" only "requiring support" (level 1), including for example Asperger syndrome and pervasive developmental disorder not otherwise specified of *DSM-IV-TR* [2]. Low-functioning autism (LFA) with co-occurring intellectual

G. Vannucchi
CREA, Research and Clinical Center, San Sebastiano Foundation, Florence, Italy

NEUROFARBA Department, University of Florence, Florence, Italy

Psychiatry Unit 2, Clinical and Experimental Medicine Department, University of Pisa, Pisa, Italy

G. Perugi
Department of Clinical and Experimental Medicine, Spedali Riuniti Santa Chiara, Psychiatry Unit 2, AOUP-Pisa, University of Pisa, Pisa, Italy
e-mail: giulio.perugi@med.unipi.it

G. Masi (✉)
Department of Child Psychiatry and Psychopharmacology, IRCCS Stella Maris, Scientific Institute of Child Neurology and Psychiatry, Pisa, Italy
e-mail: gabriele.masi@fsm.unipi.it

R. Keller (ed.), *Psychopathology in Adolescents and Adults with Autism Spectrum Disorders*, https://doi.org/10.1007/978-3-030-26276-1_7

disability (ID) and language impairment is the form "requiring very substantial support" (level 3). The two subcategories may have different diagnostic and management issues regarding eventual co-occurring psychiatric disorders in adults.

Although in the past early diagnosis was reserved only to children with severe autistic symptoms and developmental delay, in the last few years the reconceptualization of ASD and the broadening of diagnostic boundaries increased the attention to the ASD "soft" signs, with a consistent growth of the diagnoses during childhood [3, 4]. In spite of this, the first recognition of ASD in adults seeking treatment for superimposed mental issues is still very common, a phenomenon defined by Lai and Baron-Cohen as the "identification of the lost generation of adults with autism spectrum conditions" [4].

In subjects without a childhood diagnosis of ASD, the diagnostic difficulties are mainly derived by the poor acquaintance of adult clinicians about ASD, lack of reliable developmental information, and the peculiarities of psychiatric manifestations. For example, the comorbidity of bipolar disorder (BD) and HFA often produces atypical and bizarre clinical presentations, easily misdiagnosed as schizophrenia, with relevant consequences for the treatment choice and management [5, 6].

LFA with co-occurring psychiatric disorders is exactly the opposite. Subjects are diagnosed as ASD since the childhood, but the restricted repertoire of communication skills and behaviors may impact the presentation of the comorbid disorder so considerably that psychiatric manifestations may be neglected or misconceived as symptoms proper to the basic neurodevelopmental disorder. The phenomenon is known as "diagnostic overshadowing" [7]. When challenging behaviors dominate the clinical picture and an intervention is required, usually the approach is based on the problem instead of the diagnostic precision.

BD is a common psychiatric comorbidity in both HFA and LFA and may be a significant cause of further distress and impairment [8]. The purpose of this chapter is to examine epidemiological, clinical, and therapeutic implications of comorbid BD in ASD, considering different issues on the basis of the level of functioning.

7.2 Epidemiology

Depressive symptoms and episodes of manic-depressive illness have been reported since the first descriptions of ASD [9]. Current literature is not exhaustive regarding the co-occurrence of ASD and BD in adults, and the results are mixed: this can be attributable to the heterogeneity of psychiatric presentations in ASD and methodological differences across studies [10]. Moreover, a large part of the data are related to childhood and adolescence, and it is not possible to fully generalize the results to adults: in clinical samples of very young subjects, depressive and other psychiatric symptoms may be more represented than hypomanic and manic symptoms, which could become manifest later in life [7, 11]. This is confirmed by a 2011 study of the Interactive Autism Network (IAN): the rates of BD in children and adolescents aged between 5 and 18 increased with growing age from 2.3% to 10.4% [12]. On the other hand, in the last years epidemiological research has included mainly HFA, while in LFA the detection of co-occurring BD has been complicated by atypical clinical presentations with high rates of under-recognition and mistreatment.

Few research accounts for the differential prevalence of BD in ASD according to ID level. In the IAN study, Rosenberg and colleagues estimated that in 4343 ASD children and adolescents, BD was more common in Asperger syndrome than in pervasive developmental disorder not otherwise specified and autism (8.6% vs. 5.6% and 3.0%, respectively). However, the authors suggested caution in the interpretation of the data, given the inadequacy of "classical" criteria for psychiatric disorders to depict the comorbidity in lower functioning ASD [12]. The prevalence of overall mental disorders increases from 8–13% in intellectually disabled persons to 16–30.4% when an ASD is also present, similar to the prevalence rates in HFA [13]. These studies suggest that the co-occurrence of ASD add further vulnerability to the development of another psychiatric disorder.

Rates of BD in ASD range from 1.7% to 31% in pediatric samples [14] with most studies reporting percentages around 5–8% [12, 15–17]. In samples of adults, sometimes including also adolescents, prevalence rates of BD are higher, with the lowest rate at 0.74% in adults with autistic spectrum conditions regardless the IQ level [18], and the highest at 66% in a study recruiting persons with Asperger syndrome [19]. Generally, the prevalence range was 6–40% [20, 21], with variability depending on sampling, sensitivity of diagnostic criteria, and other methodological differences, whether or not data are collected in vocational, third-level, clinical settings or the general population.

On the contrary, the prevalence of ASD in children and adolescents with bipolar spectrum conditions, including BD type I, type II, and softer BD forms, ranged from 7.3% [22] to 56.9% [23], with the majority of the studies going beyond the prevalence of 15% [14, 24–26]. Such high rates are not surprising given that early onset BD could be considered a neurodevelopmental disorder and is associated to a variety of psychiatric comorbidities. Indeed, the familial correlates and the phenotypic expression were similar in BD patients, irrespective of the association with ASD [14]. There are very few studies exploring the co-occurrence of ASD in samples of BD adults. In a recent large population-based report performed matching different Swedish national registers, including data of 54,723 BD individuals, ASD was found to co-occur in the 1.4% of BD cases vs. 0.1% of the controls from the general population, and genetics accounted for 2/3 of the correlation between the two diagnoses [27]. In a screening of autistic traits by means of the autism quotient (AQ) assessment in a sample of adults with BD type I, 36.1% of BD patients scored at or above the cut-off of clinical significance. As expected, autistic traits resulted significantly more prominent in male probands than in females (50.75% vs. 21%) [28]. Data regarding the gender distribution are actually not conclusive, but it is possible that, as in the general population, some differences might rise on the basis of the bipolar illness course and subtype. For example, in a Swedish sample of 54 HFA adult outpatients, an additional diagnosis of BD type II was made in the 9% of the cases with a slight preponderance in the female gender (11% vs. 8%) [29].

The association between ASD and BD is confirmed by familial studies [30–32]. Asperger himself was convinced that the syndromic picture he described had "by nature an important load of inheritance" [33].

Among ASD patients, a positive family history for affective disorders can be found in the 17% and 13% of the family members of autistic and Asperger subjects, respectively [34]. Several studies reported higher prevalence of depression and BD among ASD patients' relatives compared to family members of children with other types of disabilities [30, 35, 36]. Some authors suggested that familiarity for mood disorders could represent a determinant for subtyping different phenotypes or distinct classes of patients. DeLong hypothesized the existence of two "taxa" of ASDs, one constituted by high-functioning subjects, with prominent anxiety, obsessive symptoms, mood imbalance, and positive family history for major psychiatric disorders, specifically mood disorders. The other class would be made up of subjects with language and learning disorders associated to the lack of family history for mood disorders [37]. In a 1988 study DeLong and Dwyer [38] found higher rates of BD in families with an AS history compared to other ASDs (6.1% vs. 3.3%). A 1994 study showed that, in ASD children, the absence of a defined neurological disease correlated with autistic syndrome was associated with family history for affective disorders [39]. The majority of the studies on psychiatric morbidity of ASD patients' parents show that the mood disorder onset usually precedes the birth of the ASD offspring. This observation seems to suggest the prevalence of biological and genetic underpinnings in mood disorders among relatives of ASD patients, particularly HFA; on the contrary, a reactive component linked to the stress of care-giving a disabled child might have less pathogenetic weight [30, 40].

In 2005 Ghaziuddin analyzed the family history of 58 AS patients aged from 7 to 20 years and recruited from the community services. The 60.3% of first-, second-, and third-degree family members of probands reported a history of depression and other mental disorders [41]. The author noted that the lack of a specific correlation with BD might be attributable to the use of different diagnostic criteria comparing to previous studies.

Another study pertinent to the IAN project considered 988 couples of mother and child and examined the potential association between maternal history of mental disorders and high-functioning phenotypes of ASD [42]. This study found a significantly higher prevalence of both depression (47.1% vs. 39.1%) and BD (10.1% vs. 6.2%) in mothers of HFA probands than in the mothers of autistic children. Women with a mood disorder, particularly those with BD, showed higher rates of depressive recurrences; moreover, the majority of mothers affected by depression and BD reported the onset as preceding the first pregnancy. On the other hand, the history of bipolar illness in this population was associated with significantly higher risk of bearing an HFA than an autistic child (OR 2.11, CI 1.20–3.69). Similar results have been obtained in a case–control study considering four different samples. A diagnosis of bipolar illness in parents increases of 1.5 to 1.9-fold the risk of ASD in offspring. The odds ratio (OR) is near to that of general population (1.1) when ID co-occurs, whereas it is 1.7 for people with average IQ. The risk of ASD is further higher (OR 2.5) in siblings of bipolar patients [43].

In summary, epidemiological and clinical studies showed a bidirectional relationship between ASD and BD both at personal and at familial level, with rates of co-occurrence higher than in the general population. In the perspective of hereditariness, the link between ASD and BD seems to be stronger in high-functioning subtypes, suggesting larger contribution of commonly shared genetic underpinnings. However, from the clinical side, the comorbidity with BD shows similar rates in both HFA and LFA with comparable implications.

7.3 Clinical Features of Bipolar Disorder in Autism Spectrum Disorder

Consistently with our experience, Skeppar et al. [6] observed that comorbid affective disorders in adults with ASD, especially in HFA, are often diagnosed as Schizophrenia spectrum conditions. When the atypical presentation of mood symptoms together with the peculiar, sometimes odd, adaptive, and behavioral functioning of autistic persons are combined, the clinical picture considered in a cross-sectional perspective may strongly resemble what we are used to call schizophrenia. Even the premorbid functioning of HFA may be confused with a variety of cluster A and C personality disorders, corroborating the misdiagnosis [4].

Manic episodes in adult with ASD seem to be frequently characterized by irritable, instable, and dysphoric mood and hostility more than classic euphoric mood, elation, and jocularity. Other important symptoms are restlessness, anxiety, perplexity, aggression, violent behavior, and insomnia [5, 6, 11, 14, 44, 45]. To our knowledge, frequencies of mixed versus classic manic features were not systematically studied in adults with ASD.

Psychotic symptoms may be an important feature of the manic: in many cases, hallucinations, psychotic interpretations, and delusional ideas (mostly with persecutory, reference and grandiose content) may be prominent and dominate the clinical presentation [5, 6, 44, 45]. Bizarre thought contents are not rare but they have to be distinguished from odd thinking, bizarre ideas, and idiosyncratic views or feelings, which are really common among ASD subjects also during euthymia [19, 45–47]. It has been suggested that during manic episodes the peculiar way of thinking of ASD subjects becomes more prominent or that they become more prone to share their thoughts with others [6, 46]. Making a differential diagnosis should be considered a crucial point. Indeed, persons without ID and language impairment and with good adaptive skills may remain undiagnosed till a comorbidity onset. The differentiation of bizarre, "different," and concrete thinking and perceptual anomalies of autistic persons by psychotic symptoms is based on comprehending whether those symptoms are autistic core features or reactive behaviors with understandable link to the experience and specific cognitive deficits of these persons [48]. For example, there are clear differences in the peculiar pedantic and accurate language of some HFA persons from the formal disturbances in thought and language found in schizophrenic patients with prominently negative symptoms, mostly incoherence, vagueness, and circumstantiality [49]. Similarly, paranoid ideas might be dragged by difficulty in the theory of mind and social reciprocity associated with repeated negative social experiences. Concretism may also lead to misinterpretation of medical questions during the psychiatric exam.

The presence of other behavioral features typical for ASD such as rigid adherence to routines, sensory issues, and early-onset stereotypies can support the diagnostic process. As a rule, although odd thinking may become more intense during acute affective phases, it is stable and long-lasting, and in the majority of the cases, it is present since childhood without the classical rift of thinking and functioning as they are described in other psychotic conditions. In addition, "psychotic" thoughts are less interfering with daily functioning and less emotionally engrossing in ASD than in schizophrenia [46, 50]. In ASD patients with ID and language impairment, the excitatory phase may be described more appropriately by the disruption of neurovegetative patterns such as appetite, sleep, sexual activity, and the variation of psychomotricity.

The detection of hypomania in BD type II and other soft bipolar spectrum conditions is usually more difficult. Irritability, excessive mood reactivity, increase of energy and activity, psychomotor activation, and diminished need for sleep may be labile and often labeled as "simple reactions" to environmental conditions in persons which are more vulnerable to changes. Such symptoms may actually be elicited by difficulties in the modulation of arousal, for example, when routines change or during the exposition to new and/or social situations [51–53] but, when a set of recurring wax-and-waning symptoms are identified, clearly different from the usual and interfering with baseline functioning, the diagnosis has to be considered. Beyond an accurate clinical interview, the systematic use of specific assessment instruments for mood symptoms is recommended [7, 11, 54, 55]. The presence of positive familial history for BD, special abilities, early onset anxiety, and/or multiple psychiatric comorbidities and comorbid Tourette's syndrome are other important risk factors for bipolarity in ASD [12, 30, 32, 37, 56–59].

In individuals with ASD, depression may be barely recognizable, because it is frequently characterized by mild severity and long-lasting, often chronic, course. Depressive symptoms have to be specifically investigated as a clear-cut variation in personal, adaptive, and social functioning in comparison with a baseline reference point: some of the core autistic dimensions, such as blunt affect and social withdrawal, can be simply amplified during depression, and the depressive dimension remains neglected [6]. Moreover, difficulties in social communication and introspection, idiosyncratic thinking, and feelings might add difficulties in investigating or correctly interpreting the "inner" dimension of depression [6, 12]. Non-verbal typical expressions of depression may also lack [4]. To improve the capacity of detecting depression in clinical settings, the systematic utilization of specific assessment instruments, both self- and hetero-administered rating scales (e.g. MADRS, BDI), could be useful. As in the case of mania and hypomania, variations in psychomotricity and neurovegetative functioning are the best depressive diagnostic parameters (from hypersomnia to insomnia, loss of appetite) [12, 55, 60, 61]. The loss of energy may reflect in the reduction of the number and involvement in usual interests and activities. Anhedonia, apathy, feelings of worthlessness or guilt, low self-esteem, recurrent thought of death, diminished concentration, and indecisiveness are common as in other depressive patients [7, 53, 55, 56]. Stressful events preceding the onset of depression are not uncommon, especially in higher functioning subjects with problems in social adjustment but high social motivation with decrease of self-esteem and experience of personal failure [62]. Mood instability, atypical, violent and sudden affective changes, from lability to irritability, aggression, self-injuring, and agitation are not uncommon [7, 63–65]. It has to be considered that such behavioral features of depression are particularly common in persons with co-occurring ID in which psychopathology may manifest itself via challenging behaviors and the increase of core symptoms of the basic neurodevelopmental disorder, for example, stereotypies. In LFA a deterioration in cognitive performance, behavior, or activities with cyclic pattern ("alternation of good and bad times"), even in the absence of other clear mood symptoms, may be indicative of the co-occurrence of bipolarity [11]. Suicidality in ASD is not infrequent becoming a primary challenge. Any suicidal behavior including suicidal ideation, planning, suicide attempt, and completed suicide ranged from 11% to 50% in different populations, much higher than suicidal rates in schizophrenic patients (7–10%) [66, 67]. In such a case, the implications of a misdiagnosis might be severe. Suicidal ideation may be facilitated by some cognitive peculiarities of HFA such as the impairment of the capacity to understand mental and emotional states, difficulties in realizing what suicide means for their relatives, reduced flexibility, and dichotomous thinking: suicidal thoughts may become an obsession, and the person may spend lot of time searching information and planning [4].

Consistent with our experience, movement disorders and catatonia have also been frequently reported in adults with ASD [68–70]. Catatonia can be identified in the 12–17% of clinical samples of ASD adolescents and young adults [71, 72]. Catatonia seems to be equally distributed in HFA and LFA [71]. Catatonia in ASD subjects seems to be often associated with repetitive self-injuries, posturing, and negativism [69]. In those cases, while lorazepam has demonstrated a certain efficacy, electroconvulsive therapy seems to be the most and persistently successful treatment [73]. *DSM-5* recognized that both BD and ASD are independently associated with catatonia which is no more considered a sign of psychosis [1] and, in persons with ASD and BD, might be precipitated or worsened by antipsychotics [74].

7.4 Treatment

Recent studies have shown that some ASD manifestations might be partially modified by appropriate pharmacological treatments, leading to improvement in socialization, language, adaptive skills, and mood [75, 76].

Current literature on pharmacological options in comorbid ASD and BD consists of case reports or case series, and all the available treatments are not adequately studied in systematic or controlled studies.

7.4.1 Mood Stabilizers

Controlled studies regarding the use of lithium and other mood stabilizers in comorbid ASD and BD are substantially lacking, but their use is supported by numerous case reports and case-series, indicating their efficacy for mood instability and cyclicity in ASD subjects, both in childhood and in adulthood, as in neurotypical persons [77–80]. Lithium is recommended as first choice for the treatment of manic symptoms in ASD-BD patients with BD among relatives [81–83]. Positive family history [36], severe hyperactivity unresponsive to stimulants, cyclical pattern of behavioral changes, irritability, enduring outbursts of laughter, subjective dizziness, and the presence of at least some BD diagnostic criteria [84] are predictors of favorable lithium response. Lithium seems to be effective in controlling aggression and hyperactivity in some cases, even in LFA, as well as in reducing manic symptoms and mood swings [85].

An anticonvulsant may be a better choice than lithium when the patient is epileptic or significant EEG alterations have been found. Some antiepileptic drugs may also be useful when other psychopathological dimensions dominate the clinical picture (e.g., severe anxiety, impulsivity, and aggression) or the clinical psychopathological picture is particularly polymorphic with a mix of variable symptoms going from psychosis to derealization/depersonalization, depression, anxiety, and somatizations, suggesting a possible etiologic correlation with forced normalization of EEG abnormalities [86]. Valproate is the anticonvulsant with the largest number of observations in comorbid ASD and BD. Some reports suggest the effective use of valproate in adults with ASD with the reduction of non-convulsive symptoms such as hyper-arousal, irritability, dysphoria, and anxiety [87]. Valproate has been found to have promising effects when in LFA with typical and atypical forms of manic depressive illness including rapid cycling [88]. Another retrospective small study including 14 patients with HFA found valproate to be effective on affective instability, impulsivity, and aggression, independently from the presence of seizures and EEG abnormalities [89]. There are two large studies regarding persons with ID, including ASD patients, one perspective and the other retrospective: they both evidenced the efficacy of valproate in the 70% of the cases on hyperactivity, impulsivity, and stereotypies but even more on aggressiveness and self-injury [90, 91], all considered possible behavioral equivalents of mood symptoms if contextualized in a syndromic and recurrent pattern.

Like valproate carbamazepine is used in persons with intellectual and relational disabilities as anticonvulsants when epilepsy co-occurs, and it has the general indication as mood stabilizer for the treatment and prophylaxis of BD even in the case of raid cycling [92, 93]. Other targets of carbamazepine may be aggressiveness and self-mutilations especially in persons with ID in which these challenging behaviors are related to epilepsy or mood disorders [94, 95]. Few observations indicated that oxcarbazepine may be useful in combination with low doses of second-generation antipsychotic HFA adults with BD [5].

Although lamotrigine has the indication for the prophylaxis of depressive recurrences in BD in neurotypical subjects, the few available data on its use in ASD do not allow conclusive remarks [96].

7.4.2 Antipsychotics

The use of antipsychotics in ASD has been extensively studied although most studies regarded small samples of children and adolescents, and the focus of the treatment was irritability. Clinical trials may have considerable selection and referral biases mostly recruiting individuals with severe problem behavior, without a clear distinction among specific clinical phenotypes, ID presence, and severity and presence of psychiatric comorbidity. As a consequence, the results are only partially generalizable to all persons with ASD.

First-generation antipsychotics (FGA) in the past were the most prescribed drugs [97, 98]. In the 1970s, haloperidol and pimozide were extensively used given their efficacy in the decrease of stereotypies, hyperactivity, emotional outbursts, and temper tantrums [99–103]. However, their used became later not recommended because of the high rate extrapyramidal side effects and dyskinesias (5–15%) [104, 105], with the exception of co-occurring tic disorders and Tourette's syndrome. As a consequence, second-generation antipsychotics (SGA) replaced FGA in the last few decades. However, it has to be kept in mind that certain FGA, mostly chlorpromazine which have a complex pharmacodynamic profile including 5-HT2a antagonism, may represent a valid treatment option in acute manic and mixed phases to rapidly reach the remission of excitatory symptoms. Risperidone and aripiprazole are the most frequently studied and used: they are the only medications with a FDA-specific indication for the treatment of irritability in ASD children [75]. The vast amount of data on the use of risperidone in children and adolescents with ASD showed it is effective for repetitive, aggressive, and impulsive behaviors; some studies also suggested it would improve at some degree social impairment [106–109]. It has to be taken into account that it is possible that the improvement of core autistic dimensions is dragged by the improvement of co-occurring mood symptoms, reactivity, and hyperactivity more than a true "curative" effect on these dimensions. The severity of irritability and also aggressive behavior are reliable predictors of response to risperidone [110]. In spite of initial enthusiasm, risperidone prolonged or high-dosage use can often produce extrapyramidal symptoms (EPS) and tardive dyskinesia, although to lesser extent than haloperidol. Moreover, risperidone often induces weight gain, drowsiness, and hyperprolactinemia and, in many cases, would require drug discontinuation [111–115]. Some data suggested paliperidone to have similar efficacy as risperidone, also in its long-acting formulation [116]. Risperidone in the 70% of HFA children and youngsters (6–12 years old) treated produced a significant reduction in negative symptoms [117]. Risperidone is widely used, in childhood as well as in adulthood, for the treatment of manic symptoms and related behavioral problems in BD [118]. In a case-series of adults with BD and HFA, low doses of risperidone associated with anticonvulsants have shown a good efficacy [5]. In children, adolescents, and adults with ID, risperidone halves the intensity of challenging behaviors (aggressiveness, rage outbursts, and self-injury in the 50% of the persons treated) [119]. The effectiveness on challenging behaviors in LFA seems to be dose-related [120] and increases by the association to rehabilitative-educational interventions, for example, parent training [121].

Aripiprazole, the second most used medication, in a study regarding HFA children and adolescents reduced irritability, aggression, self-injury, and temper tantrums in the 88% of cases, with good short-term tolerability. Common side effects were weight gain, hyperprolactinemia, dose-dependent sedation, and sialorrhoea [122]. As in the case of risperidone, the long-term use is associated with high rate of EPS and tardive dyskinesia, requiring careful monitoring. The results regarding the treatment of aggressiveness, disruptive behavior, and severe challenge behaviors in persons with ID are less consistent than risperidone [123, 124]. Aripiprazole may be useful in the treatment of mania and psychosis even in LFA adults [92]. The long-term use of aripiprazole for maintenance treatment and prophylaxis of illness recurrences requires awareness of the peculiar pharmacokinetics of these medication and the special vulnerability of LFA persons to neurological and cognitive side effects.

Olanzapine, scarcely effective on core autistic symptoms, might be very effective in agitated manic and mixed ASD patients, but its use is burdened by side effects, such as sedation and weight gain [125, 126]. Quetiapine has not been extensively studied in ASD and showed some efficacy in the control of aggressive behavior and sleep disturbances, but did not seem to influence autistic symptoms [127–129]. For these reasons, olanzapine and quetiapine should not be considered first choice drugs in the treatment of ASD. In a clinical trial comparing the anti-manic short-term (8 weeks) efficacy of SGAs (risperidone, olanzapine, quetiapine, ziprasidone, and aripiprazole) in 151 youth with BD, the efficacy and tolerability of SGAs were similar in patients with or without ASD. More specifically, 69% of BD patients and 65% of BD + ASD patients presented an improvement of at least 30% at the Y-MRS and 47% of BD patients compared to 44% of BD + ASD had an improvement of at least 50% [25]. However, a recent study reported less encouraging results: the treatment of BD with atypical antipsychotics, alone or in combination with mood stabilizers, showed response rates ranging from poor to modest. Authors noted that the response was low even though the rates of psychotic symptoms were higher than those found in previous studies [21]. The overall response to treatment was poor to modest.

There is a body of literature indicating that antipsychotics highly selective on the serotonin transporter (5-HTT) and the 5-HT2A receptors should be considered of first choice in ASD [130–132]. The scientific rationale is represented by those molecular and biological studies that observed in ASD some alterations involving the serotonergic system such as “hyperserotonemia” [133–136], high brain tissue 5-HT concentration, especially in the cortex [137], alteration in the brain 5-HT synthesis [138, 139], reduction of the 5-HT2A receptor binding capacity [140] (negatively related to the platelet 5-HT concentration), and reduction of the 5-HTT binding capacity, especially in the anterior and posterior cingulate cortex [141].

Asenapine is an antagonist of D2 and 5-HT2A receptors approved by FDA as adjunctive therapy with lithium or valproate for manic or mixed episodes in BD type I. Although there are not RCTs in ASD patients, its pharmacodynamic profile makes it an option to be considered in collaborative patients, also given the good tolerability of long-term flexible dose of sublingual administration [142].

Lurasidone too has 5-HT2A antagonistic properties and is indicated for the treatment of depressive episodes in adult BD type I patients. A recent study demonstrated its efficacy also in children and adolescents with a similar indication [143]. In a 2016 6-week placebo-controlled study in ASD children and adolescents requiring treatment for irritability, agitation and self-injury, lurasidone demonstrated few differences at different dosages compared to placebo in ameliorating irritability [144]. However, the potential effectiveness is suggested by a case report regarding an LFA adolescent with aggressive and impulsive behavior [145]. Lurasidone should be an option mostly because of its favorable metabolic tolerability profile when other SGAs demonstrated efficacy but caused excessive weight gain and metabolic side effects.

7.4.3 Antidepressants

The use of tricyclic antidepressants (TCAs) and selective serotonin reuptake inhibitors (SSRIs) is wide in daily clinical practice with young ASD patients. However, evidences of their effectiveness in ASD are poorly reliable [146, 147]. Their use with comorbid BD has not been systematically studied, but some suggestions are derived by some case reports.

SSRI antidepressants have been studied in ASDs mainly for the treatment of anxiety, obsessive-compulsive symptoms, and depression. Some evidence of efficacy has been shown for fluoxetine, citalopram, sertraline, and paroxetine [7, 148–151]. However, results are contradictory in youth and not conclusive in adulthood [147]. In the case of ineffectiveness of an SSRI, a second attempt with a different SSRI has been reported as "often unsuccessful" [152].

Especially in children and adolescents, the use of these drugs should be carefully monitored; SSRIs may be related to activation syndrome, with agitation, aggression, self-injuring, insomnia, and suicidal and, in some cases, also homicidal thoughts [153, 154]; EPS have also been reported more frequently than in the general population evidencing a peculiar vulnerability as in the case of antipsychotics [155]. In a short-term chart review of 89 young ASD outpatients treated with SSRIs, although the 44.9% of the subjects were considered responders, the 54% showed activation that in the 35.4% of the cases needed the discontinuation of the medication [154].

In bipolar HFA caution needed are more as several observations and case series reported that antidepressants, especially SSRIs, can cause (hypo)manic switches and mixed symptoms [5, 44, 156, 157]. Antidepressant treatment may also negatively influence the long-term course of bipolar illness causing increased affective instability, chronic mixed states, and rapid cycling [154, 158].

For patients with ASD in general and HFA in particular seeking treatment for depressive or anxiety symptoms, a very careful personal and family medical history survey is required to exclude a bipolar diathesis. When an antidepressant is prescribed, the clinician should plan frequent controls to detect early eventual side effects and mood changes. The possible use of an antidepressant in combination with a mood stabilizer reduces but does not eliminate the possibility of mood switches and affective destabilization [158].

7.4.4 Stimulants

There are no controlled studies exploring the use of stimulants (methylphenidate [MPH], dexmethylphenidate, dextroamphetamine, mixed amphetamine salts, dextromethamphetamine, and lisdexamfetamine) in adults with ASD-BD. However, considering that the co-occurring of ASD and ADHD is not infrequent [159] and may require a pharmacologic approach, it is appropriate to mention the small literature regarding the use of stimulants in ASD-ADHD comorbidity. Indeed, such a comorbidity may represent a condition with increased risk to develop further psychiatric disorders during adulthood, namely BD. Data on this topic are lacking because the criterion E of *DSM-IV-TR* for the diagnosis of ADHD considered the presence of an ASD as an exclusion criterion [2]. This is also one of the reasons why ADHD-like symptoms in this population are often under-recognized and undertreated, although some patients with HFA refer to clinical setting for ADHD and not for mild autistic symptoms [160].

A recent systematic review [161] on the efficacy and tolerability of stimulants for ADHD-like symptoms in individuals with ASD, considering randomized-controlled, uncontrolled studies, and expert commentaries found that stimulants may be effective in ASD in the treatment of ADHD-like symptoms. The frequency of adverse events was higher than in children with ADHD without ASD. However, stimulants seem to be more effective and better tolerated in higher functioning than in other ASD individuals [162, 163]. Decreased appetite (with medium-high doses), difficulty falling asleep, stomach or abdominal discomfort, irritability and emotional outburst are common side effects [109, 164].

7.5 Conclusion

A consistent body of research evidences a significant association between BD and ASD in clinical samples, although it is difficult to estimate the actual prevalence in the general population. Up to 20% of HFA subjects referred to clinical settings report BD comorbidity [5, 165] and the prevalence reaches similar percentages in LFA [166].

The literature also strongly supports that ASD would be associated with familial load for mood disorders [30, 35, 36, 41] and that the most frequent association is reported with BD in first-degree relatives of persons with HFA [37, 38, 42]. This last finding suggests that it is possible that high-functioning forms of ASD may represent a more homogeneous and restricted phenotype, with possible common underpinnings with BD [27]. Further research taking into account more specific phenotypes, familial history, and patterns of psychiatric versus organic comorbidity is needed.

Many of the ASD-BD adult patients are not adequately diagnosed and appropriately treated [5, 6, 46, 167]. Although epidemiological data suggest that BD is more common in HFA than in the neurotypical population, psychiatrists may neglect ASD features [168]. The presence of ASD in adults is often not correctly identified in high-functioning individuals, and the related features are interpreted as personality and/or schizophrenia spectrum disorders [6, 46, 167, 169–171].

On the contrary, in LFA, the comorbidity with BD may be underestimated, and mood symptoms are often overlooked or attributed to the neurodevelopmental condition rather than BD, in spite of the episodic or cyclic course.

In adult patients with comorbid ASD and BDs, schizophrenia is the most frequent misdiagnosis [6]. This is mainly due to the following reasons: (1) excitatory episodes are often characterized by irritability, aggression, outbursts of anger more than signs of classic mania as euphoric mood. Moreover, psychotic symptoms are common and tend to be prominent compared to other symptoms, contributing the attention of the clinician to be shifted toward the psychotic more than the affective dimension; (2) the depressive episodes are frequently chronic and attenuated by nature. Motivation, volition, and psychomotricity are mainly involved, widely overlapping with negative and residual symptoms of schizophrenia; (3) odd thinking, bizarre ideas, and idiosyncratic views can be interpreted as delusional or psychotic thoughts.

In LFA the diagnostic process is even more complicated by the very restricted repertoire of skills and behaviors and should require a longer term of observation. The collection of information from different caregivers may be necessary and the use of specific assessing tools might facilitate this process.

A correct diagnosis of BD in ASD individuals and vice versa has relevant implications on the choice of correct psychological, psychopharmacological, and rehabilitative treatments. Notably, data from controlled trials are limited in number and generalizability. In fact, patients with atypical and complex clinical pictures, multiple comorbidities, or organic disorders are usually excluded from clinical trials. Nevertheless, literature provides some useful suggestions for clinical practice. Mood stabilizers are preferable, either in monotherapy or in combination with other drugs. Antipsychotics should be used at the lowest effective dose and for the strictly necessary period to minimize short- and long-term neurological, cognitive, and metabolic effects and the risk of precipitating catatonia. The majority of data are relative to the use of the SGAs risperidone and aripiprazole, but other antipsychotics with 5-HT2A antagonists can be effective. Antidepressants should be used with caution and careful monitoring, in the attempt of an early detection of activation and switch phenomena and to prevent negative long-term impact on the course of the affective illness. The literature on this issue is still incomplete, and long-term controlled studies on large samples are needed to enrich the knowledge in the field.

Finally, educational and training interventions regarding ASD-BD comorbidity aimed at pediatricians, neurologists, and childhood and adulthood psychiatrists are crucial point to improve knowledge on this vast field and to ensure patients to receive appropriate diagnosis and treatment. A personalized psycho-educational and rehabilitative intervention should also be provided pursuing the goodness of fit. These interventions should also be specifically designed on the basis of ASD features and differentiated from programs commonly used in other chronic and disabled patients.

References

1. Association AP. Diagnostic and statistical manual of mental disorders, fifth edition (DSM-5). 5th ed. Arlington: Author; 2013.
2. APA. Diagnostic and statistical manual of mental disorders. Text revision. (DSM-IV-TR). 4th-text revision ed. Washington, DC: American Psychiatric Association; 2000.
3. Mandell DS, Novak MM, Zubritsky CD. Factors associated with age of diagnosis among children with autism spectrum disorders. Pediatrics. 2005;116(6):1480–6.
4. Lai MC, Baron-Cohen S. Identifying the lost generation of adults with autism spectrum conditions. Lancet Psychiatry. 2015;2(11):1013–27.
5. Raja M, Azzoni A. Comorbidity of Asperger's syndrome and bipolar disorder. Clin Pract Epidemiol Ment Health. 2008;4:26.
6. Skeppar P, Thoor R, Sture A, Isakson A, Skeppar I, Persson B, et al. Neurodevelopmental disorders with comorbid affective disorders sometimes produce psychiatric conditions traditionally diagnosed as schizophrenia. Clin Neuropsychiatry. 2013;10(3–4):123–33.
7. Tantam D, Girgis S. Recognition and treatment of Asperger syndrome in the community. Br Med Bull. 2009;89:41–62.
8. Weissman AS, Bates ME. Increased clinical and neurocognitive impairment in children with autism spectrum disorders and comorbid bipolar disorder. Res Autism Spectr Disord. 2010;4:670–80.
9. Rutter M. Autistic children: infancy to adulthood. Semin Psychiatry. 1970;2:435–50.
10. Masi A, DeMayo MM, Glozier N, Guastella AJ. An overview of autism spectrum disorder, heterogeneity and treatment options. Neurosci Bull. 2017;33(2):183–93.
11. Frazier JA, Doyle R, Chiu S, Coyle JT. Treating a child with Asperger's disorder and comorbid bipolar disorder. Am J Psychiatry. 2002;159(1):13–21.
12. Rosenberg RE, Kaufmann WE, Law JK, Law PA. Parent report of community psychiatric comorbid diagnoses in autism spectrum disorders. Autism Res Treat. 2011;2011:405849.
13. Vannucchi G, Coli S, Scuticchio D, Bertelli M, editors. Autism spectrum disorder: a vulnerability factor for psychiatric comorbidity in adults with intellectual disability and autism? A literature review. In: WPA XVII World Congress of Psychiatry, Psychiatry of the 21st Century: Context, Controversies and Commitment. Berlin; 2017.
14. Joshi G, Biederman J, Petty C, Goldin RL, Furtak SL, Wozniak J. Examining the comorbidity of bipolar disorder and autism spectrum disorders: a large controlled analysis of phenotypic and familial correlates in a referred population of youth with bipolar I disorder with and without autism spectrum disorders. J Clin Psychiatry. 2013;74(6):578–86.
15. Bradley E, Bolton P. Episodic psychiatric disorders in teenagers with learning disabilities with and without autism. Br J Psychiatry. 2006;189:361–6.
16. Bryson SA, Corrigan SK, McDonald TP, Holmes C. Characteristics of children with autism spectrum disorders who received services through community mental health centers. Autism. 2008;12(1):65–82.

17. Mukaddes NM, Fateh R, Kilincaslan A. Kleine-Levin syndrome in two subjects with diagnosis of autistic disorder. World J Biol Psychiatry. 2009;10(4 Pt 3):969–72.
18. Hutton J, Goode S, Murphy M, Le Couteur A, Rutter M. New-onset psychiatric disorders in individuals with autism. Autism. 2008;12(4):373–90.
19. Ghaziuddin M, Weidmer-Mikhail E, Ghaziuddin N. Comorbidity of Asperger syndrome: a preliminary report. J Intellect Disabil Res. 1998;42(Pt4):279–83.
20. Guinchat V, Cravero C, Diaz L, Perisse D, Xavier J, Amiet C, et al. Acute behavioral crises in psychiatric inpatients with autism spectrum disorder (ASD): recognition of concomitant medical or non-ASD psychiatric conditions predicts enhanced improvement. Res Dev Disabil. 2015;38:242–55.
21. Nahar A, Thippeswamy H, Shanker Reddy MS, Kishore MT, Chaturvedi SK. Psychiatric comorbidity in persons with high-functioning autism spectrum disorders: findings from a tertiary care neuropsychiatric hospital. Asian J Psychiatr. 2019;41:50–3.
22. Axelson D, Birmaher B, Strober M, Gill MK, Valeri S, Chiappetta L, et al. Phenomenology of children and adolescents with bipolar spectrum disorders. Arch Gen Psychiatry. 2006;63(10):1139–48.
23. Pine DS, Guyer AE, Goldwin M, Towbin KA, Leibenluft E. Autism spectrum disorder scale scores in pediatric mood and anxiety disorders. J Am Acad Child Adolesc Psychiatry. 2008;47(6):652–61.
24. Johnson CR, Handen BL, Lubetsky MJ, Sacco KA. Affective disorders in hospitalized children and adolescents with mental retardation: a retrospective study. Res Dev Disabil. 1995;16(3):221–31.
25. Joshi G, Biederman J, Wozniak J, Doyle R, Hammerness P, Galdo M, et al. Response to second generation antipsychotics in youth with comorbid bipolar disorder and autism spectrum disorder. CNS Neurosci Ther. 2012;18(1):28–33.
26. Joshi G, Wozniak J, Petty C, Martelon MK, Fried R, Bolfek A, et al. Psychiatric comorbidity and functioning in a clinically referred population of adults with autism spectrum disorders: a comparative study. J Autism Dev Disord. 2013;43(6):1314–25.
27. Song J, Bergen SE, Kuja-Halkola R, Larsson H, Landen M, Lichtenstein P. Bipolar disorder and its relation to major psychiatric disorders: a family-based study in the Swedish population. Bipolar Disord. 2015;17(2):184–93.
28. Abu-Akel A, Clark J, Perry A, Wood SJ, Forty L, Craddock N, et al. Autistic and schizotypal traits and global functioning in bipolar I disorder. J Affect Disord. 2017;207:268–75.
29. Lugnegard T, Hallerbäck MU, Gillberg C. Psychiatric comorbidity in young adults with a clinical diagnosis of Asperger syndrome. Res Dev Disabil. 2011;32(5):1910–7.
30. Bolton PF, Pickles A, Murphy M, Rutter M. Autism, affective and other psychiatric disorders: patterns of familial aggregation. Psychol Med. 1998;28(2):385–95.
31. Ghaziuddin M, Greden J. Depression in children with autism/pervasive developmental disorders: a case-control family history study. J Autism Dev Disord. 1998;28:111–5.
32. Piven J, Palmer P. Psychiatric disorder and the broad autism phenotype: evidence from a family study of multiple-incidence autism families. Am J Psychiatry. 1999;156(4):557–63.
33. Asperger H. Die autistischen Psychopathen im Kindersalter. Arch Psychiatr Nervenkr. 1944;117:76–136.
34. Gillberg IC, Gillberg C. Asperger syndrome—some epidemiological considerations: a research note. J Child Psychol Psychiatry. 1989;30(4):631–8.
35. Lajiness-O'Neill R, Menard P. Brief report: an autistic spectrum subtype revealed through familial psychopathology coupled with cognition in ASD. J Autism Dev Disord. 2008;38(5):982–7.
36. Piven J, Chase GA, Landa R, Wzorek M, Gayle J, Cloud D, et al. Psychiatric disorders in the parents of autistic individuals. J Am Acad Child Adolesc Psychiatry. 1991;30(3):471–8.
37. DeLong R. Autism and familial major mood disorder: are they related? J Neuropsychiatry Clin Neurosci. 2004;16(2):199–213.

38. DeLong GR, Dwyer JT. Correlation of family history with specific autistic subgroups: Asperger's syndrome and bipolar affective disease. J Autism Dev Disord. 1988;18(4):593–600.
39. DeLong R, Nohria C. Psychiatric family history and neurological disease in autistic spectrum disorders. Dev Med Child Neurol. 1994;36(5):441–8.
40. Cohen IL, Tsiouris JA. Maternal recurrent mood disorders and high-functioning autism. J Autism Dev Disord. 2006;36(8):1077–88.
41. Ghaziuddin M. A family history study of Asperger syndrome. J Autism Dev Disord. 2005;35(2):177–82.
42. Vasa RA, Anderson C, Marvin AR, Rosenberg RE, Law JK, Thorn J, et al. Mood disorders in mothers of children on the autism spectrum are associated with higher functioning autism. Autism Res Treat. 2012;2012:435646.
43. Sullivan PF, Magnusson C, Reichenberg A, Boman M, Dalman C, Davidson M, et al. Family history of schizophrenia and bipolar disorder as risk factors for autism. Arch Gen Psychiatry. 2012;69(11):1099–103.
44. Ng B, Au M, Verhoeven M, Johnston L, Perkins C. The diagnosis of Asperger's syndrome in an adult presenting with an index episode of mania. Gen Hosp Psychiatry. 2003;25(4):295–7.
45. Raja M, Azzoni A. Thought disorder in Asperger syndrome and schizophrenia: issues in the differential diagnosis. A series of case reports. World J Biol Psychiatry. 2009;10(4 Pt 3):944–52.
46. Fitzgerald M. Schizophrenia and autism/Asperger's syndrome: overlap and difference. Clin Neuropsychiatry. 2012;4(9):171–6.
47. Loveland KA, Pearson DA, Tunali-Kotoski B, Ortegon J, Gibbs MC. Judgments of social appropriateness by children and adolescents with autism. J Autism Dev Disord. 2001;31(4):367–76.
48. Van Schalkwyk GI, Peluso F, Qayyum Z, McPartland JC, Volkmar FR. Varieties of misdiagnosis in ASD: an illustrative case series. J Autism Dev Disord. 2015;45(4):911–8.
49. Tebartz van Elst L, Pick M, Biscaldi M, Fangmeier T, Riedel A. High-functioning autism spectrum disorder as a basic disorder in adult psychiatry and psychotherapy: psychopathological presentation, clinical relevance and therapeutic concepts. Eur Arch Psychiatry Clin Neurosci. 2013;263(Suppl 2):S189–96.
50. Abell F, Hare DJ. An experimental investigation of the phenomenology of delusional beliefs in people with Asperger syndrome. Autism. 2005;9(5):515–31.
51. Leibenluft E. Severe mood dysregulation, irritability, and the diagnostic boundaries of bipolar disorder in youths. Am J Psychiatry. 2011;168(2):129–42.
52. Leibenluft E, Charney DS, Towbin KE, Bhangoo RK, Pine DS. Defining clinical phenotypes of juvenile mania. Am J Psychiatry. 2003;160(3):430–7.
53. Mazzone L, Ruta L, Reale L. Psychiatric comorbidities in Asperger syndrome and high functioning autism: diagnostic challenges. Ann Gen Psychiatry. 2012;11(1):16.
54. Dejong S, Frazier JA. Bipolar disorder in children with pervasive developmental disorders. In: Geller B, DelBello MP, editors. Bipolar disorder in childhood and early adolescence. New York: Guilford Press; 2003. p. 51–75.
55. Magnuson KM, Constantino JN. Characterization of depression in children with autism spectrum disorders. J Dev Behav Pediatr. 2011;32:332.
56. Ghaziuddin M, Ghaziuddin N, Greden J. Depression in persons with autism: implications for research and clinical care. J Autism Dev Disord. 2002;32(4):299–306.
57. Kerbeshian J, Burd L. Case study: comorbidity among Tourette's syndrome, autistic disorder, and bipolar disorder. J Am Acad Child Adolesc Psychiatry. 1996;35(5):681–5.
58. McElroy SL. Diagnosing and treating comorbid (complicated) bipolar disorder. J Clin Psychiatry. 2004;65(Suppl 15):35–44.
59. Sterling L, Dawson G, Estes A, Greenson J. Characteristics associated with presence of depressive symptoms in adults with autism spectrum disorder. J Autism Dev Disord. 2008;38(6):1011–8.
60. Ghazziuddin M, Zafar S. Psychiatric comorbidity of adults with autism spectrum disorders. Clin Neuropsychiatry. 2008;5:9–12.

61. Rao U, Chen LA. Characteristics, correlates, and outcomes of childhood and adolescent depressive disorders. Dialogues Clin Neurosci. 2009;11(1):45–62.
62. Ghaziuddin M, Ghaziuddin N, Greden J. Depression in adults with autism: implications for research and clinical care. J Autism Dev Disord. 2002;32:299–306.
63. Lainhart JE, Folstein SE. Affective disorders in people with autism: a review of published cases. J Autism Dev Disord. 1994;24(5):587–601.
64. Naidu A, James I, Mukaetova-Ladinska E, Briel R. Diagnosis of Asperger syndrome in a 66-year-old male presenting with depression. Int Psychogeriatr. 2006;18(1):171–3.
65. Spencer L, Lyketsos CG, Samstad E, Dokey A, Rostov D, Chisolm MS. A suicidal adult in crisis: an unexpected diagnosis of autism spectrum disorder. Am J Psychiatry. 2011;168(9):890–2.
66. Upthegrove R, Abu-Akel A, Chisholm K, Lin A, Zahid S, Pelton M, et al. Autism and psychosis: clinical implications for depression and suicide. Schizophr Res. 2018;195:80–5.
67. Toal F, Bloemen OJ, Deeley Q, Tunstall N, Daly EM, Page L, et al. Psychosis and autism: magnetic resonance imaging study of brain anatomy. Br J Psychiatry. 2009;194(5):418–25.
68. Takaoka K, Takata T. Catatonia in high-functioning autism spectrum disorders: case report and review of literature. Psychol Rep. 2007;101(3 Pt 1):961–9.
69. Fink M. Rediscovering catatonia: the biography of a treatable syndrome. Acta Psychiatr Scand Suppl. 2013;441:1–47.
70. Quigley J, Lommel KM, Coffey B. Catatonia in an adolescent with Asperger's disorder. J Child Adolesc Psychopharmacol. 2009;19(1):93–6.
71. Wing L, Shah A. Catatonia in autistic spectrum disorders. Br J Psychiatry. 2000;176:357–62.
72. Billstedt E, Gillberg IC, Gillberg C. Autism after adolescence: population-based 13- to 22-year follow-up study of 120 individuals with autism diagnosed in childhood. J Autism Dev Disord. 2005;35(3):351–60.
73. Kakooza-Mwesige A, Wachtel LE, Dhossche DM. Catatonia in autism: implications across the life span. Eur Child Adolesc Psychiatry. 2008;17(6):327–35.
74. Fink M, Taylor MA, Ghaziuddin N. Catatonia in autistic spectrum disorders: a medical treatment algorithm. Int Rev Neurobiol. 2006;72:233–44.
75. Politte LC, McDougle CJ. Atypical antipsychotics in the treatment of children and adolescents with pervasive developmental disorders. Psychopharmacology (Berl). 2014;231(6):1023–36.
76. Doyle CA, McDougle CJ. Pharmacotherapy to control behavioral symptoms in children with autism. Expert Opin Pharmacother. 2012;13(11):1615–29.
77. DeLong GR, Aldershof AL. Long-term experience with lithium treatment in childhood: correlation with clinical diagnosis. J Am Acad Child Adolesc Psychiatry. 1987;26(3):389–94.
78. DeLong R. Children with autistic spectrum disorder and a family history of affective disorder. Dev Med Child Neurol. 1994;36:674–87.
79. Komoto J, Usui S, Hirata J. Infantile autism and affective disorder. J Autism Dev Disord. 1984;14:81–4.
80. Steingard R, Biederman J. Lithium responsive manic-like symptoms in two individuals with autism and mental retardation. J Am Acad Child Adolesc Psychiatry. 1987;26:932–5.
81. Brendel DH, Bodkin JA, Hauptman B, Ornstein A. "I see dead people": overcoming psychic numbness. Harv Rev Psychiatry. 2002;10:166–78.
82. Bishop DV. Autism, Asperger's syndrome and semantic pragmatic disorder: where are the boundaries? Br J Disord Commun. 1989;24:107–21.
83. Kerbeshian J, Burd L, Fisher W. Asperger's syndrome: to be or not to be? Br J Psychiatry. 1990;156:721–5.
84. Kerbeshian J, Burd L, Fisher W. Lithium carbonate in the treatment of two patients with infantile autism and atypical bipolar symptomatology. J Clin Psychopharmacol. 1987;7(6):401–5.
85. Tsai LY. Medical treatment. In: Berkell Zager DE, editor. Autism: identification, education, and treatment. 2nd ed. Mahweh: Lawrence Erlbaum; 1999. p. 199–257.
86. Krishnamoorthy ES, Trimble MR, Blumer D. The classification of neuropsychiatric disorders in epilepsy: a proposal by the ILAE Commission on Psychobiology of Epilepsy. Epilepsy Behav. 2007;10(3):349–53.

87. Tsai LY. Psychopharmacology in autism. Psychosom Med. 1999;61(5):651–65.
88. Sovner R. The use of valproate in the treatment of mentally retarded persons with typical and atypical bipolar disorders. J Clin Psychiatry. 1989;50:40–3.
89. Hollander E, Dolgoff-Kaspar R, Cartwright C, Rawitt R, Novotny S. An open trial of divalproex sodium in autism spectrum disorders. J Clin Psychiatry. 2001;62(7):530–4.
90. Ruedrich S, Swales TP, Fossaceca C, Toliver J, Rutkowski A. Effect of divalproex sodium on aggression and self-injurious behaviour in adults with intellectual disability: a retrospective review. J Intellect Disabil Res. 1999;43(Pt 2):105–11.
91. Verhoeven WMA, Tuinier S. Cyclothymia or unstable mood disorder? A systematic treatment evaluation with valproic acid. J Appl Res Intellect Disabil. 2001;14:147–54.
92. Bhaumik S, Branford D, Barrett M, Satheesh KG. The Frith prescribing guidelines for people with intellectual disability. 3rd ed. Oxford: Wiley; 2015.
93. Vanstraelen M, Tyrer SP. Rapid cycling bipolar affective disorder in people with intellectual disability: a systematic review. J Intellect Disabil Res. 1999;43(Pt 5):349–59.
94. Reid AH, Naylor GJ, Kay DS. A double-blind, placebo controlled, crossover trial of carbamazepine in overactive, severely mentally handicapped patients. Psychol Med. 1981;11(1):109–13.
95. Smith DA, Perry PJ. Nonneuroleptic treatment of disruptive behavior in organic mental syndromes. Ann Pharmacother. 1992;26(11):1400–8.
96. Uvebrant P, Bauziene R. Intractable epilepsy in children. The efficacy of lamotrigine treatment, including non-seizure-related benefits. Neuropediatrics. 1994;25(6):284–9.
97. Campbell M, Rapoport JL, Simpson GM. Antipsychotics in children and adolescents. J Am Acad Child Adolesc Psychiatry. 1999;38:537–45.
98. Martin A, Koenig K, Scahill L, Bregman J. Open-label quetiapine in the treatment of children and adolescents with autistic disorder. J Child Adolesc Psychopharmacol. 1999;9:99–107.
99. Anderson LT, Campbell M, Grega DM, Perry R, Small AM, Green WH. Haloperidol in the treatment of infantile autism: effects on learning and behavioral symptoms. Am J Psychiatry. 1984;141:1195–202.
100. Campbell M, Anderson LT, Meier M, Cohen IL, Small AM, Samit C, Sachar EJ. A comparison of haloperidol and behavior therapy and their interaction in autistic children. J Am Acad Child Adolesc Psychiatry. 1978;17:640–55.
101. Cohen IL, Campbell M, Posner BA, Small AM, Triebel D, Anderson LT. Behavioural effects of haloperidol in young autistic children. J Am Acad Child Adolesc Psychiatry. 1980;19:665–77.
102. Ernst M, Magee HJ, Gonzalez NM, Locascio JJ, Rosenberg CR, Campbell M. Pimozide in autistic children. Psychopharmacol Bull. 1992;28:187–91.
103. Naruse H, Nagahata M, Nakane Y, Shirahashi K, Takesada M, Yamazaki K. A multi-centre double-blind trial of pimozide (Orap), haloperidol and placebo in children with behavioral disorders, using crossover design. Acta Paedopsychiatr. 1982;48:173–84.
104. Campbell M, Armenteros JL, Malone RP, Adams PB, Eisenberg ZW, Overall JE. Neuroleptic-related dyskinesias in autistic children: a prospective, longitudinal study. J Am Acad Child Adolesc Psychiatry. 1997;36:835–43.
105. Perry R, Campbell M, Adams P, Lynch N, Spencer EK, Curren EL, Overall JE. Long-term efficacy of haloperidol in autistic children: continuous versus discontinuous drug administration. J Am Acad Child Adolesc Psychiatry. 1989;28:87–92.
106. Canitano R, Scandurra V. Risperidone in the treatment of behavioral disorders associated with autism in children and adolescents. Neuropsychiatr Dis Treat. 2008;4(4):723–30.
107. Jensen PS, Buitelaar J, Pandina GJ, Binder C, Haas M. Management of psychiatric disorders in children and adolescents with atypical antipsychotics: a systematic review of published clinical trials. Eur Child Adolesc Psychiatry. 2007;16(2):104–20.
108. McDougle CJ, Holmes JP, Bronson MR, Anderson GM, Volkmar FR, Price LH, et al. Risperidone treatment of children and adolescents with pervasive developmental disorders: a prospective open-label study. J Am Acad Child Adolesc Psychiatry. 1997;36:685–93.

109. McDougle CJ, Scahill L, Aman MG, McCracken JT, Tierney E, Davies M, et al. Risperidone for the core symptom domains of autism: results from the study by the Autism Network of the Research Units on Pediatric Psychopharmacology. Am J Psychiatry. 2005;162:1142–8.
110. Arnold LE, Farmer C, Kraemer HC, Davies M, Witwer A, Chuang S, et al. Moderators, mediators, and other predictors of risperidone response in children with autistic disorder and irritability. J Child Adolesc Psychopharmacol. 2010;20(2):83–93.
111. Malone RP, Maislin G, Choudhury MS, Gifford C, Delaney MA. Risperidone treatment in children and adolescents with autism: short- and long-term safety and effectiveness. J Am Acad Child Adolesc Psychiatry. 2002;41(2):140–7.
112. McCracken JT, McGough J, Shah B, Cronin P, Hong D, Aman MG, et al. Risperidone in children with autism and serious behavioral problems. N Engl J Med. 2002;347(5):314–21.
113. McDougle CJ, Scahill L, Aman MG, McCracken JT, Tierney E, Davies M, et al. Risperidone for the core symptom domains of autism: results from the study by the autism network of the research units on pediatric psychopharmacology. Am J Psychiatry. 2005;162(6):1142–8.
114. Aman MG, Arnold LE, McDougle CJ, Vitiello B, Scahill L, Davies M, et al. Acute and long-term safety and tolerability of risperidone in children with autism. J Child Adolesc Psychopharmacol. 2005;15(6):869–84.
115. Gagliano A, Germano E, Pustorino G, Impallomeni C, D'Arrigo C, Calamoneri F, et al. Risperidone treatment of children with autistic disorder: effectiveness, tolerability, and pharmacokinetic implications. J Child Adolesc Psychopharmacol. 2004;14(1):39–47.
116. Kowalski JL, Wink LK, Blankenship K, Habenicht CD, Erickson CA, Stigler KA, et al. Paliperidone palmitate in a child with autistic disorder. J Child Adolesc Psychopharmacol. 2011;21(5):491–3.
117. Rausch JL, Sirota EL, Londino DL, Johnson ME, Carr BM, Bhatia R, et al. Open-label risperidone for Asperger's disorder: negative symptom spectrum response. J Clin Psychiatry. 2005;66(12):1592–7.
118. Frazier JA, Meyer MC, Biederman J, Wozniak J, Wilens TE, Spencer TJ, et al. Risperidone treatment for juvenile bipolar disorder: a retrospective chart review. J Am Acad Child Adolesc Psychiatry. 1999;38(8):960–5.
119. Zarcone JR, Hellings JA, Crandall K, Reese RM, Marquis J, Fleming K, et al. Effects of risperidone on aberrant behavior of persons with developmental disabilities: I. A double-blind crossover study using multiple measures. Am J Ment Retard. 2001;106(6):525–38.
120. Kent JM, Kushner S, Ning X, Karcher K, Ness S, Aman M, et al. Risperidone dosing in children and adolescents with autistic disorder: a double-blind, placebo-controlled study. J Autism Dev Disord. 2013;43(8):1773–83.
121. Scahill L, McDougle CJ, Aman MG, Johnson C, Handen B, Bearss K, et al. Effects of risperidone and parent training on adaptive functioning in children with pervasive developmental disorders and serious behavioral problems. J Am Acad Child Adolesc Psychiatry. 2012;51(2):136–46.
122. Stigler KA, Diener JT, Kohn AE, Li L, Erickson CA, Posey DJ, et al. Aripiprazole in pervasive developmental disorder not otherwise specified and Asperger's disorder: a 14-week, prospective, open-label study. J Child Adolesc Psychopharmacol. 2009;19(3):265–74.
123. Hellings JA, Boehm D, Yeh HW, Butler MG, Schroeder SR. Long-term aripiprazole in youth with developmental disabilities including autism. J Ment Health Res Intellect Disabil. 2011;4(1):40–52.
124. Shastri M, Alla L, Sabaratnam M. Aripiprazole use in individuals with intellectual disability and psychotic or behavioural disorders: a case series. J Psychopharmacol. 2006;20(6):863–7.
125. Potenza MN, Holmes JP, Kanes SJ, McDougle CJ. Olanzapine treatment of children, adolescents, and adults with pervasive developmental disorders: an open-label pilot study. J Clin Psychopharmacol. 1999;19(1):37–44.
126. Kemner C, Willemsen-Swinkels SH, de Jonge M, Tuynman-Qua H, van Engeland H. Open-label study of olanzapine in children with pervasive developmental disorder. J Clin Psychopharmacol. 2002;22(5):455–60.

127. Golubchik P, Sever J, Weizman A. Low-dose quetiapine for adolescents with autistic spectrum disorder and aggressive behavior: open-label trial. Clin Neuropharmacol. 2011;34(6):216–9.
128. Findling RL, McNamara NK, Gracious BL, O'Riordan MA, Reed MD, Demeter C, et al. Quetiapine in nine youths with autistic disorder. J Child Adolesc Psychopharmacol. 2004;14(2):287–94.
129. Corson AH, Barkenbus JE, Posey DJ, Stigler KA, McDougle CJ. A retrospective analysis of quetiapine in the treatment of pervasive developmental disorders. J Clin Psychiatry. 2004;65(11):1531–6.
130. McDougle CJ, Holmes JP, Carlson DC, Pelton GH, Cohen DJ, Price LH. A double-blind, placebo-controlled study of risperidone in adults with autistic disorder and other pervasive developmental disorders. Arch Gen Psychiatry. 1998;55(7):633–41.
131. McDougle CJ, Scahill L, McCracken JT, Aman MG, Tierney E, Arnold LE, et al. Research Units on Pediatric Psychopharmacology (RUPP) Autism Network. Background and rationale for an initial controlled study of risperidone. Child Adolesc Psychiatr Clin N Am. 2000;9(1):201–24.
132. Buitelaar JK, Willemsen-Swinkels SH. Medication treatment in subjects with autistic spectrum disorders. Eur Child Adolesc Psychiatry. 2000;9(Suppl 1):I85–97.
133. Carneiro AM, Airey DC, Thompson B, Zhu CB, Lu L, Chesler EJ, et al. Functional coding variation in recombinant inbred mouse lines reveals multiple serotonin transporter-associated phenotypes. Proc Natl Acad Sci U S A. 2009;106(6):2047–52.
134. Carneiro AM, Cook EH, Murphy DL, Blakely RD. Interactions between integrin alphaIIbbeta3 and the serotonin transporter regulate serotonin transport and platelet aggregation in mice and humans. J Clin Invest. 2008;118(4):1544–52.
135. Veenstra-Vanderweele J, Muller CL, Iwamoto H, Sauer JE, Owens WA, Shah CR, et al. Autism gene variant causes hyperserotonemia, serotonin receptor hypersensitivity, social impairment and repetitive behavior. Proc Natl Acad Sci U S A. 2012;109:5469–74.
136. Janušonis S, Anderson GM, Shifrovich I, Rakic P. Ontogeny of brain and blood serotonin levels in 5-HT1A receptor knockout mice: potential relevance to the neurobiology of autism. J Neurochem. 2006;99:1019–31.
137. Azmitia EC, Singh JS, Whitaker-Azmitia PM. Increased serotonin axons (immunoreactive to 5-HT transporter) in postmortem brains from young autism donors. Neuropharmacology. 2011;60:1347–54.
138. Chugani DC, Muzik O, Behen M, Rothermel R, Janisse JJ, Lee J, et al. Developmental changes in brain serotonin synthesis capacity in autistic and nonautistic children. Ann Neurol. 1999;45(3):287–95.
139. Chugani DC. Role of altered brain serotonin mechanisms in autism. Mol Psychiatry. 2002;7(Suppl 2):S16–7.
140. Murphy DG, Daly E, Schmitz N, Toal F, Murphy K, Curran S, et al. Cortical serotonin 5-HT2A receptor binding and social communication in adults with Asperger's syndrome: an in vivo SPECT study. Am J Psychiatry. 2006;163(5):934–6.
141. Nakamura K, Sekine Y, Ouchi Y, Tsujii M, Yoshikawa E, Futatsubashi M, et al. Brain serotonin and dopamine transporter bindings in adults with high-functioning autism. Arch Gen Psychiatry. 2010;67(1):59–68.
142. Lee ES, Vidal C, Findling RL. A focused review on the treatment of pediatric patients with atypical antipsychotics. J Child Adolesc Psychopharmacol. 2018;28(9):582–605.
143. DelBello MP, Goldman R, Phillips D, Deng L, Cucchiaro J, Loebel A. Efficacy and safety of lurasidone in children and adolescents with bipolar I depression: a double-blind, placebo-controlled study. J Am Acad Child Adolesc Psychiatry. 2017;56(12):1015–25.
144. Loebel A, Brams M, Goldman RS, Silva R, Hernandez D, Deng L, et al. Lurasidone for the treatment of irritability associated with autistic disorder. J Autism Dev Disord. 2016;46(4):1153–63.
145. Millard PH, McLaren JL, Coffey DB. Lurasidone treatment in a child with autism spectrum disorder with irritability and aggression. J Child Adolesc Psychopharmacol. 2014;24(6):354–6.

146. Hurwitz R, Blackmore R, Hazell P, Williams K, Woolfenden S. Tricyclic antidepressants for autism spectrum disorders (ASD) in children and adolescents. Cochrane Database Syst Rev. 2012;(3):CD008372.
147. Williams K, Brignell A, Randall M, Silove N, Hazell P. Selective serotonin reuptake inhibitors (SSRIs) for autism spectrum disorders (ASD). Cochrane Database Syst Rev. 2013;(8):CD004677.
148. Couturier JL, Nicolson R. A retrospective assessment of citalopram in children and adolescents with pervasive developmental disorders. J Child Adolesc Psychopharmacol. 2002;12(3):243–8.
149. Hollander E, Soorya L, Chaplin W, Anagnostou E, Taylor BP, Ferretti CJ, et al. A double-blind placebo-controlled trial of fluoxetine for repetitive behaviors and global severity in adult autism spectrum disorders. Am J Psychiatry. 2012;169(3):292–9.
150. Khouzam HR, El-Gabalawi F, Pirwani N, Priest F. Asperger's disorder: a review of its diagnosis and treatment. Compr Psychiatry. 2004;45(3):184–91.
151. Steingard RJ, Zimnitzky B, DeMaso DR, Bauman ML, Bucci JP. Sertraline treatment of transition-associated anxiety and agitation in children with autistic disorder. J Child Adolesc Psychopharmacol. 1997;7(1):9–15.
152. Henry CA, Shervin D, Neumeyer A, Steingard R, Spybrook J, Choueiri R, et al. Retrial of selective serotonin reuptake inhibitors in children with pervasive developmental disorders: a retrospective chart review. J Child Adolesc Psychopharmacol. 2009;19(2):111–7.
153. Frazier JA, Biederman J, Bellordre CA, Garfield SB, Geller DA, Coffey BJ, et al. Should the diagnosis of attention deficit hyperactivity disorder be considered in children with pervasive developmental disorder? J Atten Disord. 2001;4:203–11.
154. Henry CA, Steingard R, Venter J, Guptill J, Halpern EF, Bauman M. Treatment outcome and outcome associations in children with pervasive developmental disorders treated with selective serotonin reuptake inhibitors: a chart review. J Child Adolesc Psychopharmacol. 2006;16(1–2):187–95.
155. Sokolski KN, Chicz-Demet A, Demet EM. Selective serotonin reuptake inhibitor-related extrapyramidal symptoms in autistic children: a case series. J Child Adolesc Psychopharmacol. 2004;14(1):143–7.
156. Damore J, Stine J, Brody L. Medication-induced hypomania in Asperger's disorder. J Am Acad Child Adolesc Psychiatry. 1998;37(3):248–9.
157. Todd RD. Fluoxetine in autism. Am J Psychiatry. 1991;148(8):1089.
158. Pacchiarotti I, Bond DJ, Baldessarini RJ, Nolen WA, Grunze H, Licht RW, et al. The International Society for Bipolar Disorders (ISBD) task force report on antidepressant use in bipolar disorders. Am J Psychiatry. 2013;170(11):1249–62.
159. Grzadzinski R, Di Martino A, Brady E, Mairena MA, O'Neale M, Petkova E, et al. Examining autistic traits in children with ADHD: does the autism spectrum extend to ADHD? J Autism Dev Disord. 2011;41(9):1178–91.
160. Reiersen AM, Todd RD. Co-occurrence of ADHD and autism spectrum disorders: phenomenology and treatment. Expert Rev Neurother. 2008;8(4):657–69.
161. Cortese S, Castelnau P, Morcillo C, Roux S, Bonnet-Brilhault F. Psychostimulants for ADHD-like symptoms in individuals with autism spectrum disorders. Expert Rev Neurother. 2012;12(4):461–73.
162. Di Martino A, Melis G, Cianchetti C, Zuddas A. Methylphenidate for pervasive developmental disorders: safety and efficacy of acute single dose test and ongoing therapy: an open-pilot study. J Child Adolesc Psychopharmacol. 2004;14(2):207–18.
163. Stigler KA, Desmond LA, Posey DJ, Wiegand RE, McDougle CJ. A naturalistic retrospective analysis of psychostimulants in pervasive developmental disorders. J Child Adolesc Psychopharmacol. 2004;14(1):49–56.
164. Posey DJ, Aman MG, McCracken JT, Scahill L, Tierney E, Arnold LE, et al. Positive effects of methylphenidate on inattention and hyperactivity in pervasive developmental disorders: an analysis of secondary measures. Biol Psychiatry. 2007;61(4):538–44.

165. Munesue T, Ono Y, Mutoh K, Shimoda K, Nakatani H, Kikuchi M. High prevalence of bipolar disorder comorbidity in adolescents and young adults with high-functioning autism spectrum disorder: a preliminary study of 44 outpatients. J Affect Disord. 2008;111(2–3):170–5.
166. La Malfa G, Lassi S, Salvini R, Giganti C, Bertelli M, Albertini G. The relationship between autism and psychiatric disorders in Intellectually Disabled Adults. Res Autism Spectr Disord. 2007;1:218–28.
167. Fitzgerald M. Misdiagnosis of Asperger syndrome as anankastic personality disorder. Autism. 2002;6(4):435.
168. Einfeld SL, Tonge BJ. Population prevalence of psychopathology in children and adolescents with intellectual disability: I. Rationale and methods. J Intellect Disabil Res. 1996;40(2):91–8.
169. Barneveld PS, Pieterse J, de Sonneville L, van Rijn S, Lahuis B, van Engeland H, et al. Overlap of autistic and schizotypal traits in adolescents with Autism Spectrum Disorders. Schizophr Res. 2011;126(1–3):231–6.
170. Esterberg ML, Trotman HD, Brasfield JL, Compton MT, Walker EF. Childhood and current autistic features in adolescents with schizotypal personality disorder. Schizophr Res. 2008;104(1–3):265–73.
171. Lugnegard T, Hallerback MU, Gillberg C. Personality disorders and autism spectrum disorders: what are the connections? Compr Psychiatry. 2012;53(4):333–40.

8 ASD and Intellectual Disability

Marco O. Bertelli

Autism spectrum disorder frequently co-occurs with other neurodevelopmental conditions (Wing and Potter 2002; [1]). ASD prevalence increase was associated with declines in other diagnostic categories, indicating that a diagnostic substitution had happened (Shattuck 2006). One of the most common co-occurrence is with intellectual disability, which has been renamed in the ICD-11 as disorders of intellectual developmental (DID).

8.1 Intellectual Disability: Disorders of Intellectual Development

Intellectual disability (ID) or disorders of intellectual development (DID), according to the most recent terminology [2], is a condition of difficult definition, which affects many people with many different presentations. Its main characteristic consists of a difficulty in reaching objectives, implying one or more of the many cognitive abilities that are still simplified with the term intelligence and measured, even more simplistically, with the IQ (intellectual quotient). This difficulty reduces the ability to learn, not only at a theoretical and scholastic level, but also at a practical and adaptive level. ID onsets in the first years of life and persists across the entire life span, like autism.

The former term for DID was mental retardation (ICD-10 [3]; *DSM-III* [4]), which was first introduced by the American Association on Mental Retardation (AAMR) in its 1961's manual. At the same time, the AAMR proposed objective diagnostic criteria, as well as tests and reference scores for the assessment of intelligence and adaptive skills. The main criterion was an IQ lower than 84,

M. O. Bertelli (✉)
CREA (Research and Clinical Centre), San Sebastiano Foundation, Florence, Italy
e-mail: mbertelli@crea-sansebastiano.org

R. Keller (ed.), *Psychopathology in Adolescents and Adults with Autism Spectrum Disorders*, https://doi.org/10.1007/978-3-030-26276-1_8

corresponding to one standard deviation below the average of the general population. The impairment of adaptive functioning was divided into four severity levels.

Two updates of the AAMR manual were published in 1973 and 1983; in the former, the IQ cutoff was reduced to two standard deviations below the average and the age of onset was extended to 18 years, in the latter, the IQ standard measurement error was added [5]. The *DSM-IV* [6] remained aligned to the AAMR in the definition of mental retardation, while it departed in the upper limit of the severity range, which was kept lower, and in the multiaxial rather than multidimensional classification.

In recent years, the release of the new international classification systems of mental disorders (*DSM-5* [7] and ICD-11 [2]) has boosted the scientific debate on the difficulties to define and to position ID. In fact these aspects have important implications, not only on clinical practice but also on socio-cultural and socio-health policies. There are two main approaches. The first is promoted by the AAMR (at present renamed as American Association on Intellectual Disabilities and Development—AAIDD) and sets its center on disability, characterized by significant impairments of intellectual functioning and adaptive behavior. This approach is aligned with the one followed in the international classification of functioning (ICF; WHO 2001). The second approach is supported mainly by the Section Psychiatry of Intellectual Disability of the World Psychiatric Association (WPA-SPID) and has a multidimensional, polynomial-polysemic character. It explains ID as a condition to be defined differently according to the classificatory context, i.e., as meta-syndromic grouping of intellectual development disorders in the ICD (International Classification of Diseases), as a condition of complex disability in the ICF.

The WPA-SPID suggested for the ICD also to replace the term "mental retardation" with "intellectual development disorders (IDD)" and proposed a definition and diagnostic criteria free from rigid references to IQ (intelligence quotient) reduction (Bertelli et al. 2014; Bertelli et al. 2018), adaptive skills, and age of onset (Salvador-Carulla et al. 2011). According to the WPA-SPID, ID is characterized by a deficit of one or more cognitive functions, prior to the acquisition of skills through learning, such as to interfere significantly, without the appropriate support, with individual functioning, as expressed by limitations in activities and restrictions in participation (Salvador-Carulla et al. 2011).

As mentioned above, the new ICD (ICD-11; [2]) has adopted the term "disorders of intellectual development" with reference to a group of conditions of different etiology originating during the age of development and characterized by intellectual functioning and adaptive behavior significantly lower than the average, at least two standard deviations (approximately below the percentile 2.3), as defined through an individualized assessment with adequately validated and standardized tests. Where these tests are not available, the diagnosis requires greater reliance on clinical judgment based on appropriate assessment of comparable behavioral indicators.

In the *DSM-5*, the fundamental characteristic of ID is a general intellectual functioning significantly (two standard deviations) below the average (criterion A). This characteristic must be associated with deficits in adaptive functioning, with particular reference to the sociocultural standards of personal independence and social responsibility (criterion B). Without continuous support, adaptive deficits limit functioning in at least one of the daily activities of life, such as communication, social participation or autonomy, in different contexts, such as one's own home, school, work, and community. The onset of intellectual and adaptive deficits must occur during the development period (criterion C), typically in the years prior to school education [7].

Until the publication of *DSM-5* (2013), the severity of ID (formerly 'mental retardation') was defined almost exclusively on the basis of IQ reduction: mild for values between 50–55 and 70 (50–69 in the ICD-10), moderate between 35–40 and 50–55 ("medium," 35–49 in ICD-10), severe between 20–25 and 35–40 (20–34 in ICD-10), and profound for values lower than 25–20 (<20 in ICD-10). In *DSM-5* the severity levels are defined more on the basis of adaptive functioning than on IQ, especially for the cases that fall within the lower part of the range. For this purpose, the domains of reference are represented by conceptualization, social and practical skills.

The prevalence of ID varies across studies between 1% and 2.5%, also based on diagnostic procedures, geographical and sociocultural factors (WHO 2007; van Bakel et al. 2014; McKenzie et al. 2016). The lowest rates were recorded in some northern European countries, such as Finland or the Netherlands, while the highest rates are for low-middle income countries, up to 6–8% (WHO 2007). The average prevalence is just over 1% (Maulik et al. 2011).

The causes of ID are classified in prenatal, perinatal, and postnatal. Among the prenatal causes, the main ones are genetic alterations, either chromosomal (or genomic, e.g., Down syndrome, Turner syndrome, Klinefelter syndrome, and cri du chat syndrome) or genic (or point-like, e.g., Fragile X, galactosemia, lipidosis, and phenylketonuria), maternal infections, maternal exposure to harmful chemical (e.g., lead, mercury, and drugs) or physical agents (e.g., radiation), malnutrition, gestational diabetes, hypoxia, hypoglycemia, or maternal toxemia. Among perinatal causes, some of the most common are labor complications, childbirth traumas, and the respiratory distress of newborn. Postnatal causes are mainly represented by infections, traumas, malnutrition, and poisoning by chemical substances. Also psycho-social factors seem to be able to determine an early cognitive impairment of intelligence, even if of a slight degree. Some of the most relevant psycho-social factors are the psychologically, socially, culturally, or economically poor environment, the severe alterations of intra-family relations, social isolation, and the forced inhibition of the natural tendency to exploratory behavior.

All scientific associations agree that ID represents a condition of high vulnerability, with mental disorders, physical illnesses, risk of abuse, risk of abandonment, and dissatisfied care needs significantly higher than those of the general population (Bertelli et al. 2009; Salvador-Carulla e and Bertelli 2008). These vulnerabilities seem to extend to persons with borderline intellectual functioning (BIF), who have an IQ below the average (between one and two standard deviations), but not enough to be comprised within the upper limit of ID. According to research findings, one-eighth of the population has BIF and shows, compared to people with higher IQ, greater social disadvantage, higher rates of psychiatric disorders, substance abuse and consequently greater use of psychopharmacological therapies and health services, including emergency services (Hassiotis et al. 2008; Wieland et al. 2014).

8.2 Co-occurrence and Differentiation of ASD and ID

Both ID and ASD represent meta-syndromic groups, including many different clinical (syndromic) conditions (Salvador-Carulla and Bertelli 2008), which combine cognitive and relational impairment. The two conditions often co-occur and are difficult to distinguish, especially as long as the cognitive impairment increases.

Thirty to forty percent of persons with ID have pervasive autistic features (Morgan et al. 2002; La Malfa et al. 2004; Cooper et al. 2007), as well as about 80% of persons with ASD has lower intellectual functioning compared to the general population ([8, 9]; Fombonne 2003; Hoekstra et al. 2009; Baio et al. 2018; Edelson 2006; Baird et al. 2006; Noterdaeme and Wriedt 2010; Bryson and Smith 1998). Many of the symptoms which characterize ID are quite common also in ASD, such as deficits of cognitive, social, and adaptive skills, as well as stereotypies, problem behaviors, and repetitive behaviors (Lee et al. 2008; Wilkins and Matson 2009). Reversely, many features of ASD are often seen also in ID, such as socialization-communication impairment and restricted-repetitive behaviors or interests (Briegel et al. 2009; Gillberg 2010; Horovitz and Matson 2010; Leung et al. 2010; Matson et al. 2009a, b; Smith and Matson 2010a, b, c; Lee et al. 2008; [9]).

Etiologically both syndromes are considered to result from an interaction of genetic and environmental factors with negative impact on the brain development. The subsequent impairment of logical-learning functions (ID), social-communicative functions (ASD), or both might depend on the position and the extension of this disruption of neural circuits. Recent evidence on alterations of proteins regulating synapses' growth and structure seems to confirm that ID and ASD are part of a single group of neurodevelopmental disorders (Owen et al. 2011; Owen 2012; Waltereit 2013).

The combination of ASD and ID presents many challenges and deficits across a range of behaviors and skills that are not seen in ID or ASD alone [10]. Severe IQ has been found to be associated with a higher severity of ASD and a higher rate of PB [11, 12]. The presence and severity of stereotypies tend to be related to severity of ASD [13] but not to severity of ID [1].

Differential diagnosis between ID and ASD as well as identification of co-occurrence are particularly challenging for those psychiatrists who did not receive specific training on the presentation of PD in persons with neurodevelopmental disorders (Bradley et al. 2011b; Hurley et al. 2003; Lunsky et al. 2008; [14]). Several tools are available to support clinicians in the assessment, such as PDD-MRS (Scale of Pervasive Developmental Disorder in Mentally Retarded Persons; Kraijer and de Bildt 2005), DiBAS-R (Diagnostic Behavioral Assessment for ASD—Revised; Sappok et al. 2014), ASD-DA (Autism Spectrum Disorder—Diagnosis Scale for Intellectually Disabled Adults; Matson et al. 2008), SCQ-AID (Social

Communication Questionnaire for Adults with ID; Derks et al. 2017), and SPAIDD-ASD (Systematic Psychopathological Assessment for persons with Intellectual and Developmental Disabilities—version for Autism Spectrum Disorder; Fruscoloni et al. 2018) for screening, and GARS-2 (Gilliam Autism Rating Scale-2nd Edition; Gilliam 2006), ADI-R (Autism Diagnostic Interview—Revised; Lord et al. 1994), and ADOS (Autism Diagnostic Observation Schedule; Lord et al. 1989) to complete patient evaluation. The Diagnostic Interview for Social and Communication Disorders (The DISCO) also provides a comprehensive assessment ASD across the range of IQ (Maljaars et al. 2012), as well as functioning ability and subtypes of autism (Wing et al. 2002); it also seems to be useful in differentiating between ADS, DID, and schizophrenia spectrum disorders (Unenge Hallerbäck et al. 2012). ADOS and ADI-R have shown some limits when used with persons with DID, especially with those with lower IQ and/or sensory impairment (Sappok et al. 2013; deVaan et al. 2016).

There is an increased risk of underestimating ASD in persons with ID when schizophrenia is diagnosed (Palucka et al. 2009; Savage et al. 2007; Bradley et al. 2011b). About 40% of the items used to screen for psychosis in ID commonly receive a high score when ASD is present (Helverschou et al. 2008).

The introduction of the spectrum model to the diagnosis of autism, which has been consolidated in the *DSM-5* [7], has resulted in the inclusion of subjects with subthreshold symptoms and blurred pictures. Future classification should pay more attention not to excessively increase the inclusive capacities of criteria and create all-encompassing diagnostic categories. They should also consider how a reevaluation of a dimensional approach to some core symptoms would allow a clearer definition of the disorders. The overlap between autism spectrum and other neurodevelopmental disorders has some social therapeutic and economic implications. ASD is more socially accepted and less stigmatizing than ID and receives higher individual, particularly rehabilitative, and family support. Unlike ID, ASD is considered a treatable disorder, and many mental health services are increasingly providing specific interventions. Moreover, autism gets a greater number of grants and economic benefits. A diagnosis of ID does not always offer this advantage.

8.3 Prevalence of Psychiatric Disorders in Persons with ID and ASD

As Boucher et al. [10] reported, people with both ID and ASD present several symptoms and deficits which are not seen in ID and ASD alone, and a different frequency of comorbid disorders. Research showed an inverse relationship between IQ and severity of ASD, with the rate of PB in ASD getting lower as long as IQ increases [11, 12]. Conversely, severity of ASD symptoms—and not that of ID—resulted directly associated with the rates of stereotypies [1, 13].

Although still limited and controversial, the literature on the prevalence of Psychiatric Disorders (PD) in persons with both ID and ASD indicates a higher rate in comparison with those with ID or ASD alone. Greater agreement has been identified on higher rates of PB, stereotypies and rituals, communication difficulties, and social impairment in comparison to ID alone [9, 15]. Furthermore, the co-occurrence of ASD with ID has been associated with a higher probability to be hospitalized and to receive a psychopharmacological treatment [16–18].

Lunsky and collaborators found that more than half of adults with ID and ASD have a co-occurring PD (26.1% mood disorder, 26.1% psychotic disorder, and 4.3% personality disorder). However, when compared with those with only ID, they did not show statistically significant differences except for the probability to receive a diagnosis of a psychotic disorder, which was lower in the ID+ASD group [14]. Also Melville et al. [19] found no significant rate of increase in the case of co-occurrence of ASD, but a higher number of PB. In addition, individuals with PB and ASD were less likely to receive a diagnosis of schizophrenia, whereas the latter increased if PB were absent [15]. In all cases the presence of PB had a negative impact on the overall functioning and quality of life [8, 15, 17, 20–25].

Cooper and van der Speck [26] found a lower prevalence of PD in people with ID+ASD compared to those with ID alone, but a more frequent diagnosis of schizophrenia.

The presence of ID in persons with ASD seems to negatively impact on the possibility to have an adjunctive diagnosis of PD. In a 10-year longitudinal study, Selten and collaborators found that the co-occurrence of ID in persons with ASD reversed the trend of a higher rate of diagnoses of bipolar and psychotic disorders than the general population [27].

Specific diagnostic procedure and tools seem to represent a significant determinant for the reliability of prevalence findings in persons with ID+ASD. These often include too many subjective symptoms which are not easy to identify in this group of patients and should be substituted by behavioral and observable equivalents (see Chap. 5). Different studies have found an increasing prevalence of PD as long as the specificity of their assessment tools rose. By using the PAS-ADD (Psychiatric Assessment Schedules for Adults with Developmental Disabilities), Thalen found an overall rate of 69.6% vs. 8.6% in persons with ID alone [28], and through the DASH-II (Diagnostic Assessment for the Severely Handicapped-II), Matson and Cervantes found statistically significant differences in eight out of the 12 subscales of the tools, on anxiety, mania, schizophrenia, stereotypies/tics, self-injurious behavior, eating disorders, sexual disorders, and impulse control [29].

Among specific PD, mood disorders [28, 30], anxiety disorders [21, 28, 31], somatic symptoms disorders, and impulse control disorders [20, 32–34] have been reported as the most frequent.

Higher rates of inattention, hyperactivity, and impulsive behaviors have been observed in teens with both autism and ID in comparison with those without ASD [35]. In addition, people with both conditions appear more vulnerable to sleep problems, organic syndrome, stereotypies, and tics [20].

The co-occurrence of PD has been found to be higher in males, youths, and persons with mild-to-moderate ID [14, 15, 17], although Thalen found the rate of psychoses and anxiety disorder to trend inversely to the severity of ID [28].

Some high rates of PD in persons with ID and ASD, such as that of bipolar disorder, seem to be related to behavioral dysregulation, as expressed by restlessness, agitation, or distraction, and may reflect the symptom overlap between PD, ASD, and ID rather than a true co-occurrence of PD. This is particularly probable in individuals with more severe PB [31].

8.4 Peculiarities and Challenges in Diagnosing Co-occurrent Psychiatric Disorders in ASD and ID

As mentioned above, the low-adaptive intellectual disability (or disorders of intellectual development) and the low-functioning autism spectrum disorder represent the fraction of neurodevelopmental disorders that show the greatest degree of disability, in communication, conceptualization, interpersonal relationships, and common activities of life.

These difficulties characterize at various levels the presentation of PD, making them much more complex and difficult to identify than in the general population ([8]; Lainhart 1999; Reaven and Hepburn 2003; Bertelli 2016). The symptomatology can in fact be chaotic, mixed, intermittent, atypical, masked, variable from poorly defined to extremely rigid (Reiss and Szyszko 1993; [36, 37]). These alterations also concern the nuclear elements of some syndromes, such as delusional perception or suicidal ideation, which may not be immediately identifiable, especially in persons with low communication skill (Mikkelsen and McKenna 1999). To promote a correct approach to this complexity, various conceptual references have been proposed. One of the most relevant is that of "diagnostic over-shadowing" (Sovner 1986), which refers to the difficulty for clinicians to distinguish between symptoms of PD and the manifestations of basic conditions.

Other concepts to consider are those of "intellectual distortion," related to the impact of cognitive, communicative, physical, and social dysfunction on the perception and communication of mental suffering (Sovner and DesNoyers Hurley 1986), "evolutionary inappropriateness," or the mismatch between the level of individual development expected for the chronological age and the level of actual individual development (Cooper and Salvador-Carulla 2009), and the "psychosocial masking," referable to the peculiarities of cultural, environmental, and interpersonal influences (Sovner 1986). Even the neurovegetative vulnerability associated with cognitive impairment, or the greater tendency to express mental distress through organic dysfunctions, somatic symptoms, or dystonias of the nervous system, can connote the clinical presentation of PD (Costello and Bouras 2006). In people with neurodevelopmental disorders, there are also more general difficulties in the very conceptualization of the mental disorder. Here in fact the impairment of functioning and the subjective distress arising from the presence of psychiatric symptoms, which constitute in the general population the fundamental criteria for the formulation of a judgment of pathology, are difficult to identify, as they are already altered by the basic condition.

In particular, perceived distress is already remarkably high, due to a complexity of biological, psychological, and socio-environmental factors, such as reduced opportunities for participation in community life, greater exposure to traumatic experiences or lower coping skills (Sovner 1986; Martorell et al. 2009). The difficulty therefore lies in understanding whether the alterations that the clinician is observing depend directly on cognitive deficits, on the presence of a co-occurring psychiatric disorder or both. An adequate assessment of psychiatric symptomatology in this type of patient should be based on the organized observation of significant variations in basic behavior, especially in the most serious cases. The presence of visual hallucinations can be detected, for example, starting from changes in gestures that are not appropriate to the context, such as fixing a point where there seems to be nothing to see, moving around as if to defend oneself against imaginary attacks, covering one's eyes or ears with one's hands in the absence of objectively annoying sounds (Bertelli 2016). A further factor of complexity in the manifestation and in the interpretation of the psychopathological frameworks is represented by PB. PB appear as one of the most frequently encountered criticalities in people with ID and LF-ASD, with a prevalence ranging between 5% and 60% (Smith et al. 1996; Smiley 2005) and very low remission rates (Cooper et al. 2009; Totsika et al. 2008, 2009).

Their incidence seems to increase in people with more marked reduction in IQ, with greater difficulties in communication or social skills and in the absence of stable supports (Felce et al. 2009). The hypotheses put forward to explain their nature and development include a wide range of factors belonging to different fields, often combined together. In some cases it has been suggested that their function was essentially communicative, in others that they represented expressions of protest, attempts to attract attention, manifestations of fear or sadness. Some PB can be identified as specific psychiatric symptoms; in these cases, we speak of "behavioral equivalents" (Hurley 2006). The relationship between these behavioral alterations and some PD has already been suggested and investigated in many studies (Emerson et al. 1999; Felce et al. 2009; Hemmings et al. 2006; Kishore et al. 2005; Moss et al. 2000; Rojan et al. 2004). Some researchers are less likely to consider PB as behavioral equivalents of a psychiatric disorder, defining them alternatively as indicators of aspecific emotional stress (Tsiouris et al. 2003; Rojan and Meier 2009).

Against these discrepancies, a careful evaluation of the onset, of the course, of the possible extinction of the PB, and of the co-presence of other possible symptoms, appears to be of fundamental importance to define whether it can be interpreted or not as a symptom equivalent (Charlot 2005). Peculiarities of the evaluation of errors in the diagnostic process may also be due to deficits in communication skills or lack of language, often present in people with ID and/or ASD (Bertelli 2016). They can indeed present great difficulties in expressing themselves verbally, striving for compliance and attributing atypical meanings to communicative contexts. Furthermore, the limited introspective abilities are often found to determine a series of difficulties in defining life experiences and states of suffering or disturbance. Some peculiar characteristics of PD, such as the sense of desperation or uselessness, suicidal ideation, or delusional perception, require a high level of expressive language, abstract thought, memory, and self-awareness; it is therefore easy to understand how they are difficult to communicate, particularly in the most serious cases (Costello and Bouras 2006; Bertelli et al. 2015).

Conducting direct interviews with people with ID and/or ASD is made equally problematic by their frequent difficulty in understanding requests (Heal and Sigelman 1995). This aspect is much rarer, if not entirely absent, in people with mild ID or borderline intellectual functioning (BIF), who have shown themselves able to describe their own behaviors and internal states (Moss et al. 1996; Bramston and Fogarty 2000; Deb et al. 2001). However, even in these cases, some aspects related to the impairment of cognitive functioning, such as suggestibility, acquiescence, attention deficits, problems with temporal sequencing, or distractibility, can cause considerable difficulty in providing a detailed account of one's experiences. In light of these difficulties, preparing an adequate assessment setting is of fundamental importance. Particular attention must be paid to aspects such as the length and flexibility of the sessions, to be conducted preferably in the person's everyday life environment; the language used must be simple, without metaphors and idiomatic expressions, and it is advisable to offer alternative answers (Bertelli 2016).

A very important role in the assessment is that played by family members and caregivers, valuable informants in the diagnostic process, and in general in clinical practice. However, even these sources of information can be limited, contradictory, and heterogeneous. The literature indicates that the assessment by proxies is conditioned by a series of factors, which include the informants' personal characteristics, their level of knowledge of the person, and their degree of affective involvement (Pickard and Knight 2005; Petry et al. 2009). The specificity of the symptomatological processions and the relative chronological evolutions require equally specialized skills, in both the evaluation and the intervention phases, but family members and frontline personnel often do not have the adequate tools to distinguish the observed behaviors and to give them a possible psychopathological meaning (Mikkelsen and McKenna 1999; Costello and Bouras 2006). Furthermore, the widespread belief that all the problems of people with ID and/or LF-ASD are inevitable and immutable (Costello and Bouras 2006; Reiss and Szyszko 1983) often leads informants to deny the presence of psychiatric symptoms or to consider them only as their subjective interpretation, thus altering the collection of anamnestic information. A recent review of the literature has highlighted a lack of studies on the correspondence of evaluations carried out by different proxies (Bertelli et al. 2015). Some authors have found a low correspondence, often characterized by the tendency of informants to highlight greater problematic from a behavioral and psychic point of view. Integrating data from different sources seems to be the most effective way to determine any significant behavioral changes, interpret them as symptom equivalents, and increase the validity of psychiatric evaluation. In particular, the scientific community agrees that the best way to assess the presence of psychiatric disorders in people with ID and/or ASD is to use a system that includes self- and hetero-evaluations (Bertelli et al. 2015).

Another reason for the persistent lack of evidence in assessing and diagnosing mental health problems in people with ID and/or ASD is the substantial inadequacy of current diagnostic systems for the general population. In common use manuals, in fact some criteria are formulated on the verbal level and therefore difficult to apply to people with ID and/or ASD, which rather express symptoms through behaviors. Of equally difficult application are the clinical specifications and extensions that often accompany the diagnostic categories, as there is almost always no precise information on the psychopathological situation of the person being evaluated (Cooper and Salvador-Carulla 2009). Moreover, despite the aforementioned frequency of PB in people with cognitive deficits, the manuals do not consider them classifiable symptoms. In order to address the critical issues related to the use of standard diagnostic criteria, in recent years changes have been proposed to be implemented in the classifications used for the general population (Cain et al. 2003; Marston et al. 1997; Ross and Oliver 2003; Szymanski and King 1999).

Specifically, the objective was to exemplify and convert preexisting criteria into behavioral equivalents (Charlot 2005; RCPsych 2001). From this attempt the two manuals Diagnostic Criteria for Learning Disability (DC-LD; RCPsych 2001) and Diagnostic Manual—Intellectual Disability (DM-ID; Fletcher et al. 2007), were produced, respectively, by the Royal College of Psychiatrists and the National Association for Dual Diagnosis. They consist essentially of adaptations and integrations of the tenth edition of the International Classification of Diseases (ICD-10; [3]) and of the revision of the fourth edition of the Diagnostic and Statistical Manual of Mental Disorders (DSMIV-TR; APA 2000), created for the general population. Recently, the second edition of the DM-ID (DM-ID 2; Fletcher et al. 2016) was published, corresponding to the adaptation of the DSM-5 [7].

Although further improvements are needed, the two manuals have proved to be very useful in clinical practice. In the field trials conducted in the United States of America for the first edition of the DM-ID, approximately 36% of clinicians indicated that the adapted criteria had enabled them to make much more valid diagnoses than they could have made using DSM-IV-TR and about 60% found very useful specifications for avoiding inaccurate diagnoses, such as those defined as "not otherwise specifiable." The group of disorders with the highest number of changes of diagnosis in favor of disorders belonging to other groups was that of psychotic disorders, while the group with most changes within the same group was that of mood disorders [38]. In addition to all the major diagnoses that are found in the DSM-5, the DM-ID 2 includes two additional chapters, which deal with assessment and diagnostic procedures as well as the behavioral phenotypes that are associated with genetic disorders, which is intended to aid in the understanding of how a disorder's genotype affects its behavioral expression.

The DC-LD provides diagnostic criteria for PD adapted for adults with moderate to severe learning disabilities; if you work with people with mild disabilities, it can also be used in combination with ICD-10 and DSM.

8.5 Assessment Tools for Co-occurrent Psychiatric Disorders in ASD and ID

Similarly to what emerged for the diagnostic criteria, also the application to people with ID and/or ASD of the assessment scales developed for the general population has shown considerable validity problems [36]. In the last 30 years, the scientific community of this field has shown a growing interest in this issue, and various studies have been conducted that aimed to develop specific tools, analyze their psychometric properties, and investigate their clinical utility. However, those supported by a consistent database are still few.

The most common tools currently used are those of general screening, designed to provide information on all the diagnoses compatible with the symptoms and behavioral equivalents found in a person, but there are also tools for specific psychopathological areas. There are few standardized diagnostic interviews, which are complex, time-consuming, and less useful for multidisciplinary collaboration. With the same psychometric qualities, the tools must be chosen on the basis of the specific purpose, the characteristics of the person to be evaluated, the training required, the administration time, and the resources available.

As mentioned above, the standardized interviews for psychopathological diagnosis in ID and ASD are few and addressed exclusively to people with good communication and introspective skills (Heal and Sigelman 1995). The best known is the Psychiatric Assessment Schedule for Adults with Developmental Disabilities (PAS-ADD), developed by Stephen Moss and collaborators (Moss 2011; Moss, Ibbotson and Prosser 1994; Moss et al. 1993) for adults with ID, which uses the ICD-10 diagnostic categories and criteria. It derives from the Schedules for Clinical Assessment in Neuropsychiatry (SCAN), semi-structured clinical interviews produced by the World Health Organization in 1994, starting from the Present State Examination (PSE; Wing, Cooper and Sartorius 1974), and used by specially trained clinicians as a support for the diagnosis of PD in adults.

PAS-ADD was designed to be used by doctors and includes 145 questions that originally referred to seven subscales corresponding to the main acute PD. Personality disorders and many less frequent PD are not detected. Direct questions on autism spectrum disorders and ADHD are not included, but it is possible to reach these diagnoses thanks to the presence of specific sections in the supplementary instruments. The PAS-ADD is available in two versions: one for cases in which it is possible to directly interview the person with ID, the other for cases in which information is provided by a proxy, that is, by an individual who is familiar with the person under evaluation.

The authors compared the scores obtained with the two versions of the instrument and found a low correspondence (41%). To increase the diagnostic sensitivity, Moss and collaborators have therefore suggested to always administer both versions of the instrument. The psychometric properties of PAS-ADD were examined by Costello, Moss, Prosser, and Hatton (1997). The concordance between assessors of the person-directed version was measured by a session in which different clinicians filled out many questionnaires in a rigorously autonomous manner after following as many interviews recorded on videotape. The concordance was low for both individual items and diagnostic groups (kappa = 0.65 and 0.66, respectively). The factor analysis gave good results, identifying a factor for each of the subscales, and also the concordance with the clinical diagnoses was high, equal to about 76%. No information on internal consistency and test-retest was provided. The experience of many researchers and clinicians suggests that PAS-ADD is more useful for screening for mental health problems in general than for identifying a specific psychiatric disorder. Compared to the Mini and Checklist versions, the PAS-ADD should be preferred in cases where you are faced with a person with ID who has language skills, you want to get a precise ICD-10 or DSM-IV (TR) diagnosis and/or you suspect a psychotic disorder, as the instrument is particularly sensitive to diagnoses in this area. A decade ago PAS-ADD has also been adapted to use with children and adolescents, with the name of Child and Adolescent Psychiatric Assessment Schedule (ChA-PAS; Moss, Friedlander and Lee 2013).

A more recent production interview is the Psychopathology Checklists for Adults with Intellectual Disability (P-AID; Hove and Havik 2008). It is a battery of instruments to be used with informants, designed to identify ten different PD and eight types of PB according to the DC-LD (Royal College of Psychiatrists, 2001). The P-AID showed acceptable internal consistency, reliability, and inter-rater, 8 units orthogonal to the factor analysis, while the sensitivity and specificity are still to be investigated (Hove and Havik 2008). Compared to PAS-ADD, it has the advantage of including a detailed assessment of the main PB, but the disadvantage of not being able to be used directly with the person with ID or LF-ASD.

Another semi-structured interview is the Schedule for the Assessment of Psychiatric Problems Associated with Autism (and Other Developmental Disorders) (SAPPA; [39]). This was also developed in the United Kingdom and includes items derived from the Research Diagnostic Criteria of Spitzer, Endicott and Robins (1978). The SAPPA is based on interviews with the client and/or an informant and helps in identifying each autistic individual's unique baseline of behaviors as well as changes from it, which may represent one or more symptoms of a new onset psychiatric disorder. SAPPA differentiates between those disturbances that were long-standing and those that were episodic and assesses if these disturbances met clinical criteria for PD.

The criteria employed to evaluate an episode of behavior change include (1) psychotic symptoms (delusions, hallucinations, catatonia, etc.); (2) a change in behavior outside the range of normal variation for the individual; and (3) definite diminution in level of social functioning as shown by at least two of the following: loss of interest in play/favourite activities, loss of self-care, loss of social involvement, loss of initiative, and need for change in supervision and/or placement [39].

Episodes of changed behavior are explored further to obtain systematic standardized information on symptoms. A symptom is deemed clinically significant if (1) it is outside the range of normal behavior for that individual; (2) it intrudes into, or disrupts, the individual's ordinary activities; (3) it is of a degree that is not readily controlled by the individual or caregivers; and (4) it is sufficiently pervasive to extend into at least two activities.

In addition, the onset and the duration of each episode is determined in the context of other circumstances (e.g., life events such as loss, bereavement, medication changes, or medical concerns such as seizures) occurring in the person's life. The symptoms during an episode that meet diagnostic criteria and the pattern of the episodes are used to establish a psychiatric diagnosis. Episodic PD identified using the SAPPA interview include mood, anxiety, and psychotic disorders. A full SAPPA evaluation requires a face-to-face clinical interview with the client and/or the caregivers (informants) for non-verbal clients. In the first part of the interview, inquiry is also made as to the family history of PD. The second part of the SAPPA interview deals with behaviors and disorders that do not follow an episodic course (e.g., some self-injurious, hyperkinetic, obsessive, compulsive, and other anxiety-type behaviors, tics, stereotypies, and other nonspecific challenging behaviors) [30].

The tool was used in a number of studies (Bolton et al. 2011; [21, 30, 40, 41]), predominantly with people with ASD and for research purpose, often with some modifications. An attempt to adapt to use in clinical practice was recently performed by Battaglia, Detrick, and Fermandez [42]. A study on the validity and other psychometric characteristics of the instrument has never been performed.

To date, the most used scales for psychopathological screening in people with ID and LF-ASD are the Psychopathology Instrument for Mentally Retarded Adults (PIMRA) (Kazdin et al. 1983; Matson et al. 1984, 2012), the Psychiatric Assessment Schedule for Adults with Developmental Disabilities Checklist (PAS-ADD) (Moss 1993), and the Diagnostic Assessment for the Severely Handicapped (DASH) (Matson et al. 1991). Although some high-quality studies support its effectiveness, these tools seem to have some limits in sensitivity, especially in reference to schizophrenic spectrum disorders, reproducibility between different evaluators and consideration of clinical anamnestic information [37].

Further limits of these and the other currently available tools are the applicability to all levels of intellectual impairment, above all to the most serious ones, the interdisciplinary usability and the possibility of managing, with the same system of symptomatological equivalence, each phase of the clinical intervention, i.e., general psychopathological screening, specific categorical diagnosis, dimensional diagnosis, and monitoring of symptoms over time. An attempt to overcome all these limits is represented by the Systematic Psychopathological Assessment for persons with Intellectual and Developmental Disabilities (SPAIDD), a comprehensive tool battery including a "G" version for the "General" screening [43], specific tools for psychopathological area (mood disorders, psychotic disorders, anxiety disorders, autism spectrum disorder, etc.), a module for psychopathological dimensional orientation and a module for symptoms' monitoring (follow-up). All the tools use the same set of adapted symptoms, are based on behaviors or other observable aspects and therefore applicable also to persons with severe impairment of communication skills and conceptualization of intrapsychic suffering. All the SPAIDD tools have been built on the DSM diagnostic criteria and constantly updated to its evolutions. The specific tools for psychopathological area also evaluate the chronology of symptoms, supporting clinicians in the differential diagnosis and in prognostic judgment. All SPAIDD instruments are subjected to in-depth assessments of psychometric characteristics. Particular attention is paid to the validity of the facade, in order to improve the motivation of the informants to use the test.

The SPAIDD-G has undergone numerous evaluations of its psychometric properties [36, 37]. The last one was performed recently on a sample of 395 persons, selected from a wider sample of 944 on the basis of the completeness of data (cases with more than one item without score were excluded). The age range of this sample was 16 and 91 years (M = 51.5; DS = 15.4) and the male-female ratio 73/27. Forty-five percent had a comorbid psychiatric diagnosis (additional to that of ID). The Kuder-Richardson coefficient (KR20) was 0.84 for the full scale and ranged from 0.14 to 0.81 for the 18 subscales. The subscales with a lower internal consistency were "identity disorder" and "sexual disorder," as expected for the low number of items, while those with higher values were "psychotic disorder," "mood disorder—depression," and substance-related disorder.

The inter-rater reliability, estimated through the calculation of Cohen's *K* coefficient, was never less than 0.76, confirming an error variance linked to the scoring criteria and the subjectivity of the rater as a whole not significant. All the raters involved in the validation studies indicated that the tool is clear and easy to use. This judgment was strengthened after the introduction of the description and the exemplification of the items. The SPAIDD-G was judged of great utility by most of the professionals who used it, even in the absence of specific training, immediately understandable and quick to fill out, about 32 min (range 25–42). In the direct comparison with the DASH-II, the SPAIDD-G showed higher face validity, easiness of use, applicability, and syndromic sensitivity. It also required a significantly lower compilation time [43]. The tool is going to be validated in English and German.

8.6 Psycho-pharmacological Therapies

People with ID and LF-ASD receive far more psychoactive drugs than the general population, both in the number of prescribed drugs and in the average prescribed dosage, with rates ranging between 32% and 89%, particularly in adolescents and adults (Bachmann et al. 2014; Merikangas et al. 2013; Steinhausen and Bisgaard 2014; de Kuijper et al. 2010; Doan et al. 2013; Holden and Gitlesen 2004; Stolker et al. 2002; Deb et al. 2015). Drugs are often prescribed to manage PB, without previous assessments of their psychopathological nature and therefore without specific indication. The extensive use also reflects the pressure exerted on clinicians by family members and other assistants of the person with ID to "do something" to quickly alleviate the undefined individual suffering and the negative behavioral changes, which often cause in turn severe distress and destabilization throughout the family and the whole relationship network.

Once prescribed, drugs tend to maintain for a long time, becoming an integral part of the long-term intervention program. On the contrary, an attempt should be made at each stage of monitoring to revisit and reevaluate the formulation and the pharmacotherapeutic plan, aiming at using the lowest possible dose for the minimum duration. Non-medication-based management strategies and the withdrawal of medication should always be considered at regular intervals [44]. Some of the main reasons of long-term treatment are carers' concern of relapse and inaccurate report of efficacy. After months or years of treatment, suspension attempts are reported to be successful only in a limited number of cases (Ahmed et al. 2000).

The most frequently prescribed drugs are antipsychotics, followed by antidepressants (SSRIs and tricyclics), mood stabilizers, and benzodiazepines.

The literature on the psychopharmacological intervention for people with ID and LF-ASD does not offer relevant support to clinicians: studies on the rationale for use, dosages, and safety are few and show great heterogeneity of results, methods, and outcome criteria (Baasland and Engedal 2009; Tyrer et al. 2014). The main hurdles for research are represented by the heterogeneity of the reference population, the indefiniteness of the intervention aims, and the ethical issues, particularly the inability of consensus in participating in randomized controlled trials (RCT) (Feldman et al. 2014). Moreover, the above-mentioned difficulties in identifying PD in persons with communication impairment has aggravated the lack of specific research on drugs with a more general lack of investigations on epidemiology, evaluation tools and procedures, specific clinical presentation, and therefore the definition of therapeutic goals. The lack of research has determined in turn a very low availability of drugs indicated for use with persons with ID and has polarized the prescriptions on the few molecules already approved. At present psychopharmacology for persons with ID and LF-ASD is stuck in a vicious circle; the acts aimed at protecting people with neurodevelopmental disability from inadequate treatments obstacle the development and implementation of appropriate ones.

Only 2% of pharmacological studies include people with ID, and more than 90% are designed to determine their automatic exclusion (Feldman et al. 2014). This trend seems set to continue in the coming years.

SSRI, such as fluoxetine, fluvoxamine, sertraline, citalopram, escitalopram, and paroxetine, are the most prescribed antidepressants due to their greater safety profile than tricyclic antidepressants (TCA), even if studies' results on their efficacy are contradictory and provide evidence of intermediate level (Aman et al. 2000; Deb et al. 2015; Ji and Findling 2016). TCA have also been widely used, both for the treatment of symptoms related to ID or ASD themselves and for the associated psychiatric and behavioral disorders. Clomipramine is the most studied drug of this class, with many reports of efficacy on repetitive behaviors, whether they are attributable to stereotypes or obsessive-compulsive symptoms, co-occurrent to the neurodevelopmental disorder (Gordon et al. 1993; Hurwitz et al. 2012).

Venlafaxine, a selective serotonin and norepinephrine reuptake inhibitor, has shown some beneficial effects in the treatment of hyperactivity, self-injury, and repetitive behaviors in children, adolescents, and adults with ASD. However, studies are very limited (Hollander et al. 2000; Carminati et al. 2006).

Trazodone, a heterocyclic antidepressant, seems to be effective in reducing aggression and self-injurious behavior, but there are only case reports (Gedye 1991).

Benzodiazepines (BDZ) have been found to be scarcely useful in the management of PB and in some cases seem to have even led to significant aggravations (Kalachnik et al. 2002). Their long-term use may increase the risk of tolerance and dependence (with withdrawal symptoms), as well as adjunctive cognitive difficulties, which have frequently been documented in older adults (Puustinen et al. 2012).

BDZ are indicated for catatonia, even at high doses in acute phases. Catatonia represents a potentially fatal psychiatric and medical urgency that is more frequent in persons with ID and ASD than in the general population, especially in late adolescence and in those with more severe disability (Gillberg and Steffenburg 1987; Wing and Shah 2000; Palm, Forsthoff et al. 2011; Ghaziuddin, Dhossche et al. 2012; Torr and D'Abrera 2014; Winarni, Schneider et al. 2015).

The use of antipsychotics (AP) in persons with ID and LF-ASD requires some specific precautions in addition to the usual rule of "go slow and stay low" valid for any psychotropic drug in this population. These precautions are connected to the particular vulnerability to side effects and to frequent comorbidities. Catatonic syndromes and seizures are frequent. In some genetic syndromes, such as Down Syndrome, the central nervous system is subject to early aging and consequent anticipation of the risk increase of cerebrovascular adverse events of some AP (olanzapine, risperidone, aripiprazole and quetiapine), identified in the general population. The use of second-generation antipsychotics (SGA) has also been associated with an increase of cardiovascular morbidity and mortality in elderly persons with ID of different kinds (de Winter, van den Berge et al. 2016; Vigod et al. 2016).

Among the first-generation antipsychotics (FGA), the most used are chlorpromazine and haloperidol. Although some efficacy in the management of PB, especially aggressiveness, FGA should not be considered first-choice therapy, due to limited tolerability (Anderson et al. 1984; La Malfa et al. 2006). For the same reason, they should be used at low dosage and for the minimum possible time. Haloperidol is indicated as an adjunctive therapy in the short term for the management of psychomotor agitation, excitement, and impulsive and violent behaviors (Bhaumik, Branford et al. 2015). Few observational and small open-label studies have shown some efficacy on hyperactivity, aggression, stereotypy, emotional lability, and anger (Naruse et al. 1982; Campbell M 1999). One of the most important studies performed on children with aggressive behaviors showed no differences between risperidone, haloperidol, and placebo (Tyrer et al. 2008).

SGA have been widely introduced in clinical practice. They present a better tolerability profile and a greater number of RCT than FGA. However, studies have been conducted almost exclusively in people with ASD. In addition to risperidone and aripiprazole, there are data on olanzapine, quetiapine, paliperidone, ziprasidone, and asenapine (Advokat et al. 2000). Compared to FGA, SGAs have diversified receptor profiles that seem to impact less on the cognitive and neuromuscular vulnerability of people with ID (de Leon et al. 2009). Some authors claim that they would also have advantages in terms of efficacy, safety, and adherence to treatment, in children, adolescents, and adults (Deb and Unwin 2007).

Despite the lack of solid evidence-based indications specific for ID, anticonvulsants are widely used in clinical practice. In fact, about 20% of people with ID suffer from some kind of epilepsy, a greater number have a history of seizures and electroencephalographic alterations (Robertson, Hatton et al. 2015). Furthermore, some anticonvulsants are currently used as mood stabilizers both in the treatment of acute mania and in the prophylaxis of bipolar disorder. In people with ID, anticonvulsants are used for the control of PB even when a precise psychiatric diagnosis has not been formulated, especially in patients with lower functioning. In many cases, epilepsy co-occur together with PB and PD, indicating some kind of causal link, although evidence upon this is controversial (Arshad, Winterhalder et al. 2011). Also clinical experience indicates a wide range of outcomes: sometimes a good control of epilepsy is associated with the improvement of the general functioning and with the attenuation of any neuropsychiatric and behavioral alteration, in other cases an effective treatment of seizures is followed by worsening of PB and PD. The choice of the anticonvulsant agent seems to play a role in these different results (Deb, Chaplin et al. 2008). Thus, the prescription of anticonvulsants to treat mood disorders and related PB should be made with caution and after a thorough assessment of the neurological comorbidities.

Psychostimulants are the first-choice drugs in children with attention deficit and hyperactivity disorder (ADHD), with a response rate of 70–80% (Greenhill, Swanson et al. 2001). Symptoms of hyperactivity, impulsivity, and inattention are frequently found in the context of other neurodevelopmental disorders including ID and ASD, with rates between 6% and 80% (Frazier, Biederman et al. 2001; Capone, Goyal et al. 2006; Dykens 2007; Rommelse, Franke et al. 2010). In persons with ID and ASD, the co-occurrence of ADHD or ADHD-like symptoms can negatively impact on the outcomes of behavioral interventions and on overall individual quality of life.

Some clinicians hesitate to use methylphenidate in persons with ID for the risk of lowering the seizure threshold in patients who are already more vulnerable than the standard population. A recent study compared the data of more than 18,000 people treated with stimulants with those of almost 55,000 untreated, highlighting that stimulants do not increase the number of hospitalizations related to seizures, even when epilepsy is associated with infantile cerebral palsy, congenital anomalies of the central nervous system, or ID (Liu, Carney et al. 2017).

Atomoxetine appears to be more effective in adults than in children, which is probably due to the different maturation of the dopaminergic and noradrenergic systems in the prefrontal cortex. The drug presents a kinetic of action completely different from the stimulants, developing its therapeutic effect in a period comprised between 1 and 2 months. RCT and open-label studies conducted in children with ASD and ADHD have given unreliable results regarding efficacy on ADHD nuclear symptoms, irritability, verbal and motor stereotypes, PB, and social withdrawal; safety and tolerability were pretty good across studies, with the most common side effects being represented by gastrointestinal alteration, fatigue, palpitations, hyporexia, irritability, and sleep problems (Jou, Handen et al. 2005; Arnold, Aman et al. 2006; Posey, Wiegand et al. 2006; Troost, Steenhuis et al. 2006; Charnsil 2011; Zeiner, Gjevik et al. 2011;

Harfterkamp, van de Loo-Neus et al. 2012). A recent review of the literature has underlined that the quality of the studies in this area is modest, and the results are not very generalizable to the whole autism spectrum (Ghanizadeh 2013). In persons with LF-ASD, atomoxetine seems to be less effective, especially in children, and to determine a higher rate of side effects (Cheng, Chen et al. 2007; Ghanizadeh 2013; Fernandez-Jaen et al. 2010; Kilincaslan et al. 2016).

References

1. Matson JL, Kozlowski AM. The increasing prevalence of autism spectrum disorders. Res Autism Spectr Disord. 2011;5(1):418–25.
2. World Health Organization. ICD-11 international classification of diseases (11th rev.). 2018. https://icd.who.int/ (l.v. 10/3/2019).
3. World Health Organisation. International classification of diseases and related health problems (10th rev., ICD-10). Geneva: World Health Organisation; 1992.
4. APA—American Psychiatric Association. Diagnostic and statistical manual of mental disorders (3rd edition) (DSM-III). Washington, DC: American Psychiatric Association; 1980.
5. Greenspan S, Switzky HN. Forty-four years of AAMR manuals. In: Switzky HN, Greenspan S, editors. What is mental retardation?: ideas for an evolving disability in the 21st century. Washington, DC: AAMR; 2006.
6. APA—American Psychiatric Association. Diagnostic and statistical manual of mental disorders (4th edition; DSM-IV). Washington, DC: American Psychiatric Association; 1994.
7. APA—American Psychiatric Association. Diagnostic and statistical manual of mental disorders (5th edition; DSM-5). Washington, DC: American Psychiatric Association; 2013.
8. Ghaziuddin M. Mental health aspects of autism and Asperger syndrome. London: Jessica Kingsley Publishers; 2005.
9. Matson JL, Shoemaker M. Intellectual disability and its relationship to autism spectrum disorders. Res Dev Disabil. 2009;30(6):1107–14.
10. Boucher J, Bigham S, Mayes A, Muskett T. Recognition and language in low functioning autism. J Autism Dev Disord. 2008;38:1259–69.
11. Murphy O, Healy O, Leader G. Risk factors for challenging behaviors among 157 children with autism spectrum disorders in Ireland. Res Autism Spectr Disord. 2009;3:474–82.
12. O'Brien G, Pearson J. Autism and learning disability. Autism. 2004;8(2):125–40.
13. Goldmon S, Wang C, Salgado MW, Greene PE, Kim M, Rapin I. Motor stereotypies in children with autism and other developmental disorders. Dev Med Child Neurol. 2009;51:30–8.
14. Lunsky Y, Gracey C, Bradley E. Adults with autism spectrum disorders using psychiatric hospitals in Ontario: clinical profile and service needs. Res Autism Spectr Disord. 2009;3(4):1006–13.
15. McCarthy J, Hemmings C, Kravariti E, Dworzynski K, Holt G, Bouras N, Tsakanikos E. Challenging behavior and co-morbid psychopathology in adults with intellectual disability and autism spectrum disorders. Res Dev Disabil. 2010;31(2):362–6.
16. Cowley A, Newton J, Sturmey P, Bouras N, Holt G. Psychiatric inpatient admissions of adults with intellectual disabilities: predictive factors. Am J Ment Retard. 2005;110(3):216–25.
17. Tsakanikos E, Costello H, Holt G, Bouras N, Sturmey P, Newton T. Psychopathology in adults with autism and intellectual disability. J Autism Dev Disord. 2006;36:1123–9.
18. Tsakanikos E, Sturmey P, Costello H, Holt G, Bouras N. Referral trends in mental health services for adults with intellectual disability and autism spectrum disorders. Autism. 2007;11:9–17.
19. Melville CA, Cooper SA, Morrison J, Smiley E, Allan L, Jackson A, et al. The prevalence and incidence of mental ill-health in adults with autism and intellectual disabilities. J Autism Dev Disord. 2008;38:1676–88.

20. Bradley EA, Summers JA, Wood HL, Bryson SE. Comparing rates of psychiatric and behavior disorders in adolescents and young adults with severe intellectual disability with and without autism. J Autism Dev Disord. 2004;34:151–61.
21. Hutton J, Goode S, Murphy M, Couteur AL, Rutter M. New-onset psychiatric disorders in individuals with autism. Autism. 2008;12(4):373–90.
22. La Malfa G, Lassi S, Salvini R, Giganti C, Bertelli M, Albertini G. The relationship between autism and psychiatric disorders in intellectually disabled adults. Res Autism Spectr Disord. 2007;1(3):218–28.
23. LoVullo SV, Matson JL. Comorbid psychopathology in adults with autism spectrum disorders and intellectual disabilities. Res Dev Disabil. 2009;30(6):1288–96.
24. Matson JL, Nebel-Schwalm MS. Comorbid psychopathology with autism spectrum disorders in children: an overview. Res Dev Disabil. 2007;28:341–52.
25. Mouridsen SE, Rich B, Isager T, Nedergaard NJ. Psychiatric disorders in individuals diagnosed with infantile autism as children: a case study. J Psychiatr Pract. 2008;14:5–12.
26. Cooper SA, van der Speck R. Epidemiology of mental ill health in adults with intellectual disabilities. Curr Opin Psychiatry. 2009;22:431–6.
27. Selten JP, Lundberg M, Rai D, Magnusson C. Risks for nonaffective psychotic disorder and bipolar disorder in young people with autism spectrum disorder: a population-based study. JAMA Psychiatry. 2015;72(5):483–9.
28. Thalen M. Comorbidity in adolescents and adults with intellectual disability (ID). Masterthesis Orthopedagogiek; 2011.
29. Cervantes PE, Matson JL. Comorbid symptomology in adults with autism spectrum disorder and intellectual disability. J Autism Dev Disord. 2015;45(2):3961–70.
30. Bradley E, Bolton P. Episodic psychiatric disorders in teenagers with learning disabilities with and without autism. Br J Psychiatry. 2006;189(4):361–6.
31. Bakken TL, Helverschou SB, Eilertsen DE, Heggelund T, Myrbakk E, Martinsen H. Psychiatric disorders in adolescents and adults with autism and intellectual disability: a representative study in one county in Norway. Res Dev Disabil. 2010;31(6):1669–77.
32. Gadow KD, Devincent CJ, Pomeroy J, Azizian A. Comparison of DSM-IV symptoms in elementary school-age children with PDD versus clinic and community samples. Autism. 2005;9:392–415.
33. Hill J, Furniss F. Patterns of emotional and behavioural disturbance associated with autistic traits in young people with severe intellectual disabilities and challenging behaviours. Res Dev Disabil. 2006;27:517–28.
34. McCarthy J. Children with autism spectrum disorders and intellectual disability. Curr Opin Psychiatry. 2007;20:472–6.
35. Bradley EA, Issacs BJ. Inattention, hyperactivity, and impulsivity in teenagers with intellectual disabilities, with and without autism. Can J Psychiatr. 2006;55:598–606.
36. Bertelli M, Scuticchio D, Ferrandi A, Ciavatta C, La Malfa G, Mango F, Porcelli C, Monchieri S. Psychopathology of people with intellectual disability: a multicentre study of a new instrument, the SPAID-G. Ital J Psychopathol. 2010;16(1):53–63.
37. Bertelli M, Scuticchio D, Ferrandi A, Lassi S, Mango F, Ciavatta C, Porcelli C, Bianco A, Monchieri S. Reliability and validity of the SPAID-G checklist for detecting psychiatric disorders in adults with intellectual disability. Res Dev Disabil. 2012;33(2):382–90.
38. Fletcher R, Havercamp S, Ruedrich S, Benson B, Barnhill J, Cooper S-A, Stavrakaki C. Clinical usefulness of the diagnostic manual-intellectual disability for mental disorders in persons with intellectual disability: results from a brief field survey. J Clin Psychiatry. 2009;70(7):967–74.
39. Bolton PF, Rutter M. Schedule for assessment of psychiatric problems associated with autism (and other developmental disorders) (SAPPA): informant version. Cambridge; London: University of Cambridge; Institute of Psychiatry; 1994.
40. Hutton J. Cognitive decline and new problems arising in association with autism. Doctor of Clinical Psychology Thesis, Institute of Psychiatry, University of London; 1998.

41. Raznahan A, Joinson C, O'Callaghan F, Osborne JP, Bolton PF. Psychopathology in tuberous sclerosis: an overview and findings in a population based sample of adults with tuberous sclerosis. J Intellect Disabil Res. 2006;50:561–9.
42. Battaglia M, Detrick S, Fernandez A. Multidisciplinary treatment for adults with autism spectrum disorder and co-occurring mental health disorders: adapting clinical research tools to everyday clinical practice. J Ment Health Res Intellect Disabil. 2016;9(4):232–49.
43. Bertelli M. SPAIDD-G, systematic psychopathological assessment for persons with intellectual and developmental disabilities—general screening, manual. Giunti Psychometrics; 2019. In Press.
44. Deb S, Kwok H, Bertelli M, Salvador-Carulla L, Bradley E, Torr J, Barnhill J, Guideline Development Group of the WPA Section on Psychiatry of Intellectual Disability. International guide to prescribing psychotropic medication for the management of problem behaviours in adults with intellectual disabilities. World Psychiatry. 2009;8(3):181–6.

Anxiety Disorders in the Autism Spectrum: Update and Multi-Case–Control Study on Clinical Phenotypes

9

Leonardo Zoccante

9.1 Introduction

Anxiety disorders are nosographic pictures listed in the Diagnostic and Statistical Manual of Mental Disorders, Fifth Edition (DSM-5). They are characterized on cognitive, behavioral, and pathophysiological levels by an excessive perception of threat in lived situations. According to the DSM-5, fear is an emotional response to an impending danger, whereas anxiety is a preview of a future threat that is responsible for a state of tension and alertness in preparation for actual danger [1]. This condition may affect the general population and be present in numerous and heterogeneous clinical pictures (Table 9.1).

According to the DSM-5 [1], people with level 1 Autism have noticeable issues with communication and social skills. It may be difficult for them to maintain back-and-forth banter during a conversation, and they may find it hard to reach out and make new friends. People who receive a diagnosis of level 1 Autism require support, but often maintain a high quality of life with little support. During school-age, people with a previous diagnosis of Autism spectrum disorders (ASD) report a recurrent presence of anxiety and related worries, which suggests a one-to-one relationship between anxiety disorders and deficits in social skills [2]. Up to 80% of children with ASD also suffer from one or more anxiety disorders. In particular, separation anxiety disorder (SAD) has the highest rate of comorbidity with ASD (38%), followed by obsessive compulsive disorder (OCD) at 37%, generalized anxiety disorder (GAD) at 35%, and social phobia at 30% [3]. In turn, these disorders increase the seriousness of basic ASD phenomenology and may have consequences for social retreat, the sleep/wake rhythm, family interactions, and the ability to adapt to educational activities [3]. Use of specific semi-structured interviews and clinical

L. Zoccante (✉)
Maternal-Child Integrated Care Department, Child and Adolescent Neuropsychiatry Unit, Azienda Ospedaliera Universitaria Integrata, OCM Borgo Trento, Verona, Italy
e-mail: leonardo.zoccante@aovr.veneto.it

R. Keller (ed.), *Psychopathology in Adolescents and Adults with Autism Spectrum Disorders*, https://doi.org/10.1007/978-3-030-26276-1_9

Table 9.1 Anxiety disorders[a]

Disorder	Features
Agoraphobia	Fear or pronounced anxiety concerning two or more situations, such as use of public transport, facing open or closed spaces, standing in a queue or crowd, and spending time away alone
Generalized anxiety disorder	Anxiety or extreme worry (e.g., nervous expectation), shown for most days and at least for 6 months, regarding a significant number of events or activities (e.g., professional services or scholastic results)
Specific phobia	Fear or pronounced anxiety regarding an object or specific situation (e.g., heights, certain animals, seeing blood, flying)
Panic disorder	Presence of frequent and unexpected panic attacks. An attack comprises sudden onset of intense fear or annoyance which reaches a peak in a few minutes
Selective muteness	Constant incapacity of talking in specific social circumstances in which it is normally expected that a person would speak. For such people, it is possible to talk in other circumstances
Separation anxiety disorder	Fear or pronounced anxiety that is inappropriate for the developmental stage, which appears in circumstances of separation from individuals to whom a person is sentimentally close
Social anxiety disorder (social phobia)	Fear or pronounced anxiety related to one or more social contexts where an individual feels exposed to other people's possible judgment. Fear becomes more pronounced in contexts where social interactions are required, when a person feels like somebody is watching them or they are required to introduce themselves to peers

[a]Table prepared according to data obtained from the DSM-5. Obsessive compulsive disorder (OCD) is located beyond the "anxiety disorders" group in the DSM-5. Unlike in previous editions of the diagnostic manual, OCD is now presented as a separate category

questionnaires has revealed that parents' judgment of social anxiety is significantly higher compared with social anxiety reported by affected individuals. This discrepancy between judgments could be a characteristic phenomenon of ASD [4].

Adolescents with Asperger syndrome, which is a low-compromised form of Autism, show significant odds of having an anxiety disorder. This increased prevalence of anxiety may be attributable to higher cognitive functioning, which corresponds to greater awareness of the surrounding environment and therefore greater social involvement with peers [3]. Adolescents who perceive forms of separation anxiety in themselves may also present bizarre behaviors, such as a habit of storing objects for sensory comfort in situations where separation is predicted. This is a common phenomenon, especially in late adolescence, and intense distress is reported in the absence of these objects of comfort [5]. The disorder tends to disappear or considerably diminish after 40 years of age [2].

In this chapter, we examine how anxiety can have different gradients and nuances in clinical pictures of ASD, especially where there is comorbidity with Attention Deficit Hyperactivity Disorder (ADHD), Tourette's Syndrome (TS), or other conditions. We also examine various specifiers that can be useful elements for classifying anxiety disorders. Throughout the chapter, results of recent basic research on the topic are considered.

9.2 Epidemiological Aspects of Anxiety Disorder

Children with ASD have double the prevalence of anxiety disorders compared with children in the general population. They also present variability of anxiety disorders based on different types of ASD. On an epidemiological level, Van Steensel, Bögels, and Perrin identified at least 40% comorbid anxiety disorders in children and adolescents with ASD [6]. In fact, nearly 40% of these children and adolescents showed clinically high levels of anxiety or had an actual anxiety disorder. Specific phobia was the most common disorder (30% of individuals), followed by OCD (17%), social anxiety disorder and agoraphobia (about 17%), GAD (15%), SAD (9%), and panic disorder (almost 2%) [6]. A close relationship between the social environment and anxious symptomatology also emerged, especially regarding forms of level 1 ASD [6, 7]. Another study highlighted that there was a greater frequency of abuse in both school and family environments in children diagnosed with Asperger syndrome or non-verbal disorder, with an overall prevalence of such episodes of about 94% of the studied population [7]. In that study, three-quarters of the parents reported that their children suffered at least one episode of abuse from peers in the year of the investigation; there were reports of bullying (75% of cases), physical or verbal attacks (10%), and real aggression with references to genitalia (15%). Children with low social skills or a diagnosis of Asperger syndrome were the most frequent victims of episodes caused by peers [7].

Prevalence studies indicate that between 11% and 84% of children with ASD suffer significant impairment attributable to anxiety [8]. It has also been noted that depending on the position on the Autism Spectrum, anxiety disorders varied in the degree of impairment and frequency, with a higher prevalence in those with Asperger syndrome and PDD-NOS (pervasive developmental disorder-not otherwise specified). These two groups also suffered panic attacks and specific phobias. Anxiety disorders had a lower prevalence among those who had been diagnosed with ASD with higher clinical impairment [6, 8]. In addition, the problems related to anxiety were more common in those with Asperger syndrome than in actual ASD [8].

White et al. [8] reported that social phobia and OCD were rarely diagnosed in the ASD population. There was a general agreement among clinicians that these symptoms could be explained by ASD; however, new neurological research has considered these disorders as possible comorbidities, highlighting reciprocal relationships between anxiety, sensory overload, and impairment of social skills [8].

It is difficult to identify and measure the symptoms of anxiety disorders in ASD, especially in those with limited verbal skills [9]. It is therefore essential to identify behavioral variations in sleep, changes in appetite, or sudden increases in the expenditure of physical and mental energies. Currently, this is difficult because specific measurement questionnaires are lacking. There is no common agreement among the scientific community about the correct way to measure anxiety or mood disorders in individuals with ASD [9]. A common hypothesis is that patients who prefer ritual activities characterized by high repetition also present baseline levels of greater anxiety. However, no precise relationships between these variables have been demonstrated. In contrast, relationships between anxiety symptoms and behavioral interferences mediated by recurrent provocative attitudes and negative automatic thoughts have been shown. However, behavioral interferences and automatic thoughts are largely variable and influenced by the environmental context. There may also be a particular frequency of gastrointestinal disorders and a reduced quality of sleep due to the occurrence of specific somatization disorders in individuals with ASD characterized by high levels of anxiety [6, 9, 10].

9.3 Possible Predisposing and Etiological Factors

In current clinical practice, it is often difficult to diagnose and distinguish anxiety disorders starting from the basic inventory of ASD symptoms. It is equally difficult to identify etiological and predisposing factors that are peculiar to ASD per se, but independent from those relating to anxiety disorders. Expressions of anxiety in pediatric age groups are essentially behavioral in nature and can therefore be erroneously traced back to comorbidities, such as oppositional defiant disorder or ADHD [9]. Conversely, in young adulthood, we find greater compensation strategies that tend to contain anxious expressions through strict or schematic adaptive reactions. In ASD cases that present with the onset of anxiety disorder during early childhood, the symptomatology of the two conditions often intensifies following their mutual enhancement [6]. It is therefore essential to extend future research to clearly identify clinical markers that could allow us to differentiate between pure ASD and comorbid ASD and anxiety disorders.

Specific consideration has been given to genetic factors and their etiological role in the expression of both ASD and anxiety disorders. In genetic research, studies on ASD and anxiety disorders follow different branches, although both disorders share some basic genetic factors [11]. Recent progress in molecular biology [12] has highlighted that ASD has a complex and elaborate genetic architecture in which inheritable genes are found [13]. Broadly, these consist of a thousand genes with marked locus heterogeneity [14] whose expression in clinical phenotypes follows complex polymorphisms that can also be determined by environmental epigenetic influences, as demonstrated by studies with monozygotic twins [15]. Many of these genes have yet to be defined with certainty. However, some could explain the alterations in social communicative skills, and others could be related to the development of narrow interests and stereotyped activities [16]. ASD is a polygenic disorder, which could be caused by directly responsible genes or by genes related to anxious manifestations with relative degrees of expression [17–19]. Today, an academic focus is considering factors predisposing gene expressions that vary according to existing environmental influences [20, 21]. It is widely known that there is a continuous mutual interaction between genetic and environmental elements [22]. Parents' social and educational factors and the patient's own behavioral profile could play a role in the expression of the clinical phenotype. As an example, some children with ASD favor selected living environments that require less empathy and social skills because of a profile lacking flexibility or reduced planning capability. However, the cognitive development of these children is influenced by the environments that they chose [23]. Environmental interactions may explain the marked variance and direct repercussion on specific brain functions [24, 25].

A previous study [26] suggested there was a relationship between neuroimaging volumetric data and anxiety or depression scores reported by parents in a sample of children with ASD that were specifically recruited and underwent magnetic resonance imaging (MRI). Significant correlations between the volume of the right amygdala and anxious symptomatology were identified, highlighting static linear relationships. The study concluded that there were possible connections between anxiety/depression symptoms and right amygdala volume [26, 27]. Shen et al. [28] suggested that compared with controls, people with ASD show an increased volume of cerebrospinal fluid. In the cases they reported, a 15% increase in average fluid content was obtained after standardization of weight, age, and sex. Strong associations between this fluid increase and sleep disorders and deficits in non-verbal skills were reported that were possibly connected with an anxiety disorder. However, an above-average cerebrospinal fluid volume can be found in healthy children at risk for developing ASD. Shen et al. also noted a relative increase in head circumference among the ASD group compared with controls [28]. Further studies are required to determine if there is an etiopathological link between increased cerebrospinal fluid volume and volumetric data for the amygdala.

A recent hypothesis concerns the particular role played by environmental interactions that represent the basis of higher cognitive functions and social skills. The focus of underlying deficits in multisensory integration allows greater characterization and understanding of ASD. Alterations in multisensory processing and integration can be heterogeneous within the Autism Spectrum; specific identification will allow us to investigate the underlying foundations of the disorder and its variants [3]. Two abnormal functional profiles have been identified in relation to sensoriality in patients with ASD: hyper-sensory and hypo-sensory profiles. Forms with a sensoriality that can be evoked by slight stimuli or lower sensory thresholds may be associated with concomitant anxiety disorders, most likely related to sensory overload added to previous social discomfort. Therefore, in clinical forms characterized by hyper-sensoriality, aspects related to anxiety should be carefully monitored and specific therapeutic programs defined.

Another hypothesis linked the presence of ligamentous hyperlaxity to anxiety disorders. Recent studies have concluded that at least 70% of people with hyperlaxity also presented with an anxiety disorder, about 70% of people with anxiety disorder, and 62% with panic disorder also had generalized hyperlaxity syndrome [29]. Ligamentous hyperlaxity may represent a somatic component that shows a peculiar frequency in anxiety and irritable temperament disorders. The relationship between hyperlaxity and anxiety disorder has been considered in both the developmental stage and adulthood [30]. Some authors suggest that the presence of a central connectivity disorder is the source of both hyperlaxity and ASD, where at the same time, there is a reduction in long-range connectivity and an increase in short-range connectivity [31]. Other researchers have related hyperlaxity to alterations in motor coordination and proprioceptive sensitivity.

9.4 Specifiers Influencing Clinical Expression

Age: In the general pediatric population, primary school (age 6–10 years) is the period in which the onset of anxiety disorder symptoms is more frequent, and anxiety often manifests as associated with difficulties in social skills. In the presence of ASD, the onset of anxiety disorders tends to be delayed, particularly during middle school, reaching peak intensity in later years and stabilizing in adulthood [2]. In people with ASD, adolescence may also be undermined by bipolar disorder, which in this age group presents its most typical onset. Borderline personality disorder, especially the early onset forms, is also frequently comorbid with ASD [3]. It has been observed that in ASD the "age" factor may be directly correlated with the magnitude of anxiety symptoms. As patients' average age increases, an increasing level of anxiety and a higher frequency of anxiety disorders are observed [6]. Conversely, other anxious expressions, such as separation anxiety, present with a decreasing frequency with increasing chronological age [2, 6]. It is possible that the expression of anxiety at an earlier age manifests itself more through behavior, and the intensity of repetitive activities may be accentuated by the anxious component.

Intelligence quotient (IQ): A significant anxious component is often present in people with ASD with high clinical impairment and low IQ scores. Although not expressed verbally, this may be associated with behavioral stereotypies or irritability in situations of environmental perturbation. Even in forms of level 1 ASD with low impairment, the manifestations of anxiety may be predominant in various functional areas and greatly affect the individual's life. Detection of low IQ scores has been associated with expressions of anxiety that are more related to social contexts [6]. Anxiety linked to social contexts would be inversely proportional to the individual's social skills and assertiveness [32]. In school age, difficulties reported in social skills often lead to deterioration in interactions with peers. Furthermore, in forms of ASD with low clinical impairment, the inhomogeneity of the cognitive profile (i.e., evidence of bias between verbal IQ and non-verbal IQ) has a direct correlation with the basal level of anxiety. However, this is not observed in high-impairment clinical forms, where the greater homogeneity of the cognitive profile makes it more difficult for the person to implement adaptive skills according to their environment and develop more routinized and standardized living environments. In these conditions, simple modifications to the routine are sufficient to determine an accentuation of behavioral rigidity and provoke irritability or aggressive reactions, from which depressive outcomes can result.

In conditions where cognitive observation has documented discrepancy between verbal and non-verbal skills (i.e., higher performance in verbal skill tests than non-verbal skill tests), there is often an association with depression + anxious disorder. Longitudinal observations from a 6-year survey by Kim et al. [9] reported the development of significant anxiety and mood problems in subjects with a previous discrepancy in cognitive tests [9]. In the school setting, parents' previous finding of sustained levels of anxiety also had a predictive value in terms of worse school performance in teacher evaluations and related family repercussions (depression, findings of impaired affectivity). In contrast, low levels of anxiety were found to have a predictive value in terms of better school performance independently of reported IQ values [8]. Similar observations allow us to hypothesize that the association with depression + anxious disorder in people with ASD may represent a negative prognostic indicator for the purpose of clinical development in childhood.

Sex: It is known that ASD has a significantly higher prevalence in males than females, with a male:female ratio of about 3:1 [33, 34]. However, it is estimated that in females, there may be a bias involving a sub-diagnosis of ASD in relation to sex-related factors. Females tend to have greater emotional empathy that results in the underestimation of clinical signs characteristic of ASD [35]. It is also known that in the general population, anxiety disorders typically present a high prevalence in females. In ASD, anxiety disorders have a female:male ratio of 3:2 [2].

Moreover, in people with ASD, anxiety disorders are associated with a high frequency of hoarding behaviors in different life contexts, especially among females [5]. In particular, the tendency to hoard is associated with forms of ASD comorbid with ADHD; this tendency may be characterized by difficulties in attention shift, self-regulation disorders, and spatiotemporal planning and organization deficits. This supports the hypothesis of a positive correlation between "pathological hoarding" and anxiety traits, obsessive-compulsive traits, and social impairments [5]. The inability to discard unnecessary objects may be directly proportional to the magnitude of ADHD symptoms detectable in the individual case and may lead to a distinct environmental disorder with disabling effects on daily life, particularly in domestic environments. Preliminary research data suggests that hoarding disorder presents a peculiar association with ASD and with the severity of symptoms such as anxiety/depression [5]. However, in males, anxiety disorder presents more contained hoarding behaviors and less pervasiveness.

9.5 Clinical Phenotypes and Possible Comorbidities

ASD presents a widely heterogeneous repertoire of clinical manifestations. It is known that anxiety may be a symptom inherent to ASD. There is a biunivocal relationship between the social communication deficits responsible for the basic condition and the adaptive alert and thoughts that it involves. True predominant phenotypes can be identified when the anxious symptomatology assumes characteristics such as becoming a group of specific symptoms that impact on clinical expression and have permanence over time. By excluding anxiety conditions that are a common reflection of ASD, we can identify anxious entities to create a comorbid disorder. The proposed interpretative model is based on three main variables: type, intensity, and duration of anxiety symptoms [6].

Various expressions of anxiety can be classified into three main frameworks: (1) social anxiety, (2) anxiety with phobias or excessive worries, and (3) anxiety with obsessive-compulsive traits or repetitive/ritualized behaviors. Varying individual degrees of expressiveness can be highlighted in each clinical picture, from forms limited in intensity and duration to forms with greater interference in daily activities. A clinical picture of comorbid anxiety disorder can be highlighted if four criteria are met: (a) permanence over time (in the absence of transience), (b) pervasiveness, (c) impact on adaptive skills, and (d) refractory nature to treatments.

Corresponding comorbidities that can be identified are:

- ASD + SAD
- ASD + specific phobia disorder or panic attacks
- ASD + OCD with/without repetitive and ritualized behavior

Figure 9.1 presents a diagram of the three levels of ASD impairment according to the DSM-5, considering the most representative anxiety disorder in each level and taking into account both the condition in which anxiety is reflexively associated with the basic clinical picture, and that in which anxiety flows from a transitory state into permanence, interfering in different neurofunctional areas, thus configuring anxiety disorder comorbidity.

A close relationship between temperament and social anxiety can be highlighted in people with level 1 ASD. In those with temperaments characterized by high empathy, the degree of perception and awareness of others' judgments of behavior that deviates from normality is also more relevant. As the empathy of people with level 1 ASD increases, a linear increase in social anxiety can be observed, particularly in the first decades of life. In temperaments with reduced empathy, particularly in adolescence, there is often a tendency to underestimate or neglect social

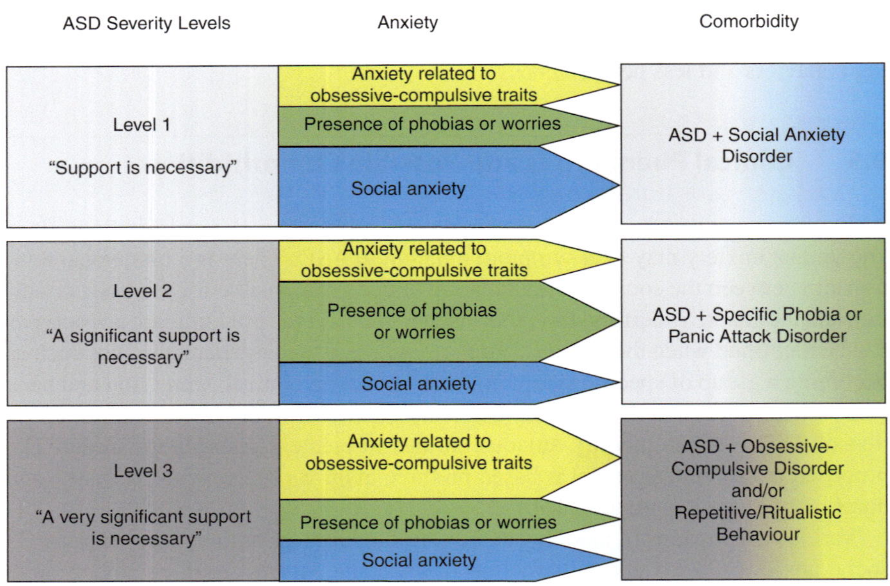

Fig. 9.1 On the left are the main diagnostic levels. At the center are clinical expression pictures with greater relative frequency, represented by the size of the colored arrows (arrow sizes are not statistically related to any data, but are purely explanatory of prevalence). On the right are anxiety disorders that take on a clinical picture of comorbidity

judgment on the part of other people. In addition, presence of the "anxiety disorder + depression" cluster may negatively influence the basic clinical picture, with deterioration in the executive functions and appearance of pathological avoidance. Psychiatric disorders with components of anxiety, obsessions, phobias, and alterations in sleep and mood are frequently found [36]. This phenomenon can be explained in relation to the secondary effects that involve the overlap of diagnostic criteria for different neuropsychiatric disorders described by the DSM-5 [1], even in level 1 forms. However, high levels of social anxiety are present in all of these different conditions. The ability to manage one's emotions is known to contribute to a greater degree of behavioral flexibility and more efficient ability to adapt responses to environmental feedback [32]. A greater awareness of discomfort and the adoption of adaptive compensations within daily occupations and interactions with peers over time [2, 8] are clinically important. As a person ages, a downward trend in social anxiety scores can usually be observed.

The diagnostic criteria for specific phobia/panic attacks are the same for individuals with or without ASD. However, it may be difficult to distinguish conditions in which the symptoms are indicative of an ASD diagnosis, or conditions in which they are due to a specific phobia or panic attack disorder diagnosis. Symptoms of phobia and anxiety are more common in people with ASD than in controls or syndromic children [8]. Factors such as cognitive and attentional deficits, and mood and behavior disorders may explain an altered perception of danger. In addition, in particular situations of risk, there may be a non-perception of danger, which is an indication of greater cognitive impairment; excessive fear can also be detected for common situations or objects in apparently calm situations [6]. For example, it is not clear how much food hyper-selectivity or rigidity toward certain foods can be explained in terms of taste, consistency, a specific phobia, or by the co-presence of several factors.

The presence of a specific phobia in ASD has greater relevance in forms that are the most cognitively compromised. According to parents' and teachers' reports, psychiatric clusters are often identified in ASD in relation to social phobia and specific phobias or to ritualistic and repetitive behavior that may or may not be associated with movement disorders (e.g., motor or vocal tics) [8]. A low cognitive profile may mask and make diagnosis of specific phobias difficult. Overall, specific phobia is the most frequent comorbidity among people with ASD, with a higher prevalence among females [37].

A restricted activity pattern and repetitive behavior is the most representative mode of anxiety disorder with obsessive-compulsive or repetitive-ritualistic traits in ASD. In highly compromised forms, this pattern supports or favors social isolation, as the expressions of anxiety have a predominantly behavioral character in these cases. Strong routines are often found with numerous and persistent daily rituals that support the chronicization of compulsive behavior. These phenomena can only partly be traced back to cognitive deficits that are an expression of ASD, but are explained in highly compromised forms through biunivocal enhancement between cognitive deficits and the poverty of behavioral expressions. It is difficult to differentiate behavioral patterns on an anxious basis compared with those linked to level 1

ASD. Careful observation can highlight an “anxious routine” pattern when it is more associated with changes in mood and irritability. Other elements that can be traced back to this expressive modality of anxiety include the tendency toward isolation and fixity toward common objects or environmental situations that can provide a feeling of reassurance and immutability, but in a way that determines interference by rituals in everyday life. In these cases, difficulty in separating from objects of little use is often reported. These characteristics compromise the level of adaptability to the environment and may lead to progressive difficulty in emotional regulation associated with resistance to change and the need for continuous reassurance [5].

9.6 Connectivity Disorders and Anxiety Disorders

Many studies have noted that some neurodevelopmental disorders can be described as an “abnormal connectivity spectrum disorder” (ACSD) based on the alterations observed at the neural connections network level. This group includes three developmental disorders: ASD, ADHD, and TS. These clinical conditions have extended overlapping and heterogeneity of clinical phenotypes. New evidence suggests that these disorders have significant similarities. For example, experimental studies have identified similarities in reduced long-range connectivity and high short-range connectivity in different brain areas [38]. This new perspective builds understanding about the severity of clinical manifestations through a gradient of altered connectivity. Supported by a neurobiological basis, these three conditions share common symptoms, such as social communication deficits, obsessive traits, Attention Deficit/Hyperactivity, and impulsivity. Diagnosis is usually formulated at preschool age and is more common in males, with deficits in functional and scholastic activity and significant behavioral, emotional, and psychosocial disorders. In cases where two of these disorders co-occur (e.g., ASD/ADHD), functional impairment in the quality of life is more evident than in individuals with a single diagnosis [3]. The co-presence of ASD/ADHD is a particular determinant of clinical levels of anxiety. In parental interviews, threshold scores were a negative predictor for the development of social skills deficits. Kim et al. [9] also found a significant correlation between social interaction difficulties and anxiety/mood disorders; the latter were not correlated with the development of language skills, which is a discriminating element of different ASD levels. Currently, the presence of anxiety disorders associated with depression in ASD is considered a major specifier of the comorbid clinical phenotype and no longer an emotional display of the underlying disorder. The specifier is analyzed through specific entries on structured parental questionnaires. Comorbid conditions are characterized by differences in cognition, motivation, and social awareness, as well as restricted interests and behavioral repetition. More aggressive and oppositional behavior has been documented in the presence of mixed conditions. In 45% of children with ASD, particularly in cases of ASD/ADHD, disruptive behavior disorder or oppositional provocative disorder may appear [39].

Epidemiologically, TS has higher comorbidity in people with ASD than in the general population; 4.6% of patients with TS also have a pervasive development disorder. However, 22% of patients with ASD show motor tics or Tourette-like symptoms, possibly attributable to the common neurobiological basis that causes a synaptic imbalance overlap [3]. In most commonly used questionnaires, parents of children with ASD report a higher frequency of obsessive thoughts related to technologies (e.g., transport vehicles, television, or computers) than obsessive thoughts about social relationships (e.g., gossip, beliefs). In TS, the content of obsessive thoughts reported by parents is more related to sensory phenomena and, in particular, to passive perceptions of environmental stimuli or sensations related to voices or auditory stimuli [6]. Obvious deficits in social communication and pragmatic skills seem to be largely associated with symptoms of ADHD found in people with ASD [10].

Recent experimental evidence that documents a connectivity disorder is mainly from the neurophysiological and neuroradiological (functional MRI) domain. Clinical phenotypes that show similarities in neuropsychological attention, stereotyped behaviors, and reduced social skills profiles [38, 40] are part of the new set categorized as ACSD. Specific associations between connectivity alteration and cognitive performance alteration have also been documented in correlation with executive functions, attentive processes, and communication skills. In ACSD, connectivity anomalies are linked to white matter anomalies. This can be related to aberrances in afferent sensory pathways reaching the brain, with consequent difficulty in central elaboration [38]. In particular, neurodevelopmental disorders have focused on alterations of the frontal lobes (site of control and regulation of impulses), which leads to atypical regulation and modulation of information from the environment.

The co-presence of reduced long-range connectivity (frontoparietal areas and inter-hemispheric connection) and high short-range connectivity (occipital and orbital-frontal areas) was highlighted by electroencephalographic spectral analysis involving large numbers of people with ASD. Moreover, the same analysis in people with ADHD and TS showed close correlations with dysfunctional symptoms and difficulty in sensory motor modulation [41].

Neuroimaging studies have confirmed the altered connectivity hypothesis. Autism Brain Imaging Data Exchange (ABIDE) data [41] appear to confirm evidence of short-range hyper-connectivity in parietal sites and fibers directed to subcortical nuclei and evidence of long-range hypo-connectivity in cortical-connected or interhemispheric fibers [42, 43]. These experimental results remain of little known value today and need to be contextualized. MRI research has confirmed that in comparison with control subjects, signs of abnormal structural and functional connectivity can be attributed to microglial activation zones. Recently this phenomenon has been investigated on a cellular level, with the hypothesis that connectivity is related to oxidative or toxic-inflammatory stress on myelinated or long-axon fibers of large-caliber neurons (e.g., Purkinje cells). From this perspective, neuronal networks of the dopaminergic or serotoninergic type would be more susceptible as they are normally used to transmit messages over distance through continuous pruning and sprouting processes. Microglial interface areas, rich in glial–axonal junctions, may also be more susceptible because synaptic connections require greater energy expenditure. According to recent hypotheses, the organization of the network of connectome may not only be confined to cerebral nerve tissue, but may involve other regulatory systems, such as the neuroendocrine and immune systems [44], that are modulated by peptidergic antigens and emotional or antigenic stressors. Molecules in continuous interchange through the blood–brain barrier can influence the activity of immunity cells by determining adaptive or defense responses to the surrounding environment [45, 46].

ACSD may therefore represent an interpretative model of the clinical heterogeneity of neurodevelopmental disorders. In particular, the literature indicates that the overlap among these disorders is high [38]. We have considered "anxiety" in relation to ASD and other two diagnostic categories (ADHD and TS) that belong to the same spectrum, with the aim of better characterizing the phenotypes [39, 47]. We conducted a study that examined anxiety disorders in three groups of patients (ASD, ADHD, and TS) who had received diagnoses according to the current diagnostic criteria.

The objectives of the study were to (1) verify the actual co-presence of anxiety symptoms in different diagnostic groups in relation to a control population and (2) establish how much anxiety coincides with internalizing or externalizing problems in the different clinical pictures. The study used the *Child Behavior Checklist* (CBCL), which is a standardized tool to identify emotional and behavioral problems in school-age children (age 6–18 years) [48].

Similar pictures to those discussed above can be found in the general population. However, the primary objective of our study was to verify if anxiety disorders can have specificity in neurodevelopmental disorders due to the presence of altered connectivity compared with control subjects. The secondary objective was to demonstrate whether there were associations between levels and types of anxiety with an evolution in an internalizing or externalizing way.

A nationwide survey in the United States found a greater presence of anxiety disorders in populations of children who showed neurological disorders than among their peers without this type of disorder [48]. That survey aimed to determine if there were higher levels of anxiety in populations with neuronal disorders, but did not delve into the way in which these symptoms occurred (i.e., externalizing or internalizing). The presentation of symptoms is important, as it can inform the design-specific treatments. However, another study showed that children with Autism tend to show a higher level of anxiety and internalizing symptoms, whereas children with ADHD showed more externalizing symptoms [49]. Although that study considered how the symptoms were presented, it did not consider TS.

Given the findings of the two studies mentioned above, we aimed to verify if anxiety disorders have specificity in neurodevelopmental disorders compared with control subjects on the basis of an altered connectivity model. We also aimed to demonstrate if there were associations between levels and types of anxiety with evolution of clinical problems.

9.7 Methods and Research Design

We analyzed anxiety disorders in three groups of patients who were diagnosed according to current clinical diagnostic scales. The standardized CBCL for school-age children (aged 6–18 years) was used to identify emotional and behavioral problems [50]. The CBCL is a 118-item measure of parental perceptions of a child's emotional and behavioral functioning over the last 6 months and has sound psychometric properties [50]. The self-report questionnaire is completed by both parents and requires them to rate how true statements regarding the behavior of their child (in the last 6 months and currently) are on a 3-point scale (0 = not true, 1 = somewhat or sometimes true, 2 = very true or often true). There was no difference in administering the checklist to the different groups of patients.

The CBCL allows evaluation of behavioral problems through an "empirically derived" scale that provides information about different syndromic frameworks and a "DSM-oriented" scale that orients professionals toward diagnosis of some disorders according to DSM-5 criteria. The individual items are divided into groups and allow identification of eight clinical frameworks/syndromes: anxious/depressed, withdrawn/depressed, somatic complaints, social problems, thought problems, attention problems, rule-breaking behavior, and aggressive behavior. These frameworks were grouped according to their belonging to a clinical dimension into three main subscales that provide a dimensional and quantitative measurement of the framework itself: internalizing (anxious/depressed, withdrawn/depressed, somatic complaints), externalizing (rule-breaking behavior, aggressive behavior), and a third subscale representing neither one nor the other. Items for the anxious/depressed scale include *cries a lot, fears, fears school, fears doing bad, must be perfect, feels unloved, feels worthless, nervous/tense, fearful/anxious, feels too guilty, self-conscious, talks about suicide,* and *worries.* On the DSM-oriented scale, items relating to anxiety problems include *dependent, fears, fears school, fears doing bad, nervous/tense, nightmares, fearful/anxious, self-conscious,* and *worries.*

This exploratory study aimed to show the continuity between the different connectivity disorders and the way in which they generate an impact on daily life through the levels of anxiety experienced. With the aim of understanding and verifying similarities and differences in the manifestation of anxiety disorders in the three selected diagnostic groups, we conducted an observational multi-case–control study using four patient samples. Eligibility criteria were:

- A diagnosis of one of the three connectivity disorders (i.e., scores above the cut-off for ASD, ADHD, or TS)
- Aged 6–18 years (according to the CBCL validation scale)
- An IQ above 80
- Agreed to participate in the study

Patients with level 1 ASD were recruited to obtain a homogeneous group in terms of the cognitive profile. Patients with ADHD and TS were recruited according to current diagnostic criteria. In addition, a group of subjects without any diagnosis and with the same age range and IQ was recruited as a control group. At the beginning of the study, 34 patients with ASD (27 males, seven females), 33 with ADHD (28 males, five females), 33 with TS (27 males, six females), and 35 control subjects (15 males, 20 females) were recruited to obtain a sufficient sample size. There were 19 dropouts following the evaluation of the inclusion and exclusion criteria and CBCL testing. This resulted in the effective recruitment of 21 patients with ASD, 31 with ADHD, and 29 with TS. In total, 116 participants were recruited, 84 males and 32 females. Initially, we expected to have a similar number of females and males in each group, but early detection of ASD, ADHD, and TS in females in sufficient numbers at an early age is not yet achieved, as the general prevalence of these disorders is lower among females.

All tests were administered in the Child Neuropsychiatry Department of Verona University Hospital, in specific outpatient areas for neurodevelopmental disorders. The tests were conducted from January 1, 2018 to November 30, 2018 (Fig. 9.2).

Table 9.2 reports the demographic characteristics of the sample and means of the results for the clinical scales in the different groups.

Descriptive statistics were calculated as means and standard deviations for continuous normally distributed variables and median and inter quartile range (IQR) for non-normally distributed variables. Frequencies and percentages were used for categorical variables. To compare the means of the considered variables among the different groups, we used a one-way (case–control status) analysis of variance (ANOVA) and a two-way (case–control status and sex) ANOVA. Post hoc tests were also performed comparing each case status with the control group. For each group (case–control status), the mean adjusted by age was calculated. The analyses were not adjusted for age, as this variable was not clinically different among the groups. The selected threshold level for statistical significance was $p < 0.05$. All analyses were performed using Stata 14 (www.stata.com).

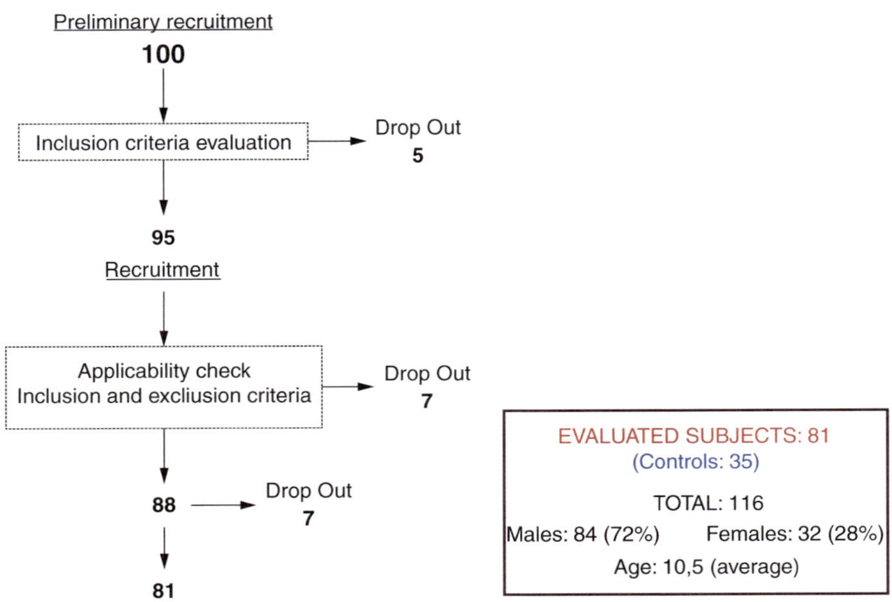

Fig. 9.2 Flowchart detailing the recruitment process, eligibility selection, and dropouts

Table 9.2 Sample characteristics

	ASD	Attention Deficit Hyperactivity Disorder	Tourette's Syndrome	Controls	
Patients, *n* (%)	21 (18.1)	31 (26.7)	29 (25.0)	35 (30.2)	
Variables					***p*-value**
	Mean (SD)				
Age, years	10.46 (2.16)	9.9 (2.13)	10.19 (1.92)	11.44 (2.34)	**0.026**
Sex					**<0.001**
Male	17 (81.0)	27 (87.1)	25 (86.2)	15 (42.9)	
Female	4 (19.0)	4 (12.9)	4 (13.8)	20 (57.1)	
Total IQ	93.75 (15.59)	95.29 (16.48)	94.04 (19.47)*	105.47 (12.33)*	**0.013**
CBCL scale					
	Median (IQR)				
Anxiety/ depression	70 (66–78)	69 (59–74)	66 (60–72)	57 (51–66)*	**<0.001**
Anxiety disorders	70 (65–82)	70 (58–76)	67 (61–76)	57 (51–68)*	**<0.001**
Internalizing problems	71 (68–74)	68 (58–73)	66 (61–71)	59 (54–66)*	**<0.001**
	Mean (SD)				
Externalizing problems	60.48 (11.48)	63.26 (10.36)	60.62 (10.14)	53.26 (7.71)*	**<0.001**

CBCL Child Behavior Checklist, *IQ* intelligence quotient, *SD* standard deviation
Note: In this table "Autism" means: level 1 Autism
Bar charts: *p*-values for the groups of patients vs. controls. * <0.05
If there is no sign above the bar in any group, it means that there was no statistically significant difference between that group and the controls

9.8 Discussion of the Findings

In relation to the "anxiety/depression" and "anxiety problems" subscales, two representative graphs are shown below that present the scores recorded in the database. Comparison of the three diagnostic groups with the control group showed a significant difference confirming a functional profile that overlapped on the anxiety/depression axis. In Figure 9.3, we consider the scores for the CBCL subscale that considers symptoms of anxiety (e.g., school phobias, perfectionism, and devaluation of self) and depressive symptoms (e.g., guilt, excessive worry, crying, and excessive jealousy). As the group of symptoms reflected on this subscale is broad and heterogeneous, it may justify the significance in all three groups. Although the significant difference reached a slightly higher range in the ASD group, it confirmed a direct correlation between the type of disorder, underlying neurobiological conditions, and the extent of the manifestation, and resulted in extensive overlap in the three groups.

Figure 9.4 shows the distribution of scores for the CBCL "anxiety problems" subscale. In this case, it can be observed that the prevalence of anxiety problems was

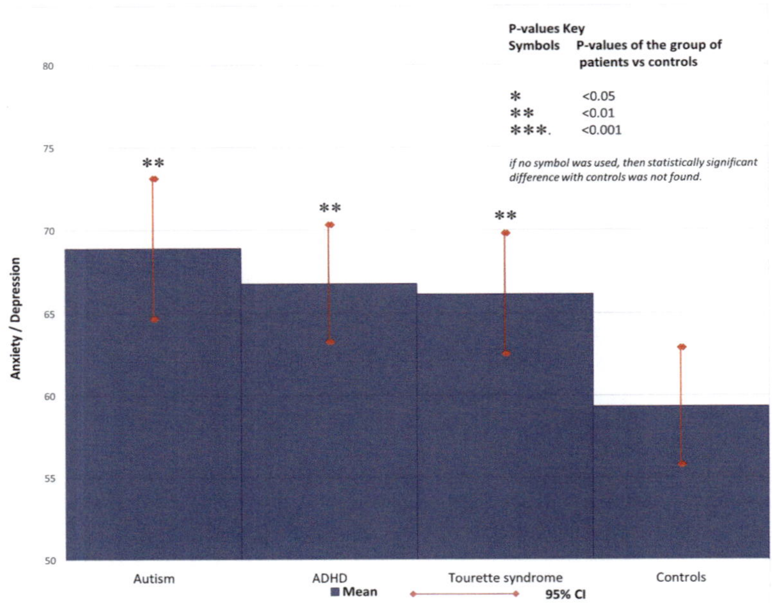

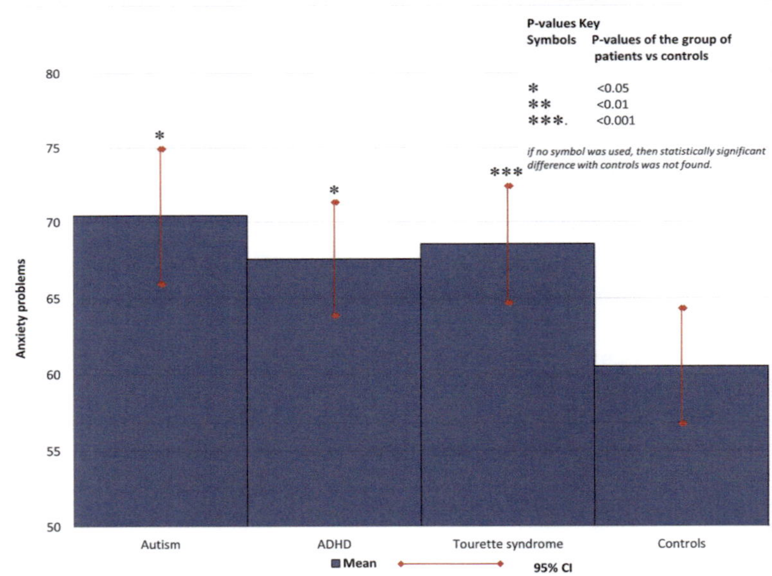

Figs. 9.3 and 9.4 [In these Figures, "Autism" means level 1 Autism]: The values on the *y*-axis indicate the range of the *T* points within which the median scores obtained by the different reference samples fall in relation to the areas (anxiety/depression) or macro-areas (internalizing, externalizing) considered. Up to 65 *T* points, the score is considered standard, a score from 65 to 70 is considered borderline, and scores of 70 and above are considered clinically significant. Such scores may indicate specific problems in each area and provide indications on different syndromic frameworks. Sex-adjusted means and 95% confidence intervals for each group

higher in the three neurodevelopmental disorder groups compared with the control group. In particular, these anxiety problems were associated with self-belittlement, which is a typical repertoire for people with TS. In fact, the reduced fluidity of thought in this condition gives rise to awareness of its own limits, which is followed by either dysfunctional anxiety or addictive behaviors and actions conditioned by obsessive-compulsive traits (e.g., fixation with objects, especially technological objects) [48]. As mentioned in the "Clinical phenotypes and possible comorbidities" section, an anxiety disorder significantly interferes with children's daily school activities, with direct repercussions in different areas of life with psycho-social value.

Anxiety disorders can present internalizing or externalizing profiles. In the first case, the disorder is associated with symptoms of inhibition and in the second with greater impulsivity. Our hypothesis was that depending on the type of comorbid clinical picture, anxiety can be managed with a turn toward withdrawal in some cases and a turn toward action in others. In ADHD, ASD, and TS, externalizing manifestations prevail in the presence of the impulsive component. What unites these two manifestations, which appear to be placed at the two extremes, is that both may be atypical reactions sustained by anxiety. In the first case, this assumes characteristics of inhibitory and conversional type, and in the second it assumes characteristics of short response latency or uncontrollable type, or a manifestation of an abnormal management of the response to environmental stressors. The internalizing and externalizing variants justify heterogeneous and overlapping manifestations within an abnormal connectivity disorders condition.

Specifically, in the ASD group, the internalizing component is supported by social anxiety, in which school and social phobia components are more prevalent than the obsessive component. In the TS group, the obsessive trait or reduced fluidity of thought and reduced tolerance of change that are typical of this condition penalize social empathy, thereby recovering social and school anxiety via another pathway. The presence of a significant difference in externalizing symptoms in the TS group may be a consequence of the percentage of patients that present a major component in overlap with ADHD, where the impulsive component prevails over the obsessive component [51].

The results of our study were consistent with those of other works, especially in that the average scores on the CBCL "anxiety problems" subscale were higher in the ASD and TS groups [48]. Furthermore, the average score related to "internalizing problems" was higher in the ASD group, and the average score related to "externalizing problems" was higher in the ADHD group [49, 52]. Comparisons between our analysis of "anxiety/depression" and "anxiety problems" subscale scores (with the three ACSD-related disorders as the reference) and other works are limited, as most of the previous studies considered only two of the three groups we examined (e.g., ASD and TS, or ASD and ADHD). Furthermore, anxiety problems in some previous studies were evaluated using different scales [49].

An important element of our study was the presence of high comorbidity; that is, those conditions in which ASD was associated with other neurodevelopmental disorders [53]. Approximately 30–50% of patients with ASD also show typical ADHD symptoms; conversely, 66% of patients with ADHD show characteristics of the Autism Spectrum [9]. The addition of two or more neurodevelopmental disorders may also significantly enhance the phenomenological expression of the underlying disorder, especially in the condition of a simultaneous presence of "anxiety disorder" + "comorbidity of neurodevelopmental disorder" + "mood disorder" (Figs. 9.5 and 9.6).

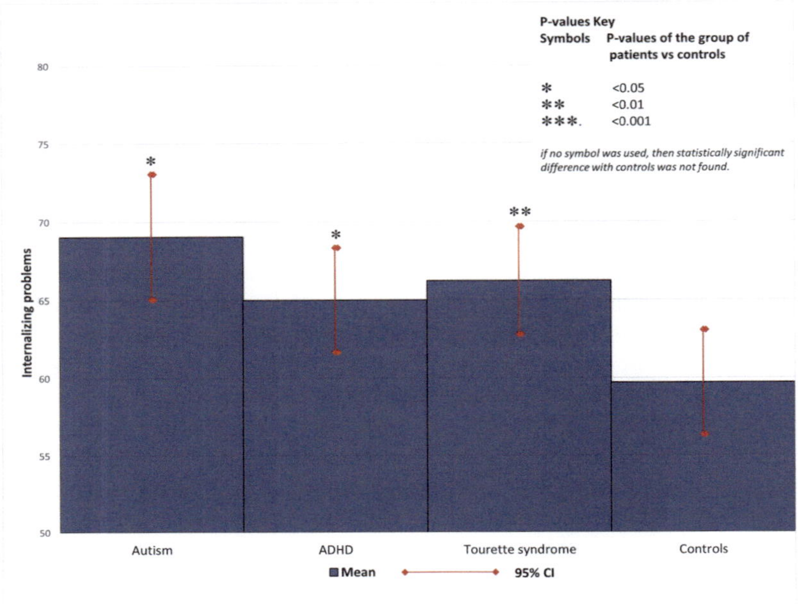

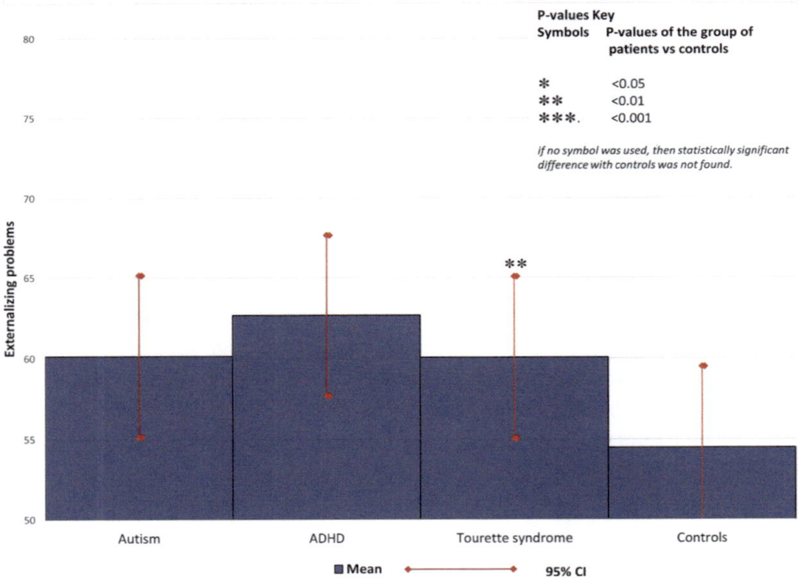

Figs. 9.5 and 9.6 [In these Figures, "Autism" means level 1 Autism]: The values on the y-axis indicate the range of the T points within which the median of the scores obtained by the different reference samples fall in relation to the areas (anxiety/depression) or macro-areas (internalizing, externalizing) considered. Up to 65 T points the score is considered standard, a score from 65 to 70 is considered borderline, and scores of 70 and above are considered clinically significant. Such scores may indicate specific problems in each area and provide indications on different syndromic frameworks. Sex-adjusted means and 95% confidence intervals for each group

9.9 Criticism and Limitations of This Study

In our observational study, we found significantly higher levels of anxiety in the continuous group of neurodevelopmental disorders than in the control group. In addition, we observed some subtle differences between the different disorders. For example, the ASD group showed a significantly higher level of anxiety problems than the other groups. Regarding the form of presentation of symptoms, the groups of children with ASD and TS showed a higher level of internalizing symptoms. Those with ADHD also had a slightly higher level of internalizing symptoms than the control group, but lower than the ASD and TS groups. The TS group showed the highest prevalence of externalizing symptoms, with the ASD and ADHD groups having slightly lower levels. All three groups had a higher prevalence of externalizing symptoms than the control group, which was consistent with previous investigations.

A limitation of our study was that we considered the three diagnostic groups without identifying subdivisions between the pure conditions and comorbidities. The initial aim of our study was to consider overlapping conditions, based on the new definition of ACSD. However, from a diagnostic perspective, the current criteria satisfied the purposes of the definition and inclusion of subjects in the specific diagnostic frameworks. Another limitation was the use of structured interviews completed by parents rather than by patients themselves. A strength of this study was the specific definition of the priority clinical picture, despite the known levels of comorbidities. In particular, in the ASD group, we only selected patients who required low level of support (defined as level 1 according to the DSM-5) to obtain homogeneous samples for language and cognitive profiles.

Another limitation of this study was the number of participants. It is necessary to collect information from larger groups so that the trends are clearer and provide more useful information to determine appropriate support mechanisms for each case. However, only a small number of females were recruited in our study, partly because of the difficulty in early diagnosis in females. Many females with ASD receive a late diagnosis, making it difficult to include them in the studies of children and adolescents. A better system for the early detection of neurodiversity in females is recommended, especially during school age.

The identification of anxiety disorders in different diagnostic groups with the same cognitive and neurofunctional profile, as implemented in this study, allows us to observe how much the anxiety disorder itself, even in people with ASD, represents a condition that stands out and overlaps with the basic symptomatological core. Treatment for the anxiety disorder may also reduce the severity of the general picture, thus allowing a the individual to experience a better quality of life.

9.10 Therapeutic Perspectives

The treatment of anxiety disorders in ASD includes individualized approaches to cognitive-behavioral and pharmacological therapy [54]. Careful clinical observation with a multi-dimensional survey is required to provide a global reading of dysfunctional behaviors and obtain the best therapeutic results. Currently, there are several tests that can be administered to parents, and extended to operators who work daily with the child. Although several questionnaires are used to detect anxiety disorders in people with ASD, few have been specifically defined for the Autism Spectrum [55].

Numerous studies have shown positive results with cognitive-behavioral therapy (CBT) [55–57]. In CBT, removal of anxiety stimuli and phobias is planned, taking care not to reinforce previous avoidance behaviors. A second phase is then scheduled where the patient is gradually exposed to feared stimuli and contexts, so that rituals or avoidance behaviors can be disfavored. CBT has shown particularly encouraging results in developing adaptive and spontaneous strategies for anxiety symptoms [56]. For anxiety management, three essential modalities are usually adopted: a psycho-educational approach, a cognitive approach, and an anxiety stimuli and phobic thoughts hierarchy approach.

The psycho-educational approach aims to make the patients more informed about the nature of their anxiety disorder, allowing them to obtain gradual and progressive adherence to the proposed therapeutic program. The cognitive approach favors restructuring thoughts, so that the patients can question their own fears and concerns. The third approach starts with the classification and hierarchization of phobic sources based on their anxiogenic properties, followed by gradual and repeated exposure of the patients to these sources to obtain spontaneous and natural reduction of anxiety symptoms. Better results are achieved in CBT when different protagonists are involved, for example, parents, educators, teachers, and other operators who are in close contact with the child with ASD. To achieve a more precise and stable clinical impact on the anxiety disorder over time, the program must be jointly established by a multidisciplinary team. In this way, control and reduction of anxiety can be obtained, promoting greater flexibility with regard to social dynamics. CBT results in an improvement of interactions and finding a modulation more in keeping with the frustrations and unexpected events imposed by daily life and usual conversations [56].

A meta-analysis by Ung et al. [55] also reported positive results of CBT, suggesting that future research on CBT should consider the differences between specific anxiety disorders in individuals with ASD and different pharmacological treatments in individual cases. In a review of patients treated with CBT, Warwick et al. [56] found percentages of positive responses up to 60% and showed that, in many cases, there was inconsistent discussion of the results obtained and questionable comparisons between the different studies. Those authors identified how results were sometimes reported separately based on the individual anxiety disorder and sometimes presented on the basis of anxiety disorders considered as part of a diagnostic group. Apparent differences or similarities in the results obtained can be derived from difficulties in comparing data sets [57]. Although in a majority of cases the responses to CBT were positive, the nature of this therapy requires a medium-long implementation time. In the presence of symptoms that are acute or need to be managed in the medium term, it may still be necessary to resort to traditional psychopharmacological treatments.

Drugs belonging to the selective serotonin reuptake inhibitor or serotonin-norepinephrine reuptake inhibitor categories are at the forefront of psycho-pharmacological treatment for anxiety disorders. These drugs have proven efficacy for symptoms related to anxiety that cause functional impairment. These drugs have few secondary effects and are free of cardiotoxicity. As second-line drugs, benzodiazepines may be used in specific situations and are especially useful for treating acute GAD and depression-associated forms. The use of drugs from other categories (e.g., antipsychotics, beta-blockers) is rarely considered because of adverse effects on behavior. However, individual responses to these drugs should be carefully monitored by a specialized doctor, so that contraindications or side effects can be identified [56]. Common side effects are sleep abnormalities, anxious paradoxical reactions, or uncontrolled increases in appetite and body weight. Appropriate initial psycho-pharmacological treatment may allow more adequate participation in CBT programs or other possible therapeutic approaches for anxiety disorders in ASD.

9.11 Conclusion

Anxiety disorders affect a significant percentage of the ASD population, presenting predominant characteristics according to the levels of impairment reported by the DSM-5. An "anxiety" symptom, in relation to its gradient, could also represent a transient or reactive condition of the ASD framework or assume an increasingly specific connotation to the point of constituting a comorbid anxiety disorder. Comorbid anxiety disorders have been identified as social anxiety, anxiety with specific phobias or panic attacks, or anxiety with obsessive-compulsive or repetitive-ritualistic traits. The presence of a comorbid anxiety disorder affects the individual's clinical evolution.

It is important that the assessment process for people with ASD uses standardized tools that are shared by the scientific community and precociously recognizes the presence of comorbidity. The identification and management of these problems during the developmental stage could reduce the risk for developing chronicity in adulthood. Containment of the disabling effects of these conditions on individual life paths could eventually allow a better quality of life for individuals with ASD.

Considering the different clinical dimensions (e.g., level of impairment, type of anxiety disorder, presence of comorbidity, degree of empathy, and correlated capacity for emotional management), anxiety in people with ASD tends to show specific behavioral manifestations toward internalizing rather than externalizing problems. In level 1 Autism cases, it is more frequent to find worries and feelings of inadequacy, which are accentuated in social contexts.

Finally, the presence of overlap in ASD with other neurodevelopmental disorders, in addition to characterizing different phenotypic expressions, may sustain or accentuate the anxiety itself, justifying a more complete perspective, according to an ACSD model (Fig. 9.7).

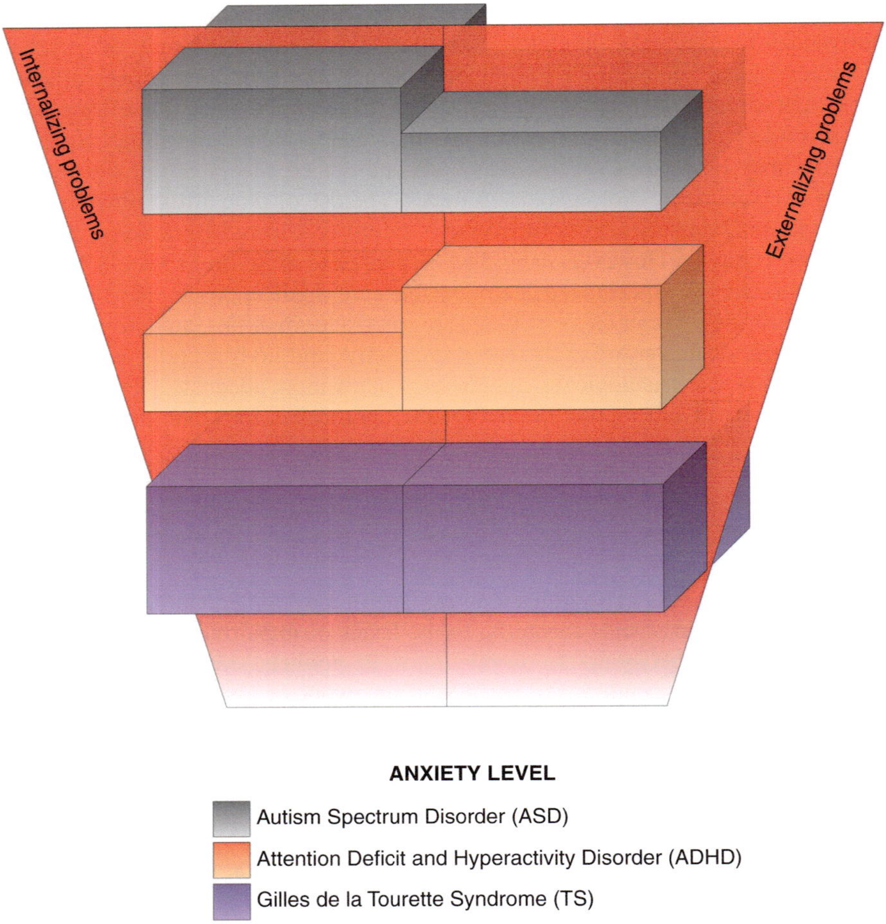

Fig. 9.7 Level of anxiety and predominance of internalizing/externalizing problems in relation to the disorders currently included in abnormal connectivity spectrum disorder (ACSD). Sizes and heights of the figures are not related to any data and are purely explanatory of level and predominance

Acknowledgments We thank the staff at Edanz Group (www.edanzediting.com/ac) for critically reviewing a draft of this manuscript.

References

1. American Psychiatric Association. Manuale diagnostico e statistico dei disturbi mentali DSM-V. Milano: Raffaello Cortina Editore; 2014.
2. Maddox B, White S. Comorbid social anxiety disorder in adults with autism spectrum disorder. J Autism Dev Disord. 2015;45(12):3949–60.

3. Sharma S, Gonda X, Tarazi F. Autism spectrum disorder: classification, diagnosis and therapy. Pharmacol Ther. 2018;190:91–104.
4. Gillott A, Furniss F, Walter A. Anxiety in high-functioning children with autism. Autism. 2001;5(3):277–86.
5. La Buissonière-Ariza V, et al. Presentation and correlates of hoarding behaviors in children with autism spectrum disorders and comorbid anxiety or obsessive-compulsive symptoms. J Autism Dev Disord. 2018;48(12):4167–78. Springer.
6. Van Steensel FJA, Bögels SM, Perrin S. Anxiety disorders in children and adolescents with autistic spectrum disorders: a meta-analysis. Clin Child Fam Psychol Rev. 2011;14:302–17.
7. Little L. Middle-class mothers' perceptions of peer and sibling victimization among children with Asperger's syndrome and nonverbal learning disorders. Issues Compr Pediatr Nurs. 2002;25:43–57.
8. White SW, et al. Anxiety in children and adolescents with autism spectrum disorders. Clin Psychol Rev. 2009;29:216–29.
9. Kim JA, et al. The prevalence of anxiety and mood problems among children with autism and Asperger syndrome. Autism. 2000;4(2):117–32.
10. Factor R, et al. Does the presence of anxiety and ADHD symptoms add to social impairment in children with autism spectrum disorder? J Autism Dev Disord. 2017;47(4):1122–34. New York: Springer.
11. Ronald A, Happe F, Plomin R. The genetic relationship between individual differences in social and nonsocial behaviours characteristic of autism. Dev Sci. 2005;8(5):444–58.
12. Geschwind DH. Genetics of autism spectrum disorders. Trends Cogn Sci. 2011;15(9):409–16.
13. Klei L, Sanders SJ, Murtha MT, Hus I. Common genetic variants acting additively are a major source of risk for autism. Mol Autism. 2012;3(1):9. https://doi.org/10.1186/2040-2392-3-9.
14. Morrow EM, Yoo SY, Flavell SW, Kim TK. Identifying autism loci and genes by tracing recent shared ancestry. Science. 2008;321(5886):218–23.
15. Jablonka E, Lamb MJ. The inheritance of acquired epigenetic variations. Int J Epidemiol. 2015;44(4):1094–103.
16. Berg JM, Geschwind DH. Autism genetics, searching for specificity and convergence. Genome Biol. 2012;13(7):247. https://doi.org/10.1186/gb4034.
17. Smoller J. The genetics of stress-related disorders: PTSD, depression, and anxiety disorders. Neuropsychopharmacol Rev. 2016;41:297–319.
18. Shimada-Sugimoto M, Otowa T, Hettema J. Genetic epidemiological and molecular studies in humans. Psychiatry Clin Neurosci. 2015;69:388–401.
19. Muhle R, et al. The emerging clinical neuroscience of autism spectrum disorder: a review. JAMA Psychiatry. 2018;75(5):514–23.
20. Patterson E, Anckarsater H, et al. Different neurodevelopmental symptoms have a common genetic etiology. J Child Psychol Psychiatry. 2013;54:1356–65.
21. Pennington B. From single to multiple deficit models of developmental disorder. Cognition. 2006;101:385–413.
22. Rutter M, Silberg J. Gene-environment interplay in relation to emotional and behavioural disturbances. Annu Rev Psychol. 2002;53:463–90.
23. Silberman S. Neurotribes: the legacy of autism and how to think smarter about people who think differently. London: Allen & Unwin; 2015.
24. Eapen V, Crnčec R, Walter A. Exploring links between genotypes, phenotypes and clinical predictors of response to Early Intensive Behavioral Intervention in Autism Spectrum Disorder. Front Hum Neurosci. 2013;7:567.
25. Murdoch JD, State MW. Recent developments in the genetics of Autism Spectrum Disorders. Curr Opin Genet Dev. 2013;23(3):310–5.
26. Juranek J, et al. Association between amygdala volume and anxiety level: magnetic resonance imaging (MRI) study in autistic children. J Child Neurol. 2006;21(12):1051–8.
27. Cauda F, Keller R, et al. Grey matter abnormality in autism spectrum disorder: an activation likelihood estimation meta-analysis study. J Neurol Neurosurg Psychiatry. 2011;82(12): 1304–13.

28. Shen M, et al. Extra-axial cerebrospinal fluid in high-risk and normal-risk children with autism aged 2-4 years: a case-control study. Lancet Psychiatry. 2018;5(11):895–904. Elsevier.
29. Baeza-Velasco C, et al. Joint hypermobility and the heritable disorders of connective tissue: clinical and empirical evidence of links with psychiatry. Gen Hosp Psychiatry. 2015;37(1):24–30. https://doi.org/10.1016/j.genhosppsych.2014.10.002.
30. Smith T, et al. Do people with benign joint hypermobility syndrome (BJHS) have reduced joint proprioception? A systematic review and meta-analysis. Rheumatol Int. 2013;33(11):2709–16.
31. Kaur M, Srinivasan S, Bhat A. Comparing motor performance, praxis, coordination, and interpersonal synchrony between children with and without Autism Spectrum Disorder (ASD). Res Dev Disabil. 2018;72:79–95.
32. Bellini S. Social skill deficits and anxiety in high-functioning adolescents with autism spectrum disorders. Focus Autism Other Dev Disabil. 2004;19(2):78–86.
33. Lai MC, Lombardo MV, Baron-Cohen S. Autism. Lancet. 2014;383(9920):896–910.
34. Loomes R, Hull L, Mandy WPL. What is the male-to-female ratio in autism spectrum disorder? A systematic review and meta-analysis. J Am Acad Child Adolesc Psychiatry. 2017;56(6):466–74.
35. Ryland HK, Hysing M, Posserud MB. Autistic features in school age children, IQ and gender effects in a population-based cohort. Res Autism Spectr Disord. 2014;8(3):266–74.
36. Hollocks MJ, Jones CRG, Pickles A, Baird G, et al. The association between social cognition and executive functioning and symptoms of anxiety and depression in adolescent with Autism Spectrum Disorders. Autism Res. 2014;7(2):216–28.
37. Davis T III, Ollendick T. Fear: autism spectrum disorder and/or specific phobia. In: Davis III T, White S, Ollendick T, editors. Handbook of autism and anxiety. Autism and Child Psychopathology Series. Cham: Springer; 2014.
38. Kern J, et al. Shared brain connectivity issues, symptoms and comorbidities in autism spectrum disorder, attention deficit/hyperactivity disorder, and Tourette syndrome. Brain Connect. 2015;5(6):321–35.
39. Mayes SD, et al. Disruptive mood dysregulation disorder (DMDD) symptoms in children with a, and neurotypical development and impact of co-occurring ODD, depression, and anxiety. Res Autism Spectr Disord. 2015;18:64–72.
40. Palumbo D, Maughan A, Kurlan R. Tourette syndrome is only one of several causes of a developmental basal ganglia syndrome. Arch Neurol. 1997;54:475–83.
41. Lenroot RK, Yeung PK. Heterogeneity within a Autism Spectrum Disorders, what have we learned from neuroimaging studies. Front Hum Neurosci. 2013;7:733.
42. Kana RK, Libero LE, Moore HS. Disrupted cortical connectivity theory as an explanatory model for autism spectrum disorders. Phys Life Rev. 2011;8(4):410–37.
43. Vissers ME, Cohen MX, Geurts HM. Brain Connectivity and high functioning autism, a promising path of research that needs refined models methodological convergence and stronger behavioural links. Neurosci Biobehav Rev. 2012;36(1):604–25.
44. Paolelli E. Il concetto di Psiche e Psichiatria in medicina funzionale. M.F. medicina funzionale. 2000;3:18–22.
45. Mannion A, Leader G. Comorbidity in autism spectrum disorder: a literature review. Res Autism Spectr Disord. 2013;7(12):1595–616.
46. Middleton E, et al., editors. Allergy: principles and practice. 4th ed. St Louis: Mosby; 1993.
47. Cath DC, et al. Symptom overlap between autism spectrum disorder, generalized social anxiety disorder and obsessive-compulsive disorder in adults: a preliminary case-controlled study. Psychopathology. 2008;41:101–10.
48. Whitney D, et al. The contribution of neurologic disorders to the national prevalence of depression and anxiety problems among children and adolescents. Ann Epidemiol. 2018;29:81–4.
49. van Steensel FJA, Bögels SM, de Bruin EI. Psychiatric comorbidity in children with autism spectrum disorders: a comparison with children with ADHD. J Child Fam Stud. 2013;22:368.
50. Achenbach TM, Rescorla LA. Manual for the ASEBA school-age forms & profiles. Burlington: University of Vermont, Research Center for Children, Youth, & Families; 2001.

51. Gillberg C, et al. Co-existing disorders in ADHD—implications for diagnosis and intervention. Eur Child Adolesc Psychiatry. 2004;13(Suppl 1):80–92.
52. Gadow KD, et al. Comparative study of children with ADHD only, autism spectrum disorder + ADHD, and chronic multiple tic disorder + ADHD. J Atten Disord. 2009;12:474–85.
53. Wood JJ, Gadow KD. Exploring the nature and function of anxiety in youth with autism spectrum disorders. Clin Psychol Res Pract. 2010;17:281–92.
54. Hagopian L, Jennett H. Behavioral assessment and treatment for anxiety for those with autism spectrum disorder. In: Davis III T, White S, Ollendick T, editors. Handbook of autism and anxiety. Autism and Child Psychopathology Series. Cham: Springer; 2014.
55. Ung D, et al. A systematic review and meta-analysis of cognitive behavioral therapy for anxiety in youth with high-functioning autism spectrum disorders. Child Psychiatry Hum Dev. 2014;46(4):533–47.
56. Warwick H, et al. Complete recovery from anxiety disorders following Cognitive Behavior Therapy in children and adolescents: a meta-analysis. Clin Psychol Rev. 2016;52(2017):77–91.
57. Stern T, et al. Psychopharmacology and neurotherapeutics. Massachusetts General Hospital. New York: Elsevier; 2016.

Personality Disorders and ASD

10

Francesca De Cagna, Edoardo Squillari, Matteo Rocchetti, and Laura Fusar-Poli

10.1 What Is Personality?

There are many definitions of personality, depending on the theoretical approaches. Millon [1] conceived personalities as varieties of successful and failed efforts in attempting to balance three essential bipolarities that comprise the goals of life: existential survival (avoiding death/pain and enhancing life/pleasure), ecological adaptation (environmental accommodation/passive and environmental modification/active), and species replication (maximizing reproduction/self and nurturing progeny/others). Roberts [2] defined personality traits as the relatively enduring patterns of thoughts, feelings, and behaviors that reflect the tendency to respond in certain ways under certain circumstances. In 1993, a model of the development of normal and deviant personality as a dynamic self-organizing system modeled on family and socio-cultural influences was formulated. According to the authors' perspective, personality can be defined as the dynamic organization, within an individual, of the psychobiological systems that modulate adaptation to a changing environment. They developed a test for personality assessment called "Temperament and Character Inventory" (TCI), a self-report tool that deconstructs personality in seven dimensions of temperament and character [3].

Temperament refers to those aspects of an individual's personality that are often regarded as the result of biological evolution, initially constitutionally based rather than learned [4]. Even though there are many definitions of character, it has been theorized as less heritable, later developing, influenced by processes of maturation, and representing individual differences in self-object relationships [5].

F. De Cagna · E. Squillari · M. Rocchetti
Department of Brain and Behavioral Sciences, University of Pavia, Pavia, Italy

L. Fusar-Poli (✉)
Department of Clinical and Experimental Medicine, Section of Psychiatry, University of Catania, Catania, Italy

R. Keller (ed.), *Psychopathology in Adolescents and Adults with Autism Spectrum Disorders*, https://doi.org/10.1007/978-3-030-26276-1_10

Psychoanalytic theorists focused on the importance of early childhood experiences and their influence on the development of "character styles" and disorders of adaptation. In the psychogenetic hypothesis, early events determine the formation of defensive systems that may remain in adult life conditioning the reactions of the individual to new situations as if they were the same events occurred in childhood [6].

10.2 Personality Traits in Individuals with Autism Spectrum Disorder

Personality, temperament, and character are of course present in all people, including those with autism spectrum disorder (ASD). Findings about temperament, character, and broad personality traits among autistic population are, not surprisingly, consistent with the heterogeneous clinical picture of ASD. In fact, there might be a genetic effect behind the phenotypic covariation between neurodevelopmental disorders and personality [7]. Nevertheless, separating clinical features of ASD which are largely neurobiologically derived and early onset in childhood from possible overlapping pathological personality traits is important both for nosographic clarity and for clinical usefulness. Distinguishing personality disorders (PD) from abnormal personality trait patterns assumes also a relevant meaning in ASD-correlated personality evaluation.

Kraepelin defined the "*autistic temperament*" as a pre-psychotic state that could evolve in dementia praecox. In Kraepelin's observation children of this temperament "*frequently exhibited a quiet, shy, retiring disposition, made no friendship, and lived only for themselves.*" They were disinclined to be open or to become involved with others, were reclusive, and had difficulty adapting to new situations. They showed little interest in what went about them, often refrained from participating in games and other pleasures, seemed resistant to influence, and were inclined to withdraw increasingly in a world of their own fantasies [8].

Using the TCI, several studies correlated ASD positively with harm avoidance, negatively with sociability, novelty seeking, reward dependence, self-directedness, and cooperativeness both in adults and children [7, 9, 10]. According to these studies, ASD-specific social and communication impairments correspond with low reward dependence (temperament), less extraversion and agreeableness (five-factor model traits), schizoid and avoiding traits. A recent meta-analysis of Big Five personality traits in ASD [11] indicates that ASD is associated with lower openness, conscientiousness, extraversion, agreeableness, and emotional stability. Many studies examining the relationship of personality traits to ASD had as primary purpose the facilitation of diagnosis and identification of individuals with ASD. However, Big Five traits showed heterogeneous presentation in ASD and in our opinion clinicians should carefully consider the theoretical framework in which the construct was originally theorized. For these reasons we do not recommend the use of this approach for ASD diagnosis per se. It is our opinion that personality trait measurement should be considered as a potential resource to enhance rather than replace traditional diagnostic tools.

Almost all researches about personality in the autistic spectrum include high-functioning autistic individuals, although rarely in these studies intelligence quotient (IQ) is specified. In part, this could be explained by the difficulty of describing personality in subjects with intellectual disability (ID). In general, people with ID experience more failure, rejection, and social deprivation leading to personality traits that may further impede their ability to learn [12]. Individuals with ID might also have more rigid or extreme personality traits, such as particularly high or low expectations for success, a more limited range of skills and solutions to negotiate difficult situations and difficulties with problem-solving or cognitive flexibility [13, 14].

10.3 A Definition of Personality Disorders

As reported above, the term "personality" refers to the relatively constant pattern of thinking, feeling and relating to reality of a person: it represents the individual's peculiar way to adapt to intrapsychic and environmental reality, having the potential to strongly impact the subject's well-being. A pervasive, stiff and maladaptive pattern of cognitive, emotional, and behavioral responses is what is called a personality disorder (PD). These patterns develop early, typically in adolescence, becoming during the life course a rigid way to feel, think, or act to interpersonal and social experiences, causing significant distress and disability. The Diagnostic and Statistical Manual for mental disorder (DSM-5) [15] lists ten different types of personality disorders: paranoid, schizoid, schizotypal, antisocial, borderline, histrionic, narcissistic, avoidant, dependent, and obsessive-compulsive personality disorder. The DSM-5 now classifies these conditions in the same way as other mental diseases, rather than on a different axis, as in the previous editions of the manual [16]. A second change occurred in the last version of DSM is that PD are considered both from a categorial and a dimensional point of view, in two different sections. A consequence of adopting a hybrid categorial-dimensional classification is to consider PD less as discrete entities sharply separated from normal personality and more as a maladaptive extension of the same traits that describe a healthy personality. The introduction of an "Alternative DSM-5 Model for Personality Disorder" in Section III of the latest DSM version explains, on one hand, the person's degree of functioning impairment, considered both as a general quality of life reduction and as impairment of a specific personality domain (identity, self-direction, empathy, and intimacy) [15]. On the other hand, the Alternative Model offers a dimensional description of personality traits, derived from the five-factor model of personality, which can be assessed with several psychometric tests. The five broad trait domains are: negative affectivity (vs. emotional stability), detachment (vs. extraversion), antagonism (vs. agreeableness), disinhibition (vs. conscientiousness), psychoticism (vs. lucidity).

Including functioning and personality traits in PD diagnosis implies that an abnormal personality trait pattern alone doesn't constitute a personality disorder by itself. Rather, the relationship between personality and social context and the ability to adapt to environmental demands are considered, from a dimensional point of view, factors determining a personality disorder.

10.4 ASD and Personality Disorders as a Clinical Conundrum

In general, considering the relationship between ASD and personality disorders implies to clarify the nature of a certain personality trait in the context of an autistic person's functioning. More precisely, we can summarize three situations:

1. A certain abnormal personality trait can be considered as (or derives directly from) a typical clinical feature of ASD (no personality disorder).
2. A certain personological pattern reminds both an ASD clinical manifestation and a certain personality disorder in neurotypical people (differential diagnosis between ASD and PD).
3. Pathological personality traits develop during life as consequence of a complex interaction of multiple factors: person's temperament, early environmental response to his/her temperament, past and present life experiences, social demands, etc. Resulting cognitive, affective, or behavioral symptoms are a source of further distress and disability and are not a direct manifestation of the autistic symptomatology (comorbidity ASD-PD).

In the next paragraphs, we will focus on differential diagnosis, clinical features in common between autism and certain types of personality disorder and the feature of comorbid PD and ASD.

The diagnosis of personality disorder (PD) in the lowest-functioning part of the spectrum is particularly controversial. In fact, some clinicians are convinced that it is not possible to make a diagnosis of PD in individuals with ID, given the severity of the comorbid mental health problems [17]. Other authors suggest that individuals with ID are more vulnerable to PD and that more efforts are needed to meet the necessities of this population [13, 18]. In recognition of the limitations of the standard diagnostic systems (i.e., DSM and ICD), two alternative classification systems have been developed:

- Diagnostic Criteria for Learning Disability (DC-LD) [19],
- The Diagnostic Manual for ID (DM-ID) [20].

Considerable problems regarding PD in ID are: the absence of a sufficiently developed personality in individuals with severe or profound ID; the difficulty in making a diagnosis prior to the age of 21 because of immaturity and delayed personality development; diagnosis should be provisional as a change of environment may lead to consequent change in behavior and attitudes; diagnosis of schizoid, dependent and anxious/avoidant PD is not recommended in DC-LD and DM-ID recommends they should only be diagnosed with care when traits are extreme [13]. Bertelli et al. [21] proposed the SPAID (Psychiatric Instrument for the Intellectually Disabled Adult) as a potential useful scale for the diagnosis of comorbid psychopathological conditions, including PD, in people with ID.

10.5 ASD and Personality Disorders: From Differential Diagnosis to Comorbidity

Several psychiatric disorders are often mistaken for ASD in adults. Differential diagnosis is particularly challenging for psychiatrists who did not receive a specific training on psychopathology in adults with neurodevelopmental disorders [22]. A comprehensive evaluation performed by professionals with expertise in ASD is thus essential in making a differential diagnosis [23, 24].

Many PD, particularly those belonging to cluster A or C of DSM-IV-TR [16], share several features with ASD. As for psychotic disorders, a determination of the onset is critical, since personality disorders usually become evident at least since adolescence or early adulthood and they are usually not diagnosed before the age of 18 years. On the contrary ASD must be present in early development, although sometimes not recognized until adulthood [23, 25]. Moreover, it should be excluded that a PD is a manifestation or consequence of any other mental disorder (criterion E of PD diagnosis in accordance with DSM-5), in this case a manifestation or consequence of ASD. Similar to PD, ASD becomes most evident in social contexts and usually involves multiple areas of life, such as employment and relationships [26]. Furthermore, both ASD and PD patients often perceive their symptoms as highly ego-syntonic compared to patients with other psychiatric disorders. Therefore, it is difficult to make a differential diagnosis.

It is worth mentioning that more than 70% of individuals with ASD have concurrent medical, developmental, or psychiatric conditions. The high frequency of comorbidity could be a result of shared pathophysiology, secondary effects of growing up with autism, shared symptom domains and associated mechanisms, or overlapping diagnostic criteria [27]. Few studies analyzed the prevalence of PD in ASD, and all of these considered a sample of high-functioning autistic subjects. A recent meta-analysis estimated the prevalence of PD in adults with ASD around 12.6%, while the prevalence increased to 20.6% when researchers included only studies based on clinical interviews [28]. In their study Lugnegard et al. [29] suggested that approximately 50% of adults with ASD fulfilled criteria for a PD. Looking at patients with Asperger Syndrome, Hofvander et al. [30] found that 68% met DSM-IV criteria for at least one PD and according to Anckarsater et al. [31] 75% of the 174 subjects for whom the SCID-II was completed met criteria for at least one personality disorder, and 46% fulfilled criteria for more than one category of personality disorder.

10.5.1 ASD and Cluster A Personality Disorders

Personality disorders (PD) can be classified into three clusters of patterns of thinking and behavior. Cluster A personality disorders are characterized by odd, eccentric thinking or behavior, including schizoid, schizotypal, and paranoid personality disorders [15]. Schizoid and schizotypal personality disorders are characterized by long-standing patterns of detachment from social relationships and social anxiety. Although the impairment of social and interpersonal competences occurs in both disorders, each disorder has their own characteristic symptoms.

Symptoms of schizotypal personality disorder can include severe social anxiety, thought disorder, paranoid ideation, derealization, transient psychotic symptoms, and often unconventional beliefs (paranormal and superstitious beliefs are common). The DSM-5 defines the schizotypal personality disorder as a "*pervasive pattern of social and interpersonal deficits marked by acute discomfort with, and reduced capacity for, close relationships as well as by cognitive or perceptual distortions and eccentricities of behavior, beginning by early adulthood and present in a variety of contexts.*" Diagnostic criteria include thought and perception disorders (ideas of reference, strange beliefs or magical thinking, paranoia, abnormal perceptions), behavioral oddness (strange thinking and speech, strange behavior or appearance), and social and interpersonal impairment (inappropriate or constricted affect, lack of close friends, excessive social anxiety). Exclusion criterion is the co-occurring diagnosis of schizophrenia or ASD [15].

Symptoms of schizoid personality disorder include a high preference of conducting a solitary sheltered lifestyle, lack of understanding of social cues, an apparent little desire for intimate relations or sexual relationships, apathy and lack of motivation in everyday activities. Diagnostic features include pervasive mood/affect abnormalities (lack of pleasure in most/all activities, emotional coldness, detachment or flattened affectivity) and social-relational impairment (poor interest in close relationship, tendency to solitary life, indifference toward others' praise or criticism, lack of interest in sexual experiences) [15].

Still controversial is the linkage between those two conditions and schizophrenia: some experts suggest that schizotypal personality disorder might be a mild form of schizophrenia, whereas other researchers argue that the two conditions strongly differentiate from each other from clinical, genetic, and neuropathological point of view [32]. The concepts of autism and schizophrenia have common roots. Bleuler defined autism as a detachment from reality associated with rich fantasy life [33]. He considered autism as a pathognomonic feature of the whole schizophrenia spectrum, including the schizoid and "*latent*" cases. He described a wide set of clinical manifestations of autism: poor ability to get in touch with others, withdrawal, inaccessibility (even negativism), indifference, rigid attitudes and behaviors, deranged hierarchy of values and goals, inappropriate behavior, idiosyncratic logic, and a propensity to delusional thinking [34]. This first effort to describe the autistic phenomenon was focused mainly on observable "*external*" behaviors or signs, rather than on patients' inner life. A deeper phenomenological investigation of the autistic feature was conducted by Minkowski [35]*:* he considered mental states as an expression of the more basic experiential and existential alterations (for example, changes in temporalization or in the relatedness to the world). He named those primary changes at the base of pathological mental states "*troubles générateur*" (generative disorder), considering autism to be the generative disorder of schizophrenia [36]. In his description, autism is not simply a withdrawal to solitude or an attitude to daydreaming, but a deficit in the basic attunement between the person and his world, i.e., a lack of *"vital contact with reality"* [37]. Minkowski defined the vital contact as the capacity of "resonating with the world" and empathizing with others. In this perspective, autistic attitudes are either direct manifestations of the lack of vital contact or compensating personality traits: they comprise "*morbid rationalism*" (viewing all human moves as driven by purely logical rules), excessive preoccupations with symmetry and numerical aspects of the world ("*geometrism*"), excessive fantasy life, and peculiarly lifeless patterns of stereotyped regrets or moodiness [37]. As previously said, those first descriptions of the autistic phenomenon were referred to patients who are today classified within the schizophrenic spectrum rather than the autistic spectrum. Nevertheless, several phenomenological and clinical features seem to belong to both categories.

Within the current research on ASD, several studies focused on delimiting difference and overlays between ASD and schizophrenia spectrum. In particular, the comparison between the milder manifestations of both continuums (i.e., schizoid and schizotypal personality and high-functioning ASD) shows a partial clinical overlapping and often represents a further diagnostic challenge.

Indeed, both spectra involve altered and impaired social and communicative functioning [38, 39], which has suggested to some authors that ASD and schizotypy spectrum conditions overlap in their etiologies [40, 41]. On the other hand, shared clinical features often have different diagnostic relevance in the two conditions. For example, impairments in social reciprocity, communication, and behavioral flexibility are more central features of the autism spectrum than they are of schizoid-schizotypic personalities.

A common approach to addressing the relationship between ASD and schizotypy spectrum conditions has been the compared analysis of the psychometric questionnaires currently used to assess both conditions, collected from clinical or nonclinical populations. Most of the studies focused on cognitive and behavioral features, most notably in the realm of social dysfunction: in fact, if the presence of positive symptoms (i.e., hallucinations, paranoia, thought disorder, referential thinking, or delusions) constitutes a significative criterion for differential diagnosis, indeed it could be a feature of schizotypy, but not classically related to autism [42]; negative symptoms, like social withdrawal, flattened affect, apathy and alogia, tend to co-occur in both spectra [43] and appear most directly related to social and communication deficits.

Trying to summarize the current hypotheses on the relationship between autism and schizotypy at both etiological and phenotypic level, three different models could be identified [44]:

1. Under the "independence model," autism and schizoid-schizotypic personality disorders are distinct conditions which do not share common etiology and differ in many clinical and phenomenological aspects. In support of this hypothesis, there is the evidence of different developmental trajectories and age of onset of the two conditions. Moreover, the lack of evidence for an increased prevalence of schizophrenia in autistic populations [45], and, in reverse, the evidence of a strongest linkage between schizotypy and schizophrenia, have shaped the view that the etiologies underlying the two disorders are independent [46].
2. Conversely, the "*overlapping model*" asserts that overlapping phenotypes between autism and schizotypy could reflect common etiologies. That hypothesis emerges from several neuropsychological and psychometric evidences: both spectra are characterized by reduced performances across a range of social-cognitive abilities, including theory of mind and emotion recognition, as well as corresponding impairments in overall social functioning. Psychometric tools as the Autism-Spectrum Quotient (AQ) [47] and the Schizotypy Personality Questionnaire (SPQ) [48] showed, in different studies conducted on both clinical and nonclinical populations, a strong positive association between the two tests scores [41, 49, 50], especially between negative schizotypy and AQ social skills, and between disorganized schizotypy and AQ communication. According to this model, the authors interpreted these trait associations as indicating that autism and schizoid-schizotypy conditions may overlap on a single spectrum, rather than existing as two distinct nosologic entities as currently implied by DSM categories.
3. A third model places autism and schizotypy on opposite ends of an axis of social cognition. By this "diametric model" [44, 51], the phenotypes of autism spectrum develop around a core constituted by an under-developed social cognition, whereas positive schizotypal and schizophrenic spectrum phenotypes involve manifestations of over-developed social cognition, such as "hyper-developed" theory of mind in paranoid symptoms or an exaggerated sense of self and agency in referral or megalomanic delusions. Under the diametric model, social deficits and lack of interpersonal competences as assayed by psychometric data could manifest similarly (for example, as social withdrawal or disinterest), but such similarities may reflect highly diverse or diametrically different causes between ASD and schizotypy conditions. Some studies provide evidences in support of the model: after statistically removing the overlap between the AQ and the SPQ, which, as previously said, is mainly referred to the similarity between negative schizotypy and autistic-like interpersonal features, an autism-schizotypy phenotypic axis will emerge where autistic features negatively predict positive schizotypal [44, 52].

In conclusion, autism and schizoid and schizotypic personality disorders partially share their clinical manifestations, and a phenotypic overlap has been empirically highlighted, especially between the negative symptoms of schizoid-schizotypal PD and the social-communicative deficits that are central to autism. Generalized deficits, such as abnormal social functioning, comprise a broad range of mental disease and likely reflect a multitude of complex causal factors, such that phenotypic similarities inferred from psychometric and behavioral data are not sufficient to infer shared etiologies, sustaining the DSM-5 choice to keep these conditions separate. Moreover, recent research suggests that focusing on more constitutive factors, as social cognition and theory of mind, the two conditions tend to place at the two ends of an axis.

Unfortunately, we could not extensively discuss the linkage between ASD and paranoid personality disorder. Paranoid personality disorder is characterized by paranoia and a pervasive and generalized suspiciousness and mistrust of others. People with this PD habitually relate to the world by a vigilant scanning of the environment for clues or suggestions that may validate their suspects [15]. Given the deficit in social cognition and theory of mind of ASD individuals, subtle social clues might be difficult to interpret for them, thus provoking higher levels of paranoia [53]. Unfortunately, literature describing the overlapping symptomatology, as well as the possible co-occurrence, between ASD and paranoid personality disorder, another PD belonging to cluster A, is underrepresented.

However, according to the aforementioned observations, it is our opinion that the possible overlapping manifestation of cluster APD and ASD poses a complex conundrum regarding the possibility of actual comorbidity. This is especially true for those conditions in which a series of negative experiences with other people could bring to a paranoid style of thinking [54]. More practically, we highlighted the differences between these conditions, as from an accurate assessment different therapy approaches could be derived. For differential diagnosis purposes we suggest exploring the whole range of symptoms that could manifest in these conditions, and to carefully consider the subjective point of view, the insight and the personal perception of the behaviors. Finally, as always in ASD assessment, the developmental perspective could help in the differential diagnosis.

10.5.2 ASD and Cluster B Personality Disorders

Borderline personality disorder (BPD) is a frequent psychiatric disorder since it affects 10% of psychiatric out-patients and 20% of in-patients [55]. It is characterized mainly by marked instability in various areas of psychic life and behavior, including affect regulation, interpersonal relationships, impulse control, and self-image, often accompanied by self-harm and suicidal ideation [56]. It has been suggested a significant overlap between BPD and ASD, particularly for what concerns the highest-functioning side of the autism spectrum. ASD and BPD could share some behavioral manifestations: acting out instead of verbalizing emotions, especially through self-injurious behavior, the presence of intense relationships and superficial friendships, miscommunications associated with impairments in social functioning (especially incorrectly assumed intentions), and emotionally charged meltdowns. This potential overlap between the two disorders could be possibly related with similar—but not identical—neurocognitive functioning. In fact, neuropsychological studies targeting the recognition of emotions in faces and tone of voice have found that both subjects with ASD and BPD have similar difficulty in theory of mind and in accurate interpretation of emotions [57]. Dell'Osso et al. [58] showed that patients with BPD have higher autistic traits than healthy individuals. Moreover, higher levels of autistic traits were found to relate to a history of physical or sexual abuse and to lifetime suicidality among subjects suffering from BPD [58]. During the past ten years there has been a growing interest in mentalizing. Both in autism and in PD research, the term "mentalization" is referred to the implicit and explicit understanding of other persons' act as motivated by inner mental process such as beliefs, wishes, and fears [59, 60]. Clinical and empirical evidence suggests that there is a common ground in defect mentalizing skill both in PD and ASD [61, 62]. However, failure in mentalizing due to BPD is considered to be intermittent, often triggered by an emotional climate that the subject experienced as too intense. In ASD a low mentalizing skill is considered as one of the possible mechanisms underlying the interpersonal difficulties, but, in contrast to BPD, it appears more as a "trait condition," relatively stable in time and across situations, rather than a "state condition."

The co-occurrence of ASD and BPD is not rare. Rydén et al. [63] found that 15% of 41 female patients with BPD fulfilled diagnostic criteria for ASD. Noteworthy, the relevance of this comorbidity is supported by several clinical observations. Patients with comorbid BPD and ASD had significantly more frequent suicide attempts, more negative self-image, and lower global functioning. The association appears to be specific, as they did not seem to differ in number of comorbid axis I and II disorders with the exception of less common substance abuse [63]. Nanchen et al. [64] reported that almost half of 38 women with BPD scored beyond the ASD cut-off of the AQ. The subgroup with high autistic traits had lower scores for cognitive empathy and higher alexithymia scores. Conversely, Anckarsater et al. [31] reported a 12.2% prevalence of BPD among 74 ASD patients and Hofvander et al. [30] found that, among 122 referred adults with high-functioning ASD, 15% of females and 5% of males had comorbid BPD. Finally, Dudas et al. [65] compared 624 ASD, 23 BPD, and 16 comorbid (ASD + BPD) patients, and 2081 neurotypical controls. According to the report of this observational study, comorbid ASD and BPD patients appear to have the higher levels of autistic traits [65]. The clinical overlapping of the behavioral manifestation observed in the two conditions appears also to be present as a sub-clinical manifestation. A recent study of Chabrol and Raynal [66] examined the co-occurrence of autistic and borderline traits in a nonclinical sample of young adults and its influence on the levels of suicidal ideation, depressive symptomatology, and substance use. This study suggests that there is a significant minority of nonclinical adolescents characterized by the presence of both autistic and borderline traits, and higher levels of suicidal ideations. Taking this group into account may have implications in the understanding and prevention of suicidal behaviors [66].

Few studies analyzed the overlap between ASD and narcissistic personality disorder (NPD). It may be difficult to distinguish these disorders considering solely the behavioral level. Like individuals with ASD, patients with NPD tend to focus predominantly on themselves. NPD relationships are described as self-centered and selfish [67]. The DSM-5 states that interpersonal relationships of patients with NPD are impaired due to a disregard for the sensitivities of others. In fact, for both ASD and NPD, there is clinical and scientific evidence for reduced empathic abilities [68, 69]. However, the limitations in empathy are expressed in different ways. Whereas individuals with ASD have limited competencies in theory of mind and are therefore impaired in cognitive empathy, i.e., recognizing and defining emotional expressions [68], patients with NPD show primarily reduced emotional empathy, i.e., sympathy and compassion, and they are less motivated to make attributions for the mental states of others [69]. Therefore, patients with NPD have no difficulties in identifying the needs and feelings of others but appear to be less interested in others' mental states and probably feel less compassion.

Strunz et al. [70] revealed clear differences between the personality profile of ASD subjects and the personality profiles of NPD and BPD patients and nonclinical controls. In sum, the ASD personality profile was characterized by introversion in almost all aspects, and low openness to experience, straightforwardness, orderliness, and conscientiousness. Dissocial behavior was significantly lower in individuals with ASD than both NPD and BPD patients. Compared to ASD patients, individuals with NPD were more extroverted, more open to experience and much less organized. Compared to patients with BPD, individuals with ASD were significantly more introverted and conscientious [70].

The relationship between histrionic personality disorder and ASD has been understudied, and a recent meta-analysis reported a low rate of diagnosis of histrionic PD in comorbidity with ASD [28]. However, among cluster B personality disorders, antisocial personality disorder (APD) could present overlapping appearance with ASD. According to DSM-5, antisocial personality is referred to those individuals who habitually and pervasively ignore or violate the rights and considerations of others without remorse [15]. Therefore, people with APD may be habitual criminals, or engage in criminal behaviors; they can also be manipulative and hurt others in non-criminal, but immoral or irresponsible ways, in violation of social norms and expectations. APD is sometimes known as "sociopathy" or "psychopathy" [71]. Indeed, in the first accounts of the condition, Hans Asperger denominated ASD as "Autistic Psychopathy" [72]. While defining the clinical picture of "Autistic Psychopathy," Asperger depicted some typical and unmistakable characteristics, such as the disturbance of contact, the disciplinary difficulties, the malice, the pedantries and stereotypies, the automaton-like nature of the whole personality, the lack of ability to learn, in contrast with relatively superior spontaneous performance. Asperger also recognized unemphatic conducts and aggressive behaviors among the ASD population [73]. Notably, some of these features seem to partially overlap those of APD. However, literature have scarcely focused on the potential comorbidity between the two conditions, and the majority of research was conducted in the last few years. The overlapping symptomatology might be related to the deficits in empathy showed by individuals affected by both disorders. In particular, psychopathic tendencies appear to be associated with diminished affective empathy (i.e., the capacity to respond with an appropriate emotion to another's mental states) but not cognitive empathy or theory of mind (i.e., the ability to take another's perspective) [74]. Conversely, individuals with ASD would show deficits in theory of mind [75], but not in affective empathy [74]. In fact, in her translation and commentary on Asperger's work, Frith [73] suggests that while Asperger described some behaviors as antisocial in nature, the intent of such conducts may not have been malicious, but instead aimed at eliciting a clear emotional reaction in other people by individuals who found difficulties in interpreting the social world. It is worth mentioning that individuals with ASD have difficulty in understanding the perspective of others and consequently may react in a seemingly cold and uncaring manner in real-life situations [76]. However, if information is presented in a way that enables individuals with ASD to identify others' point of view, they appear to show as much concern and compassion as typically developing individuals. The available data thus suggest that, although both psychopathy and ASD are associated with social difficulties and a decreased emotional expression, the etiology, broad behavioral profiles, and the cognitive-affective deficits associated with these two disorders may be quite separate [74].

However, some studies showed that psychopathic tendencies could co-occur with ASD [77]. In particular, a distinct subgroup of autistic people with a stable pattern of antisocial behavior has been designated as having "callous–unemotional traits" [78], defined by a lack of empathy, a lack of guilt, a failure to put forth effort in important activities, and shallow emotions [79]. Additionally, some ASD behaviors may put them at risk of being persecuted by the criminal justice system. For instance, a disruption of routines, a lack of understanding of social situations, and poor negotiation skills might lead people with an ASD to becoming aggressive; an obsessional interest might lead someone to committing an offence in the pursuit of that interest, perhaps exacerbated by a failure to recognize the consequences of the behavior [80]. Recently, few researchers have sought to identify the presence of autistic subjects in forensic settings, finding that the proportion of people with ASD in the criminal justice system can be compared to that found among the general population, though they commit a variety of crimes and seem to have a number of predisposing features. Notably, there is poor evidence of the presence of comorbid psychiatric diagnoses (except in mental health settings) amongst offenders with ASD [80].

Conclusively, we suggest to carefully consider the clinical relevance of both possible comorbidity and differential diagnosis between cluster B personality disorders and ASD. Aside from theoretical consideration, the clinical relevance of the differential diagnosis is clear as very different care planning is required for the two conditions and similar therapeutic approaches have shown different results [81]. Furthermore, despite the common impairment in social and occupational functioning, alongside with several other clinical features, the severity of the clinical picture tends to diminish with time among patients with BPD, as opposed to what is described in ASD. Nevertheless, it is clinically crucial to correctly diagnose the presence of comorbidity as the severity of the symptoms and problem behavior appear to be more severe in this scenario.

10.5.3 ASD and Cluster C Personality Disorders

According to DSM-5 [15], cluster C personality disorders include the avoidant, dependent, and obsessive-compulsive personality disorder. Avoidant personality disorder is characterized by a pervasive pattern of social inhibition, feelings of inadequacy, and hypersensitivity to negative evaluation that begins by early adulthood and is present in a variety of contexts. Dependent personality disorder (DPD) is characterized by a pervasive and excessive need to be taken care of that leads to submissive and clinging behavior associated with fears of separation beginning in the early adulthood. The obsessive-compulsive personality disorder (OCPD) is described by pervasive preoccupation with orderliness, perfectionism, and mental and interpersonal control, at the expense of flexibility, openness, and efficiency beginning by early adulthood.

Frequently, avoidant behavior is present in individuals with ASD, and could be considered a consequence of the ASD itself. For some individuals with ASD, their disability in interpreting social cues leads to a major concern about what impression they make on others and even a disabling fear for social situations, thus increasing the risk for avoidant behavior. Moreover, elevated sensitivity to stressful environments because of visual and auditory perceptual difficulties may well contribute to avoidant behavior.

A meta-analysis by Vuijk [82], including four studies [29, 30, 83, 84], shows that avoidant PD and OCPD are among the most widespread PD in comorbidity with ASD (23% and 31%, respectively). Criteria for OCPD and ASD criteria show similarities, particularly about restricted behavior patterns. The major difference across the two categories regards the onset: for obsessive-compulsive PD, the onset of the behavior has to be at least "early adulthood," whereas for ASD, a childhood onset is stipulated [29]. However, the differential diagnosis could be difficult considering that obsessive-compulsive personality traits, even though not overtly dysfunctional, could be already present during earlier stages of life. According to Fitzgerald [85], there is a clear risk for misdiagnosis if ASD is not considered in patients with obvious obsessive-compulsive traits [85]. Nevertheless, there are features of compulsive personality disorder that are not typically seen in subjects with ASD, such as excessively high performance standards, perfectionism, a disproportionate inclination to self-criticism, and agonizing indecisiveness when the customary rules and values do not apply [86].

In his self-report, Paul [87] explored the phenomenological nature of the comorbidity between the autism spectrum disorder known as Asperger's syndrome (AS), obsessive-compulsive disorder (OCD), obsessive-compulsive personality disorder (OCPD), and major depressive disorder (MDD). The author used himself as the basis of a case study for the purpose of exploring the phenomenology of the intersections. In fact, during his life he received the diagnoses of AS, OCD, MDD, and OCPD. His hypothesis was that his AS created a "*vacuum of the mind*"—which he would define as an inner mental life that consists of abnormally few representations of real and living human beings—and that this vacuum made him susceptible to the development of obsessive-compulsive traits (OCPD) and behaviors (OCD). AS is neither a necessary nor a sufficient condition for the genesis of OCD—many persons have OCD without AS, and conversely, many persons have AS without OCD; nevertheless, AS and OCD have been found to be related to a number of clinically significant ways. Paul [87] elaborated general hypotheses potentially susceptible of investigation: one of these assumed that "*if AS and OCPD are comorbid in a given subject, then the subject's obsessive pursuit of narrow interests is more likely to be circumscribed by rules, procedures, and restrictions than in subject with AS without OCPD.*"

10.6 Conclusion

Acknowledging the heterogeneous theoretical framework about personality disorders in ASD, we still consider the evaluation of personality of extreme clinical relevance in individuals with ASD. Apart from the troublesome and essential differential diagnosis among these conditions, we also regard the dimensional investigation of individual personality as a relevant field of research where, in fact, personality traits could mirror the heterogeneity of the clinical presentations of ASD. The two groups of conditions share many psychopathological features: from oddness (cluster A), to emotional dysregulation (cluster B), to obsessiveness and social avoidance (cluster C). However, the developmental anamnestic approach is diriment and crucial especially in the adult population. For this reason, an accurate clinical evaluation made by experts in neurodevelopmental disorders, together with the administration of appropriate standardized assessment tools, appears of extreme importance while assessing adults who present overlapping symptomatology. Comorbid ID could pose significant limitations in the adoption of standardized assessment tools, and the use of reference manual is recommended in these cases. As literature reports the possible comorbidity between ASD and PD, it is always important to take into account also this occurrence, that could imply more severe clinical outcomes and require more careful treatment approach.

References

1. Millon T. Toward a new personology: an evolutionary model. Oxford: Wiley; 1990.
2. Roberts BW. Back to the future: personality and assessment and personality development. J Res Personality. 2009;43(2):137–45.
3. Cloninger CR, Svrakic DM, Przybeck TR. A psychobiological model of temperament and character. Arch Gen Psychiatry. 1993;50(12):975–90.
4. Strelau J. The concept and status of trait in research on temperament. Eur J Personality. 2001;15(4):311–25.
5. Cloninger CR, Bayon C, Svrakic DM. Measurement of temperament and character in mood disorders: a model of fundamental states as personality types. J Affect Disord. 1998;51(1):21–32.
6. Millon T. On the history and future study of personality and its disorders. Annu Rev Clin Psychol. 2012;8(1):1–19.
7. Kerekes N, Brandstrom S, Lundstrom S, Rastam M, Nilsson T, Anckarsater H. ADHD, autism spectrum disorder, temperament, and character: phenotypical associations and etiology in a Swedish childhood twin study. Compr Psychiatry. 2013;54(8):1140–7.
8. Kraepelin E. Dementia praecox and paraphrenia. Edinburgh: Livingstone; 1919.

9. Vuijk R, de Nijs PF, Vitale SG, Simons-Sprong M, Hengeveld MW. Personality traits in adults with autism spectrum disorders measured by means of the temperament and character inventory. Tijdschr Psychiatr. 2012;54(8):699–707.
10. Poustka L, Bender F, Bock M, Bolte S, Mohler E, Banaschewski T, et al. Personality and social responsiveness in autism spectrum disorders and attention deficit/hyperactivity disorder. Z Kinder Jugendpsychiatr Psychother. 2011;39(2):133–41.
11. Lodi-Smith J, Rodgers JD, Cunningham SA, Lopata C, Thomeer ML. Meta-analysis of Big Five personality traits in autism spectrum disorder. Autism. 2019;23(3):556–65.
12. Roy M, Retzer A, Sikabofori T. Personality development and intellectual disability. Curr Opin Psychiatry. 2015;28(1):35–9.
13. Pridding A, Procter NG. A systematic review of personality disorder amongst people with intellectual disability with implications for the mental health nurse practitioner. J Clin Nurs. 2008;17(21):2811–9.
14. Harris J. Time to make up your mind: why choosing is difficult. Br J Learn Disabil. 2003;31(1):3–8.
15. American Psychiatric Association. Diagnostic and statistical manual of mental disorders (DSM-5®). Arlington, VA: American Psychiatric; 2013.
16. American Psychiatric Association. Diagnostic and statistical manual of mental disorders: DSM-IV-TR. Arlington, VA: American Psychiatric; 2000.
17. Alexander R, Cooray S. Diagnosis of personality disorders in learning disability. Br J Psychiatry. 2003;182:S28–31.
18. Dosen A, Day K. In: Došen A, Day K, editors. Treating mental illness and behavior disorders in children and adults with mental retardation. Arlington, VA: American Psychiatric Pub; 2001. xv, 561-xv, p.
19. Royal College of Psychiatrists. DC-LD: diagnostic criteria for psychiatric disorders for use with adults with learning disabilities/mental retardation. London: Gaskell; 2001.
20. Barnhill J, Cooper SA, Fletcher RJ. Diagnostic manual–intellectual disability 2 (DM-ID): a textbook of diagnosis of mental disorders in persons with intellectual disability. New York: National Association for the Dually Diagnosed; 2007.
21. Bertelli M, Scuticchio D, Ferrandi A, Lassi S, Mango F, Ciavatta C, et al. Reliability and validity of the SPAID-G checklist for detecting psychiatric disorders in adults with intellectual disability. Res Dev Disabil. 2012;33(2):382–90.
22. Bertelli MO, Piva Merli M, Bradley E, Keller R, Varrucciu N, Del Furia C, et al. The diagnostic boundary between autism spectrum disorder, intellectual developmental disorder and schizophrenia spectrum disorders. Adv Mental Health Intell Disabil. 2015;9(5):243–64.
23. Wolf JM, Ventola P. Assessment and treatment planning in adults with autism spectrum disorders. In: Volkmar FR, Reichow B, McPartland JC, editors. Adolescents and adults with autism spectrum disorders. New York: Springer; 2014. p. 283–98.
24. Fusar-Poli L, Brondino N, Rocchetti M, Panisi C, Provenzani U, Damiani S, et al. Diagnosing ASD in adults without ID: accuracy of the ADOS-2 and the ADI-R. J Autism Dev Disord. 2017;47(11):3370–9.
25. Volkmar FR, Paul R, Rogers SJ, Pelphrey KA. Handbook of autism and pervasive developmental disorders, assessment, interventions, and policy. New York: Wiley; 2014.
26. Howlin P, Moss P. Adults with autism spectrum disorders. Can J Psychiatry. 2012;57(5):275–83.
27. Lai M-C, Lombardo MV, Baron-Cohen S. Autism. Lancet. 2014;383(9920):896–910.
28. Lugo-Marín J, Magán-Maganto M, Rivero-Santana A, Cuellar-Pompa L, Alviani M, Jenaro-Rio C, et al. Prevalence of psychiatric disorders in adults with autism spectrum disorder: a systematic review and meta-analysis. Res Autism Spectr Disord. 2019;59:22–33.
29. Lugnegard T, Hallerback MU, Gillberg C. Personality disorders and autism spectrum disorders: what are the connections? Compr Psychiatry. 2012;53(4):333–40.
30. Hofvander B, Delorme R, Chaste P, Nyden A, Wentz E, Stahlberg O, et al. Psychiatric and psychosocial problems in adults with normal-intelligence autism spectrum disorders. BMC Psychiatry. 2009;9:35.
31. Anckarsater H, Stahlberg O, Larson T, Hakansson C, Jutblad SB, Niklasson L, et al. The impact of ADHD and autism spectrum disorders on temperament, character, and personality development. Am J Psychiatry. 2006;163(7):1239–44.

32. Fusar-Poli P, Borgwardt S, Bechdolf A, Addington J, Riecher-Rossler A, Schultze-Lutter F, et al. The psychosis high-risk state: a comprehensive state-of-the-art review. JAMA Psychiatry. 2013;70(1):107–20.
33. Bleuler E. Dementia praecox, oder Gruppe der Schizophrenien. Leipzig: F. Deuticke; 1911.
34. Parnas J, Bovet P. Autism in schizophrenia revisited. Compr Psychiatry. 1991;32(1):7–21.
35. Minkowski E. La schizophrénie: psychopathologie des schizoïdes et des schizophrènes. Paris: Payot; 1927.
36. Minkowski E. Le Temps vécu: études phénoménologiques et psychopathologiques. Paris: J. L. L. L. d'Artrey; 1933.
37. Parnas J, Bovet P, Zahavi D. Schizophrenic autism: clinical phenomenology and pathogenetic implications. World Psychiatry. 2002;1(3):131–6.
38. Pilowsky T, Yirmiya N, Arbelle S, Mozes T. Theory of mind abilities of children with schizophrenia, children with autism, and normally developing children. Schizophr Res. 2000;42(2):145–55.
39. Solomon M, Olsen E, Niendam T, Ragland JD, Yoon J, Minzenberg M, et al. From lumping to splitting and back again: atypical social and language development in individuals with clinical-high-risk for psychosis, first episode schizophrenia, and autism spectrum disorders. Schizophr Res. 2011;131(1–3):146–51.
40. Craddock N, Owen MJ. The Kraepelinian dichotomy—going, going... but still not gone. Br J Psychiatry. 2010;196(2):92–5.
41. Hurst RM, Nelson-Gray RO, Mitchell JT, Kwapil TR. The relationship of Asperger's characteristics and schizotypal personality traits in a non-clinical adult sample. J Autism Dev Disord. 2007;37(9):1711–20.
42. Spek AA, Wouters SGM. Autism and schizophrenia in high functioning adults: behavioral differences and overlap. Res Autism Spectr Disord. 2010;4(4):709–17.
43. Konstantareas MM, Hewitt T. Autistic disorder and schizophrenia: diagnostic overlaps. J Autism Dev Disord. 2001;31(1):19–28.
44. Dinsdale NL, Hurd PL, Wakabayashi A, Elliot M, Crespi BJ. How are autism and schizotypy related? Evidence from a non-clinical population. PLoS One. 2013;8(5):e63316.
45. Volkmar FR, Cohen DJ. Comorbid association of autism and schizophrenia. Am J Psychiatry. 1991;148(12):1705–7.
46. Rutter M. Autism research: prospects and priorities. J Autism Dev Disord. 1996;26(2):257–75.
47. Baron-Cohen S, Wheelwright S, Skinner R, Martin J, Clubley E. The autism-spectrum quotient (AQ): evidence from Asperger syndrome/high-functioning autism, males and females, scientists and mathematicians. J Autism Dev Disord. 2001;31(1):5–17.
48. Raine A. The SPQ: a scale for the assessment of schizotypal personality based on DSM-III-R criteria. Schizophr Bull. 1991;17(4):555–64.
49. Barneveld PS, Pieterse J, de Sonneville L, van Rijn S, Lahuis B, van Engeland H, et al. Overlap of autistic and schizotypal traits in adolescents with autism spectrum disorders. Schizophr Res. 2011;126(1–3):231–6.
50. Russell-Smith SN, Maybery MT, Bayliss DMJP. Relationships between autistic-like and schizotypy traits: an analysis using the Autism Spectrum Quotient and Oxford-Liverpool Inventory of feelings and experiences. Personal Individ Differ. 2011;51(2):128–32.
51. Crespi B, Badcock C. Psychosis and autism as diametrical disorders of the social brain. Behav Brain Sci. 2008;31(3):241–61; discussion 61-320.
52. Del Giudice M, Angeleri R, Brizio A, Elena MR. The evolution of autistic-like and schizotypal traits: a sexual selection hypothesis. Front Psychol. 2010;1:41.
53. Blackshaw AJ, Kinderman P, Hare DJ, Hatton C. Theory of mind, causal attribution and paranoia in Asperger syndrome. Autism. 2001;5(2):147–63.
54. Mottron L, Soulieres I, Menard E. Elements of a clinical differential diagnosis between Asperger syndrome and the schizoid/paranoid personality. Sante Ment Que. 2007;32(1):367–75.
55. Korzekwa MI, Dell PF, Links PS, Thabane L, Webb SP. Estimating the prevalence of borderline personality disorder in psychiatric outpatients using a two-phase procedure. Compr Psychiatry. 2008;49(4):380–6.

56. Lieb K, Zanarini MC, Schmahl C, Linehan MM, Bohus M. Borderline personality disorder. Lancet. 2004;364(9432):453–61.
57. Mitchell AE, Dickens GL, Picchioni MM. Facial emotion processing in borderline personality disorder: a systematic review and meta-analysis. Neuropsychol Rev. 2014;24(2):166–84.
58. Dell'Osso L, Cremone IM, Carpita B, Fagiolini A, Massimetti G, Bossini L, et al. Correlates of autistic traits among patients with borderline personality disorder. Compr Psychiatry. 2018;83:7–11.
59. Gergely G. The development of teleological versus mentalizing observational learning strategies in infancy. Bull Menninger Clin. 2003;67(2):113–31.
60. Morandotti N, Brondino N, Merelli A, Boldrini A, De Vidovich GZ, Ricciardo S, et al. The Italian version of the reflective functioning questionnaire: validity data for adults and its association with severity of borderline personality disorder. PLoS One. 2018;13(11):e0206433.
61. Bateman A, Fonagy P. Psychotherapy for borderline personality disorder: mentalization-based treatment. Oxford: Oxford University Press; 2004.
62. Frith U, Frith CD. Development and neurophysiology of mentalizing. Philos Trans R Soc Lond B Biol Sci. 2003;358(1431):459–73.
63. Rydén G, Rydén E, Hetta J. Borderline personality disorder and autism spectrum disorder in females—a cross-sectional study. Clin Neuropsychiatry. 2008;22(1).
64. Nanchen K, Brodfuehrer A, Heinrichs M, Philipsen A, van Elst LT, Matthies S. Autistic traits in patients with borderline personality disorder. Z Psychiatr Psychol Psychother. 2016;64(4):247.
65. Dudas RB, Lovejoy C, Cassidy S, Allison C, Smith P, Baron-Cohen S. The overlap between autistic spectrum conditions and borderline personality disorder. PLoS One. 2017;12(9):e0184447.
66. Chabrol H, Raynal P. The co-occurrence of autistic traits and borderline personality disorder traits is associated to increased suicidal ideation in nonclinical young adults. Compr Psychiatry. 2018;82:141–3.
67. Miller JD, Campbell WK, Pilkonis PA. Narcissistic personality disorder: relations with distress and functional impairment. Compr Psychiatry. 2007;48(2):170–7.
68. Dziobek I, Rogers K, Fleck S, Bahnemann M, Heekeren HR, Wolf OT, et al. Dissociation of cognitive and emotional empathy in adults with Asperger syndrome using the multifaceted empathy test (MET). J Autism Dev Disord. 2008;38(3):464–73.
69. Ritter K, Dziobek I, Preissler S, Ruter A, Vater A, Fydrich T, et al. Lack of empathy in patients with narcissistic personality disorder. Psychiatry Res. 2011;187(1–2):241–7.
70. Strunz S, Westphal L, Ritter K, Heuser I, Dziobek I, Roepke S. Personality pathology of adults with autism spectrum disorder without accompanying intellectual impairment in comparison to adults with personality disorders. J Autism Dev Disord. 2015;45(12):4026–38.
71. Walsh A, Wu HH. Differentiating antisocial personality disorder, psychopathy, and sociopathy: evolutionary, genetic, neurological, and sociological considerations. Crim Justice Stud. 2008;21(2):135–52.
72. Asperger H. Die "Autistischen Psychopathen" im Kindesalter. Eur Arch Psychiatry Clin Neurosci. 1944;117(1):76–136.
73. Frith U. Asperger and his syndrome. In: Autism and Asperger syndrome, vol. 14. New York: Cambridge University Press; 1991. p. 1–36.
74. Blair RJR. Fine cuts of empathy and the amygdala: dissociable deficits in psychopathy and autism. Q J Exp Psychol. 2008;61(1):157–70.
75. Baron-Cohen S, Leslie AM, Frith U. Does the autistic child have a "theory of mind"? Cognition. 1985;21(1):37–46.
76. Rogers K, Dziobek I, Hassenstab J, Wolf OT, Convit A. Who cares? Revisiting empathy in Asperger syndrome. J Autism Dev Disord. 2007;37(4):709–15.
77. Rogers J, Viding E, Blair RJ, Frith U, Happe F. Autism spectrum disorder and psychopathy: shared cognitive underpinnings or double hit? Psychol Med. 2006;36(12):1789–98.
78. Frick PJ, White SF. Research review: the importance of callous-unemotional traits for developmental models of aggressive and antisocial behavior. J Child Psychol Psychiatry. 2008;49(4):359–75.

79. Kimonis ER, Fanti KA, Frick PJ, Moffitt TE, Essau C, Bijttebier P, et al. Using self-reported callous-unemotional traits to cross-nationally assess the DSM-5 'With Limited Prosocial Emotions' specifier. J Child Psychol Psychiatry. 2015;56(11):1249–61.
80. King C, Murphy GH. A systematic review of people with autism spectrum disorder and the criminal justice system. J Autism Dev Disord. 2014;44(11):2717–33.
81. Bateman A, Fonagy P. Effectiveness of partial hospitalization in the treatment of borderline personality disorder: a randomized controlled trial. Am J Psychiatry. 1999;156(10):1563–9.
82. Vuijk R, Deen M, Sizoo B, et al. Temperament, character, and personality disorders in adults with autism spectrum disorder: a systematic literature review and meta-analysis. Rev J Autism Dev Disord. 2018;5(2):176–97.
83. Anckarsäter H, Stahlberg O, Larson T, Hakansson C, Jutblad SB, Niklasson L, et al. The impact of ADHD and autism spectrum disorders on temperament, character, and personality development. Am J Psychiatry. 2006;163(7):1239–44.
84. Ketelaars C, Horwitz E, Sytema S, Bos J, Wiersma D, Minderaa R, et al. Brief report: adults with mild autism spectrum disorders (ASD): scores on the autism spectrum quotient (AQ) and comorbid psychopathology. J Autism Dev Disord. 2008;38(1):176–80.
85. Fitzgerald M. Misdiagnosis of Asperger syndrome as anankastic personality disorder. Autism. 2002;6(4):435.
86. Lehnhardt FG, Gawronski A, Pfeiffer K, Kockler H, Schilbach L, Vogeley K. The investigation and differential diagnosis of Asperger syndrome in adults. Dtsch Arztebl Int. 2013;110(45):755–63.
87. Paul JD. The vacuum of the mind: a self-report on the phenomenology of autistic, obsessive-compulsive, and depressive comorbidity. Schizophr Bull. 2015;41(6):1207–10.

Adult Attention Deficit Hyperactivity Disorder (ADHD) in ASD

11

Luana Salerno and J. J. Sandra Kooij

11.1 Introduction

The condition we currently define as "Attention Deficit Hyperactivity Disorder" or "ADHD" is a neurobiological disorder, characterized by core symptoms of inattention, impulsivity, and hyperactivity, that has received multiple definitions in the scientific literature over the course of the last century. These include among others "Defect of moral control" [1], "Hyperkinetic disease of infancy" [2], and "Minimal brain dysfunction" [3]. The term "Attention" was recognized as the central feature of the condition only since 1980s, when the Diagnostic and Statistical Manual of Mental Disorders (DSM) changed the "Hyperkinetic Impulse Disorder" into "Attention Deficit Disorder" (ADD), that was further refined as "Attention Deficit Hyperactivity Disorder (ADHD)" in 1987 [4]. Currently, the DSM-5 mentions ADHD as Attention-Deficit/Hyperactivity Disorder [5].

ADHD has been considered for a long time as a childhood condition, fading as children grew up. Instead, increased evidence demonstrated that ADHD changes its clinical presentations with age, but persists in most cases with its associated impairment [6].

While children with ADHD can be visibly hyperactive, running about or climbing in situations where it is not appropriate, the presentation of ADHD in adults is slightly different. Outward visible hyperactivity tends to decrease with age, transforming into feelings of inner restlessness, nervousness, and/or talkativeness. Therefore, adults with ADHD are less overly hyperactive and may compensate their

L. Salerno (✉)
INS—Institute of Neuroscience, Florence, Italy

J. J. Sandra Kooij
Amsterdam University Medical Center, VUMc, Amsterdam, The Netherlands

Expertise Center Adult ADHD, PsyQ, The Hague, The Netherlands
e-mail: s.kooij@psyq.nl

R. Keller (ed.), *Psychopathology in Adolescents and Adults with Autism Spectrum Disorders*, https://doi.org/10.1007/978-3-030-26276-1_11

restlessness by excessive sport activity [7]. However, they can be still slower in thinking and solving problems, disorganized and with a poor sense of time. Their mind is frequently elsewhere, lost in thoughts unrelated to tasks at hand, or they

Table 11.1 Examples of the clinical presentation of ADHD in adults

Inattention	Hyperactivity	Impulsivity	Other symptoms supporting an ADHD diagnosis
Easily distracted by noises or by own thoughts	Fidgeting with hands, legs, or feet; tapping pens; fiddling with items	Interrupting and finishing other people's sentences	Irritability
Difficulty sustaining attention except for activities of interest (chatting, videogames)	Avoiding meetings, conferences, and courses due to difficulty staying seated for long periods of time	Difficulty waiting turn	Mood lability
Disorganized, being messy	Stressed when forced to stay seated	Tendency to say what comes to mind without considering impact to others	Easily frustrated
Difficulty working in a detailed way	Inner restlessness or agitation	Impatience	Angry outbursts
Too much time needed to complete tasks	Feeling of being trapped when in a place they cannot leave	Acting without thinking of the consequences	Sleep problems
Forgetfulness	Talking too loud and too much	Risky and sensation seeking behavior	Binge eating
Lose or misplace thing (mobile phone, keys, wallet, documents)	Difficulty to relax	Interrupting others and finishing other people's sentences	
Lose a lot of time to search for things he/she needs	Pacing up and down	Difficulty delaying gratification	
Difficulty following a conversation		Starting and ending relationships quickly	
Easily bored		Tendency to spend too much	
Poor planning and organization			
Mind wandering			
Difficulty following instructions			
Procrastination			
Difficulty starting and completing tasks			
Difficulty being on time: being either too late or too early			

may experience hyperfocused periods when they are engaged in those activities they find interesting [8]. In fact, they can spend countless hours browsing the internet, watching entire TV series on Netflix, videos on YouTube, or chatting with friends. They still make careless mistakes, be forgetful and tend to lose things. They frequently act without thinking beforehand, show sensation seeking behavior, and tend to engage in risky situations [7].

Emotional dysregulation is considered a symptom supporting the diagnosis of ADHD [5]. It consists of poor self-regulation of emotions, volatility, irritability and a low tolerance to frustration [9, 10]. Table 11.1 shows some examples of the clinical presentation of ADHD in adults.

11.2 Burden of ADHD

ADHD affects approximately 2.8% of the general adult population worldwide [11] and is associated with high societal and economic burden. ADHD interferes significantly with the individual's functioning at home, in educational settings and in social and family relationships. Indeed, adults with ADHD have a frequent history of learning problems, school rejections and dropouts, peer rejection, and relationship problems [12]. Untreated ADHD is associated with increased rates of unemployment, more frequent illicit drug use and alcohol abuse, 2–3 times more frequent teenage pregnancies, higher rates of separation and divorce, intimate partner violence, increased rates of suicide attempts and suicide, home and traffic accidents, and increased mortality and criminality [7, 13–18]. The prevalence of ADHD in long-term inmates in prison was estimated at 40% [13], and it has been reported that 47% of individuals with ADHD have at least one criminal sentence [19].

People with ADHD are also more vulnerable to physical diseases. The chance of obesity is up to 70% increased in ADHD, resulting in increased rates for diabetes and cardiovascular diseases, as a consequence of their disorganized lifestyles, chronic sleep loss, and poor health habits [20–25]. People with ADHD have also an increased risk for asthma [24]. A study performed in Japan found that individuals with ADHD visited physicians 10 times more often than people without the disorder, and hospitalization rates were three times higher than in those without ADHD [26]. As a result, ADHD is associated with a lower life expectancy and a twofold increased risk of early death compared to those without the disorder [18]. The burden of ADHD is also increased by the high rate of psychiatric comorbidities [27]. The majority of adults with ADHD are suffering from chronic sleep disorders, such as restless legs syndrome, insomnia, sleep apnea, and delayed circadian rhythm sleep disorder [28, 29]. They are also three times more likely to suffer from a major depressive disorder (MDD), six times more likely to suffer from dysthymia and have twofold increased prevalence of substance abuse or dependence than the general population [11, 30].

The presence of comorbid conditions determines a more severe course of illness [31]. Early intervention can reduce most of the adverse consequences associated with ADHD, such as development of substance use disorders, criminality, and poor educational and occupational outcomes. Indeed, research showed that when people with ADHD are in treatment using medication, there is a decrease of 30–40% in motor vehicle accidents, of 60–70% in suicidality, and 30–40% of criminality rates [32–34].

11.3 ADHD and ASD: Prevalence, Distinctive and Overlapping Features

It is only since 2013, with the release of DSM-5, that it is possible to diagnose ADHD in the presence of ASD. This change was based on studies performed in children showing comorbidity rates ranging from 40 to 70% [35–38]. Moreover, an important epidemiological study performed by Simonoff et al. [39] found a rate of ADHD in ASD that was 6 times higher than the recognized prevalence of ADHD in children and adolescents worldwide [40, 41]. Of the adults with a diagnosis of ASD, 28–44% also meet criteria of ADHD [42]. Notably 15–25% of youth with ADHD also exhibit ASD traits [43, 44]. The risk of ASD and ADHD in later born siblings of a child with ASD, and vice versa the risk of ADHD and ASD in later born siblings of a child with ADHD are also increased [45], pointing to shared familial mechanisms.

The prevalence rate of both disorders changed during the last two decades. In 2011, Boyle and colleagues [46] reported that from 1997 to 2008 the ADHD prevalence increased by 33%, while that of ASD increased by 289%. This rise of prevalence rates got several explanations, such as the modification of the diagnostic definitions, the improvement of the diagnostic methods [47], but it could also reflect a greater knowledge about the clinical presentation of the two disorders over the lifespan. However, it is not possible to exclude the influence of some external factors on child development, causing a higher risk for both conditions [48].

ASD is defined by the presence of impairments in social communication and social interaction and restricted, repetitive patterns of behavior, interests, or activities [5]. ADHD is defined by a persistent pattern of inattention and/or hyperactivity–impulsivity that interferes with the individual's functioning in more than one setting [5]. However, inattentive, hyperactive, and impulsive symptoms are frequently reported in subjects with ASD [49]. On the other hand, impairments in social communication as well as repetitive and stereotyped behavior also have been described in children with ADHD [48, 50].

Studies investigating the co-occurrence of such disorders at a genetic, structural, and functional level of analysis indicate that they share common genetic risk factors, involve similar biological mechanisms, and affect the same brain regions.

Both ASD and ADHD are conditions with a high heritability of around 75% in childhood [51, 52]. Studies focusing on adults report heritability estimates ranging from 30 to 50% for both disorders [53–55]. Several large-scale genome-wide studies showed that ASD and ADHD present the same genetic susceptibility, and the overlap in the 50–70% of contributing genetic factors can explain their frequent co-occurrence [56]. ASD and ADHD share rare genetic risk variants (Copy Number Variants or CNVs) [57–59], and many family studies reported that relatives of patients with ASD or ADHD frequently display the typical symptoms of the other condition [60]. Greater within-individual and within-family associations have been found in high-functioning ASD compared to low-functioning ASD [61]. This is an important finding with several possible explanations. One of them is that low-functioning ASD is considered as a more severe ASD phenotype because of the presence of Intellectual Disability (ID), presenting a minimal aetiological overlap with other neurodevelopmental disorders as ADHD [61]. However, it may also be possible that people with ASD and ID presenting symptoms of ADHD are less likely to receive such an additional diagnosis. This is not unlikely, as the "diagnostic overshadowing" effect is frequently reported in people with ID, consisting in the tendency to attribute symptoms of other mental health conditions to the intellectual disability, causing inadequate or delayed treatment [62].

Environmental factors such as low birth weight, premature birth as well as adverse socioeconomic variables have been linked to an increased risk for the development of ADHD [63]. Although prenatal inflammation and prematurity have been reported as common risk factors for both ADHD and ASD [41], a large study performed in 2016 found that it is very unlikely that the ADHD-ASD comorbidity can be explained by shared pre- and perinatal risk factors alone [64].

A meta-analysis of cross-sectional neuroimaging studies found a decreased total brain volume in children, but not adults with ADHD; volume reductions in children were reported in the bilateral amygdala, accumbens, and hippocampus [65]. While the brain of ASD individuals has an accelerated growth stage during the first four years of life, followed by greater reductions in gray matter [66], the current conceptualization of ADHD as a neurodevelopmental disorder reflects the evidence supporting a "global perturbation" of connectivity [67] and brain maturation in ADHD, caused by a delay in the development of cortical thickness [68] as well as of the surface area [69].

From a neuropsychological point of view, the most promising candidate endophenotype of ADHD is the intra-subject variability (ISV) of reaction time (RT) [70]. There is evidence that the ISV of RT is a stable trait [71–73], that is both hereditary [74, 75] and familial [76, 77]. It seems a "task-independent anomaly" able to negatively influence the performance regardless the specific difficulties posed by a task [78]. Individuals with ADHD present with increased ISV in reaction times across a variety of cognitive tasks [79, 80]. Studies exploring the ISVs in ASD found a small increase in ISV in respect to controls, but those differentiating between individuals with ASD and individuals with ASD+ADHD found increased ISV of RT only in people with ASD+ADHD [70, 81–83]. Impaired attention switching is reported in both ADHD and ASD [84], although in tests evaluating such ability subjects with ASD were slower and more accurate than adults with ADHD [84]. The severity level of attentional dysfunction appeared greater in ADHD and ASD+ADHD groups [85]. Studies on children with ADHD showed more difficulties in sustained and divided attention tasks compared to controls, but in the presence of comorbid ASD there were more problems in tasks measuring divided attention and alertness [86].

Both ASD and ADHD are characterized by impairments in executive functions (EF), that are caused by disruption in the fronto-striatal and fronto-parietal circuits. People affected by both ASD and ADHD present the same deficits in flexibility and planning characterizing people with only ASD, and they are impaired in response inhibition as people with only ADHD [85]. The impairments in EF in both disorders are associated with different patterns of psychiatric comorbidities: the cognitive inflexibility associated with ASD predicted greater internalizing problems as well as aggressive behavior; the cognitive disinhibition characterizing ADHD predicted greater externalizing problems [87].

A study comparing the temperament profile of individuals with ASD in comparison to those with ADHD found that ASD was associated with high levels of harm avoidance and low reward dependence; instead ADHD appeared to be closely associated with novelty seeking traits [88].

11.4 The Burden of ADHD+ASD Comorbidity

The co-existence of both disorders puts a significant burden on the individual and the family. Individuals with ASD presenting ADHD symptomatology exhibit a more severe phenotype, with higher autistic traits, greater impairment in adaptive behavior, anger, tantrums, and higher levels of oppositional and conduct behaviors [44, 89]. Moreover, people with both ASD+ADHD are at increased risk for developing additional psychiatric conditions such as anxiety, depression, and sleep problems. From a neuropsychological point of view, they were characterized by lower full-scale IQ and more executive function deficits [44].

Substance Use Disorders (SUDs) are frequent comorbidities in ADHD, with prevalence rates ranging from 17% to 45% for alcohol abuse or dependence, and from 9 to 30% for illicit drugs [90]. Vice versa, 23% of individuals with SUD meet the criteria for ADHD [91]. Literature regarding the co-occurrence of SUDs in people with ASD is still scarce [92]. However, the available evidence indicates a lifetime prevalence of SUD in ASD ranging from 11 to 29% [93–95]. Risk factors for the development of SUDs in people with ASD and ADHD are similar: early onset of smoking (OR = 5.68), parental SUD (OR = 5.36), and adverse family history (OR = 2.67) [95]. Interestingly, in this study people with ADHD started smoking regularly 2 years earlier than those with ASD (mean age 14.6 for ADHD versus 16.6 for ASD). Data from cross-sectional interviews and self-report questionnaires administered to 3080 young adult Australian twins with a mean age of 31.9 years, showed an association between higher ADHD symptoms and elevated autistic traits scores, and a high level of regular smoking and cannabis use disorder [96].

Finally, ADHD exerts a negative impact on the treatment outcomes of social skills training in people with ASD [97], and children with both ADHD and ASD are more frequently bullied and victimized by peers [38, 98, 99].

11.5 The Diagnosis of ADHD

The diagnosis of ADHD is established clinically, on the basis of criteria defined by diagnostic classification systems such as the DSM and ICD. The DSM is a diagnostic classification system for mental disorders using a common framework. It provides operational criteria for psychiatric diagnoses and covers all mental health disorders affecting children as well as adults. The other one is the International Classification of Diseases (ICD), which has been developed by the World Health Organization. It includes descriptions of factors influencing health, or external causes of mortality and morbidity; its diagnostic codes are mainly used for health insurance billing [100].

The DSM-5 included ADHD in the chapter of "Neurodevelopmental Disorders." It further includes the Autism Spectrum Disorders (ASD), Intellectual Disability (Intellectual Developmental Disorder), Communication Disorders, Specific Learning Disorders, and Motor Disorders. These disorders generally begin early in life and have a chronic course during the lifespan.

On the basis of the DSM-5 criteria, the diagnosis of ADHD in adulthood is established when at least 5 current inattentive or hyperactive-impulsive symptoms are present, with several symptoms in childhood, with an onset before age 12. The symptoms should be present for at least 6 months, causing significant impairment in the individual's functioning in social, academic, or occupational domains. The clinician can specify the severity level considering the number of symptoms exceeding those required for the diagnosis. The DSM-5 recognizes three presentation types of ADHD:

- the predominantly inattentive type,
- the predominantly hyperactive/impulsive type,
- the combined type.

The further novelty in the DSM-5, as already stated above, is the possibility to make an ADHD diagnosis in the presence of ASD.

The assessment and diagnosis of ADHD should rely on information on the symptoms provided by the patient and whenever possible by collateral informants. Rating scales may help the clinician to screen for the presence of childhood and current symptoms of ADHD, but they are not sufficient to make the diagnosis. Indeed, the diagnostic process must include the following steps:

- Evaluation of impairment caused by the suspected ADHD,
- Developmental, medical, and psychiatric history,
- Assessment of any comorbidity (among others sleep-, mood-, anxiety and substance use disorders),
- Investigation of patterns of ADHD and other psychiatric disorders in the family, including sleep-, mood-, or anxiety disorders and substance abuse.

11.6 Screening and Diagnostic Tools

As for other psychiatric disorders, there is not a single test with enough predictive power to establish an ADHD diagnosis. However, several tools can assist the clinician during the diagnostic process. When possible, a collateral interview with a family member during the assessment is suggested, for gathering valuable information that the patient may not self-report.

There are several rating scales for screening ADHD symptoms in adults. The vast majority are based on DSM-IV criteria, but they can be easily adapted to the DSM-5 using the new cut-off (5 current symptoms instead of 6) and age-of-onset criterion (symptoms emerged before age 12 instead of age 7). While rating scales can be useful as a rapid screening of symptoms of adult ADHD, the symptoms may be exaggerated, but also underreported. Underreporting can happen when the individual evaluates the symptoms while taking into account settings where he/she is less impaired (such as during interesting activities) [101].

A semi-structured clinical interview is the best instrument for establishing the diagnosis of ADHD in adults, as it permits to investigate the age of onset and number of symptoms and their persistence, as well as the associated impairment in both childhood and adulthood. Among the available semi-structured clinical interviews for adult ADHD there is the Diagnostic Interview for ADHD in adults, second edition (DIVA 2.0) [102]. It is based on the DSM-IV-TR criteria, and is under revision for adaptation to DSM-5 in several languages. It has been validated in two studies [103, 104] and is available online at www.divacenter.eu and as the DIVA 2.0 app in the Google Play and App stores. The other clinical interviews are the Conners' Adult ADHD Diagnostic Interview for DSM-IV (CAADID), and the ACE+. Table 11.2 shows the most used instruments in the diagnostic process of adult ADHD. These instruments are not validated in the ASD population, but they can be useful in case of suspected adult ADHD.

Table 11.2 Most used rating scales and semi-structured interviews for adult ADHD

Rating scales	Description
Adult ADHD Self-Report Scale Symptom Checklist (ASRS) [105]	Self-report symptoms checklist, also in screener version (ASRSv1.1), both available at https://med.nyu.edu/psych/adhd-self-assessment-tools-and-information
Barkley Adult ADHD Rating Scale IV (BAARS-IV) [106]	Self-report symptom checklist with norm-referenced scores; observer rating forms for corroboration of symptomatology. Available for purchasing at www.guilford.com
Conners' Adult ADHD Rating Scales (CAARS) [107]	Self-report symptom checklist with norm-referenced scores; observer rating forms for corroboration of symptomatology. Available for purchasing at www.mhs.com
Brown Attention Deficit Disorders Scale-Adult Version (BADDS) [108]	40-item inventory with norm-referenced scores. Not based on DSM criteria. Available for purchasing at www.pearsonclinical.com
Structured diagnostic interviews	**Description**
DIVA 2.0 (will be updated to DIVA 5.0) [8]	Semi-structured clinician-administered interview, available at www.divacenter.eu in 20 languages
Conners' Adult ADHD Diagnostic Interview for DSM-IV (CAADID) [109]	Structured clinician-administered interview, available for purchasing at www.mhs.com
ACE+	Semi-structured interview for ADHD in adults available at www.psychology-services.uk.com/adhd.htm

As many individuals with ASD have a poor insight in their impairments, it is very important to obtain collateral histories as well as symptom rating from close relatives/informants, and consider school reports, if available. This may enhance the accuracy of the diagnosis.

11.7 Neuropsychological Measures

Even though persons with ADHD—considered at a group level—performed poorly in a series of executive function (EF) measures, up until now there is no ancillary neuropsychological test or test battery with enough positive predictive power to be confidently used for establishing the ADHD diagnosis at the individual level [7, 110]. However, neuropsychological testing can be of help to investigate comorbid conditions, such as a learning disability or a neurocognitive disorder. Moreover, based on the risk of informant bias and the frequent discrepancies between the different sources of information (i.e., patient *versus* parents) [111], the use of objective measures may give the clinician useful additional information. In this context, a recent study showed that the use of the Qb-Test, that combines a continuous performance test measuring inattention and impulsivity and an infra-red camera measuring hyperactivity, improved the diagnostic accuracy when used in combination with the DIVA 2.0 [103].

11.8 When to Think of ADHD in ASD

It is not simple to diagnose ADHD in individuals with ASD because of the overlapping features described above. ADHD can be easily missed in adults, particularly in those presenting with other comorbid psychiatric disorders. However, suspecting ADHD can emerge in the presence of difficulties with inhibition and problems with sustaining attention long enough to execute complex tasks [72]. Social skills acquisition in people with ASD is crucial, but inattentiveness and hyperactive/impulsive symptoms of ADHD make this process more challenging. In fact, ADHD can create problems in the learning of sequential actions and in maintaining focus during social interaction. In addition due to the lack of inhibitory control, individuals with ADHD can have more problems with respect to taking turns.

The co-occurrence of ADHD in ASD should be considered in the presence of:

- time management problems,
- disorganization,
- procrastination,
- forgetfulness (missing appointments, losing things),
- premature shifting of activities (starting an activity but quickly getting distracted by something else),
- impulsive decisions (spending too much or changing plans without reflecting beforehand),
- use of illegal drugs,
- emotional dysregulation.

Missing a diagnosis of ADHD not only leads to inadequate care, but can also result in inadequate treatment and poor outcomes.

11.9 Treatment of ADHD

The most effective treatment approach for ADHD is multimodal treatment. It comprises of psychoeducation, pharmacological treatment, cognitive behavior therapy (CBT), and coaching. Psychoeducation on the heritability of ADHD, brain dysfunctions, prevalence, symptoms of ADHD and comorbidities, and order of the treatment plan should be the first step in treatment.

The pharmacological treatment is based on two distinct drug categories: stimulants and non-stimulants. Stimulants work by acting on dopamine and noradrenaline reuptake inhibition, and presynaptic release. They are considered the first-line treatment for adult ADHD as they demonstrate highest effect sizes [112, 113]. A recent systematic review and network meta-analysis comparing the efficacy and tolerability of ADHD medications in children and adults with ADHD concluded that methylphenidate is first choice in children, but dexamphetamine in adults [114]. Unfortunately, the stimulants are not available in all countries, leading to lower response rates using medications for ADHD.

In adults, long-acting formulations are more suitable than immediate release medications, as they are better to prevent abuse or diversion. Moreover, they permit to control symptomatology during all day, without the rebound effects each time after the short acting agents wear off. Atomoxetine, which is a non-stimulant medication, permits a 24-h coverage but is associated with small effect sizes after 4 weeks of treatment that may become moderate after 6 months [115]. It acts as a noradrenaline reuptake inhibitor and inhibits the presynaptic noradrenaline transporter. Among the non-stimulants agents there are also guanfacine and clonidine, more used in children and adolescents [7], and bupropion, that may be used in patients who do not respond to the previous medications [7, 116, 117]. Although some data support the use of modafinil, a wakefulness-promoting agent in the treatment of ADHD [118], it was not effective in a study in adults affected by the disorder [119].

Regarding side effects, stimulants can among others cause increased heart rate and blood pressure, loss of appetite, and trouble falling asleep. Non-stimulants can cause sleepiness, headache, nausea, and dizziness. An increased heart rate and blood pressure may occur also with atomoxetine treatment, which is dose dependent and resolves with the cessation of therapy [120]. As atomoxetine is metabolized via the CYP2D6 pathway in the liver, it should be used with caution in individuals having mutations or deletions in the genes that codify for such enzymes. In fact, in this population atomoxetine is associated with increased side effects [121].

Although ADHD is a disorder with high response rates to the pharmacological treatment [122], this is not always sufficient to improve the individual's quality of life. Non-pharmacological interventions, such as psychoeducation, CBT, and coaching are also important. Psychoeducation is particularly useful after the diagnosis, as it provides useful information for a better understanding of the disorder, enabling patients to consciously choose their treatment and allow them to make better choices in their daily lives [8].

There is increasing evidence supporting the use of CBT in reducing ADHD symptomatology, but preferably in combination with pharmacological treatment [123–125]. In fact, until now there is insufficient evidence indicating the efficacy of CBT alone for the treatment of adult ADHD [124, 126–128]. However, when the patient does not tolerate medications, CBT should be considered [7]. Several CBT approaches have been developed for adults with ADHD and are organized in a series of modules focusing on the development of skills such as organization, time and financial management, emotional control, and problem-solving. As people with ADHD frequently have a negative self-esteem caused by their frequent experiences of failure, CBT can be useful in restructuring the dysfunctional cognitive schemas [7, 129].

Coaching is different from CBT as the relationship between a coach and client is very structured, practical, and goal-driven. The coach has an active role in the coaching process, offering suggestions, and chooses with the client the approach that might work best. There is no set model, methodology may vary, and coaching can be provided in sessions conducted in person, in groups, or by email/phone calls/apps/video chats. Although controlled studies evaluating the efficacy of coaching in the treatment of adults with ADHD are lacking, some positive outcomes have been reported in uncontrolled studies [7, 130, 131].

11.10 Treatment of ADHD in ASD

Methylphenidate and atomoxetine have been studied in people with both ASD and ADHD. They demonstrated efficacy although with lower effect sizes and a high number of side effects compared to people with only ADHD [38]. In fact, methylphenidate proved useful in managing hyperactivity and impulsivity symptoms in children [132], but was associated with an increased likelihood of social withdrawal, irritability, and depression [133]. In a recent naturalistic study investigating the effects of atomoxetine in children with ASD and ID, this agent was effective for both social withdrawal and ADHD symptoms [134]. A previous review indicated that atomoxetine may be effective in high-functioning individuals with ASD or in those with a low severity of ASD. Individuals with severe ASD had more adverse effects of atomoxetine [135].

Unfortunately, people with ADHD are known for their poor compliance and adherence to treatment [136]. Most people believe that ADHD is a problem of impaired performance only in academic or work settings. Consequently, patients with ADHD generally assume they only need pharmacotherapy from Monday to Friday, but not during the weekend or the holidays. However, based on the chronic nature of ADHD, as well as the increased risk to be involved in conflicts, substance abuse, and driving accidents [137], discontinuation of medication can lead to a suboptimal control of symptomatology and poor outcomes.

11.11 Stigma in ADHD

The stigma around ADHD is striking. A recent research examined the online databases of several Flemish newspapers on articles on ADHD and ASD published between 2010 and 2014. Authors found a twofold more often negative coverage of ADHD compared to ASD, particularly in the domains of symptomatology, diagnostic assessment, and medical treatment [138]. Stigma related to ADHD is due to:

- poor knowledge about the nature of the disorder,
- prejudice about the validity and reliability of the ADHD diagnosis,
- prejudice about aggressive behavior of individuals with ADHD in general, thought of as persons with a tendency toward violence,
- the public's skepticism toward ADHD medications [7, 139],
- the stereotype that adult ADHD is a way to mask substance abuse [140].

Training about ADHD in adults is still scarce and generally not included in university programs for aspiring doctors or psychologists. Increasing awareness of the public and systematic training of healthcare professionals is essential to reduce stigma.

Stigma impedes patients to ask for help, with serious consequences for their lives. It is necessary to increase awareness about ADHD in adults and include it in the professionals' training programs. Thus, it is possible to reduce the many barriers that people with ADHD face to access proper diagnosis and treatment.

11.12 Conclusion

ADHD is a neurodevelopmental disorder with high heritability, causing impairment to individuals and their family, and posing a high burden to society. ADHD and ASD present shared environmental as well as biological risk factors, and their co-occurrence determines a more severe phenotype. When ASD and ADHD are comorbid, each disorder is more difficult to diagnose compared to the single condition [141], and people affected have an increased risk to develop additional psychiatric conditions. The ADHD diagnosis remains clinical, based on identifying the core symptoms of ADHD, which have been present since childhood and persist into adulthood.

Pharmacological treatments for ADHD, such as methylphenidate and atomoxetine, have been studied in individuals with ADHD+ASD, demonstrating efficacy in decreasing ADHD severity although with lower effect sizes than in people with only ADHD.

There is still a large and undiagnosed population of adults with ADHD. ADHD in ASD—if untreated—can reduce the efficacy of social skill programs for ASD and increase the risk for illicit drug use. Therefore, healthcare professionals should be alert for signs of comorbid ADHD. More research is needed to better understand the needs of adults with both ADHD+ASD, including in general health, around aging, treatment options, and the development of services across the lifespan.

References

1. Still GF. Some abnormal psychical conditions in children: the Goulstonian lectures. Lancet. 1902;1:1008–12.
2. Kramer F, Pollnow H. Über eine hyperkinetische Erkrankung im Kindesalter. Monatsschr Psychiatr Neurol. 1932;82:1–40.
3. Ross DM, Ross SA. Hyperactivity: research, theory and action. New York: Wiley; 1976.
4. APA. Diagnostic and statistical manual of mental disorders (DSM-III-R). 3rd Rev ed. Washington, DC: American Psychiatric Association; 1987.
5. APA. Diagnostic and statistical manual of mental disorders—DSM 5. In: APAD-T, editor. Force. 5th ed. Washington, DC: American Psychiatric Publishing; 2013.
6. Philipsen A, Hesslinger B, Tebartz van Elst L. Attention deficit hyperactivity disorder in adulthood: diagnosis, etiology and therapy. Dtsch Arztebl Int. 2008;105(17):311–7.
7. Kooij JJS, Bijlenga D, Salerno L, Jaeschke R, Bitter I, Balázs J. Updated European Consensus Statement on diagnosis and treatment of adult ADHD. Eur Psychiatry. 2019;56:14–34. https://doi.org/10.1016/j.eurpsy.2018.11.001.
8. Kooij JJS. Adult ADHD. Diagnostic assessment and treatment. 3rd ed. London: Springer-Verlag; 2013 . ISBN 978-1-4471-4138-9. https://doi.org/10.1007/978-1-4471-4138-9.
9. Skirrow C, McLoughlin G, Kuntsi J, Asherson P. Behavioral, neurocognitive and treatment overlap between attention-deficit/hyperactivity disorder and mood instability. Expert Rev Neurother. 2009;9:489–503. https://doi.org/10.1586/ern.09.2.
10. Skirrow C, Asherson P. Emotional lability, comorbidity and impairment in adults with attention-deficit hyperactivity disorder. J Affect Disord. 2013;147(1-3):80–6.
11. Fayyad J, Sampson NA, Hwang I, Adamowski T, Aguilar-Gaxiola S, Al-Hamzawi A, Andrade LH, Borges G, de Girolamo G, Florescu S, Gureje O, Haro JM, Hu C, Karam EG, Lee S, Navarro-Mateu F, O'Neill S, Pennell BE, Piazza M, Posada-Villa J, Ten Have M, Torres Y, Xavier M, Zaslavsky AM, Kessler RC, WHO World Mental Health Survey Collaborators. The descriptive epidemiology of DSM-IV Adult ADHD in the World Health Organization World Mental Health Surveys. Atten Defic Hyperact Disord. 2017;9(1):47–65.
12. de Graaf R, Kessler RC, Fayyad J, ten Have M, Alonso J, Angermeyer M, et al. The prevalence and effects of adult attention-deficit/hyperactivity disorder (ADHD) on the performance of workers: results from the WHO World Mental Health Survey Initiative. Occup Environ Med. 2008;65(12):835–42.
13. Ginsberg Y, Hirvikoski T, Lindefors N. Attention deficit hyperactivity disorder (ADHD) among longer-term prison inmates is a prevalent, persistent and disabling disorder. BMC Psychiatry. 2010;10:112. https://doi.org/10.1186/1471-244X-10-112.
14. Østergaard SD, Dalsgaard S, Faraone SV, Munk-Olsen T, Laursen TM. Teenage parenthood and birth rates for individuals with and without attention-deficit/hyperactivity disorder: a nationwide cohort study. J Am Acad Child Adolesc Psychiatry. 2017;56(7):578–584.e3. https://doi.org/10.1016/j.jaac.2017.05.003. Epub 2017 May 11.
15. Wymbs BT, Dawson AE, Egan TE, Sacchetti GM. Rates of intimate partner violence perpetration and victimization among adults with ADHD. J Atten Disord. 2016;23:949–58. pii: 1087054716653215.
16. Young S, Gudjonsson G, Asherson P, Theobald J, Oliver B, Scott C, et al. Attention deficit hyperactivity disorder and critical incidents in a Scottish prison population. Personal Individ Differ. 2009;46:265–9.
17. Manor I, Gutnik I, Ben-Dor DH, Apter A, Sever J, Tyano S, Weizman A, Zalsman G. Possible association between attention deficit hyperactivity disorder and attempted suicide in adolescents - a pilot study. Eur Psychiatry. 2010;25(3):146–50.
18. Dalsgaard S, Østergaard SD, Leckman JF, Mortensen PB, Pedersen MG. Mortality in children, adolescents, and adults with attention deficit hyperactivity disorder: a nationwide cohort study. Lancet. 2015;385(9983):2190–6. https://doi.org/10.1016/S0140-6736(14)61684-6.
19. Torgersen T, Gjervan B, Rasmussen K. ADHD in adults: a study of clinical characteristics, impairment and comorbidity. Nord J Psychiatry. 2006;60(1):38–43.

20. Cortese S, Moreira-Maia CR, St Fleur D, Morcillo-Peñalver C, Rohde LA, Faraone SV. Association between ADHD and obesity: a systematic review and meta-analysis. Am J Psychiatry. 2016;173(1):34–43.
21. Bijlenga D, van der Heijden KB, Breuk M, van Someren EJ, Lie ME, Boonstra AM, et al. Associations between sleep characteristics, seasonal depressive symptoms, lifestyle, and ADHD symptoms in adults. J Atten Disord. 2013;17(3):261–74.
22. Spencer TJ, Faraone SV, Tarko L, McDermott K, Biederman J. Attention-deficit/ hyperactivity disorder and adverse health outcomes in adults. J Nerv Ment Dis. 2014;202(10):725–31.
23. Stickley A, Koyanagi A, Takahashi H, Ruchkin V, Inoue Y, Kamio Y. Attention- deficit/hyperactivity disorder and physical multimorbidity: a population-based study. Eur Psychiatry. 2017;45:227–34.
24. Instanes JT, Klungsoyr K, Halmoy A, Fasmer OB, Adult ADHD, Haavik J. Comorbid somatic disease: a systematic literature review. J Atten Disord. 2018;22(3):203–28.
25. Kooij JJ, Bijlenga D. The circadian rhythm in adult attention-deficit/hyperactivity disorder: current state of affairs. Expert Rev Neurother. 2013;13(10):1107–16.
26. Kirono E, Imagawa H, Goto T, Montgomery W. Sociodemographics, comorbidities, healthcare utilization and work productivity in Japanese patients with adult ADHD. PLoS One. 2015;10(7):e0132233. https://doi.org/10.1371/journal.pone.0132233.
27. Jacob CP, Romanos J, Dempfle A, Heine M, Windemuth-Kieselbach C, Kruse A, et al. Co-morbidity of adult attention-deficit/hyperactivity disorder with focus on personality traits and related disorders in a tertiary referral center. Eur Arch Psychiatry Clin Neurosci. 2007;257(6):309–17. Epub 2007 Apr 1.
28. Van Veen MM, Kooij JJ, Boonstra AM, Gordijn MC, Van Someren EJ. Delayed circadian rhythm in adults with attention-deficit/hyperactivity disorder and chronic sleep-onset insomnia. Biol Psychiatry. 2010;67(11):1091–6.
29. Vogel SWN, Bijlenga D, Benjamins JS, Beekman ATF, Kooij JJS, Van Someren EJW. Attention deficit hyperactivity disorder symptom severity and sleep problems in adult participants of the Netherlands sleep registry. Sleep Med. 2017;40:94–102.
30. Martinez-Raga J, Szerman N, Knecht C, de Alvaro R. Attention deficit hyperactivity disorder and dual disorders. Educational needs for an underdiagnosed condition. Int J Adolesc Med Health. 2013;25(3):231–43. https://doi.org/10.1515/ijamh-2013-0057.
31. Katzman MA, Bilkey TS, Chokka PR, Fallu A, Klassen LJ. Adult ADHD and comorbid disorders: clinical implications of a dimensional approach. BMC Psychiatry. 2017;17:1–15. https://doi.org/10.1186/s12888-017-1463-3.
32. Chang Z, Quinn PD, Hur K, Gibbons RD, Sjölander A, Larsson H, D'Onofrio BM. Association between medication use for attention-deficit/hyperactivity disorder and risk of motor vehicle crashes. JAMA Psychiat. 2017;74(6):597–603. https://doi.org/10.1001/jamapsychiatry.2017.0659.
33. Liang SH, Yang YH, Kuo TY, Liao YT, Lin TC, Lee Y, McIntyre RS, Kelsen BA, Wang TN, Chen VC. Suicide risk reduction in youths with attention-deficit/hyperactivity disorder prescribed methylphenidate: a Taiwan nationwide population-based cohort study. Res Dev Disabil. 2018;72:96–105. https://doi.org/10.1016/j.ridd.2017.10.023.
34. Lichtenstein P, Halldner L, Zetterqvist J, Sjölander A, Serlachius E, Fazel S, Långström N, Larsson H. Medication for attention deficit-hyperactivity disorder and criminality. N Engl J Med. 2012;367(21):2006–14. https://doi.org/10.1056/NEJMoa1203241.
35. Joshi G, Faraone SV, Wozniak J, Petty C, Fried R, Galdo M, Furtak SL, McDermott K, Epstien C, Walker R, Caron A, Feinberg L, Biederman J. Examining the clinical correlates of autism spectrum disorder in youth by ascertainment source. J Autism Dev Disord. 2014;44(9):2117–26.
36. Salazar F, Baird G, Chandler S, Tseng E, O'sullivan T, Howlin P, Pickles A, Simonoff E. Co-occurring psychiatric disorders in preschool and elementary school-aged children with autism spectrum disorder. J Autism Dev Disord. 2015;45(8):2283–94.
37. Kaat AJ, Gadow KD, Lecavalier L. Psychiatric symptom impairment in children with autism spectrum disorders. J Abnorm Child Psychol. 2013;41(6):959–69.

38. Antshel KM, Zhang-James Y, Wagner KE, Ledesma A, Faraone SV. An update on the comorbidity of ADHD and ASD: a focus on clinical management. Expert Rev Neurother. 2016;16:279–93. https://doi.org/10.1586/14737175.2016.1146591.
39. Simonoff E, Pickles A, Charman T, Chandler S, Loucas T, Baird G. Psychiatric disorders in children with autism spectrum disorders: prevalence, comorbidity, and associated factors in a population-derived sample [Article]. J Am Acad Child Adolesc Psychiatry. 2008;47:921–9. https://doi.org/10.1097/CHI.0b013e318179964f.
40. Polanczyk GV, Willcutt EG, Salum GA, Kieling C, Rohde LA. ADHD prevalence estimates across three decades: an updated systematic review and meta-regression analysis. Int J Epidemiol. 2014;43(2):434–42.
41. Taurines R, Schwenck C, Westerwald E, Sachse M, Siniatchkin M, Freitag C. ADHD and autism: differential diagnosis or overlapping traits? A selective review. Atten Defic Hyperact Disord. 2012;4(3):115–39.
42. Lai M-C, Lombardo MV, Baron-Cohen S. Autism. Lancet. 2014;383:896–910.
43. Kotte A, Joshi G, Fried R, Uchida M, Spencer A, Woodworth KY, Kenworthy T, Faraone SV, Biederman J. Autistic traits in children with and without ADHD. Pediatrics. 2013;132(3):e612–22.
44. Cooper M, Martin J, Langley K, Hamshere M, Thapar A. Autistic traits in children with ADHD index clinical and cognitive problems. Eur Child Adolesc Psychiatry. 2014;23(1):23–34.
45. Miller M, Musser ED, Young GS, Olson B, Steiner RD, Nigg JT. Sibling recurrence risk and cross-aggregation of attention-deficit/hyperactivity disorder and autism spectrum disorder. JAMA Pediatr. 2019;173:147–52.
46. Boyle CA, Boulet S, Schieve LA, Cohen RA, Blumberg SJ, Yeargin-Allsopp M, et al. Trends in the prevalence of developmental disabilities in US children, 1997–2008. Pediatrics. 2011;127(6):1034–42.
47. Yoo HJ. Recent increase in autism and ADHD: true or inflated? J Korean Med Sci. 2013;28(7):974–5.
48. Kern JK, Geier DA, Sykes LK, Geier MR, Deth RC. Are ASD and ADHD a continuum? A comparison of pathophysiological similarities between the disorders. J Atten Disord. 2015;19:805–27. https://doi.org/10.1177/1087054712459886.
49. Banaschewski T, Poustka L, Holtmann M. Autism and ADHD across the life span. Differential diagnoses or comorbidity? Nervenarzt. 2011;82:573–80.
50. Grzadzinski R, Di Martino A, Brady E, Mairena MA, O'Neale M, Petkova E, Castellanos FX. Exam- ining autistic traits in children with ADHD: does the autism spectrum extend to ADHD? J Autism Dev Disord. 2011;41:1178–91.
51. Ronald A, Hoekstra RA. Autism spectrum disorders and autistic traits: a decade of new twin studies. Am J Med Genet Pt B Neuropsychiatr Genet. 2011;156B:255–74.
52. Nikolas MA, Burt SA. Genetic and environmental influences on ADHD symptom dimensions of inattention and hyperactivity: a meta-analysis. J Abnorm Psychol. 2010;119:1–17.
53. Hoekstra RA, Bartels M, Verweij CJH, Boomsma DI. Heritability of autistic traits in the general population. Arch Pediatr Adolesc Med. 2007;161:372–7.
54. Boomsma DI, Saviouk V, Hottenga J-J, Distel MA, de Moor MHM, Vink JM, et al. Genetic epidemiology of attention deficit hyperactivity disorder (ADHD index) in adults. PLoS One. 2010;12:e10621.
55. Larsson H, Asherson P, Chang Z, Ljung T, Friedrichs B, Larsson J-O, et al. Genetic and environmental influences on adult attention deficit hyperactivity disorde symptoms: a large Swedish population-based study of twins. Psychol Med. 2013;43:197–207.
56. Chen MH, Wei HT, Chen LC, Su TP, Bai YM, Hsu JW, et al. Autistic spectrum disorder, attention deficit hyperactivity disorder, and psychiatric comorbidities: a nationwide study. Res Autism Spectr Disord. 2015;10:1–6.
57. Martin J, Cooper M, Hamshere ML, Pocklington A, Scherer SW, Kent L, et al. Biological overlap of attention-deficit/hyperactivity disorder and autism spectrum disorder: evidence from copy number variants. J Am Acad Child Adolesc Psychiatry. 2014;53:761–770, e726.

58. Williams NM, Franke B, Mick E, Anney RJ, Freitag CM, Gill M, et al. Genome-wide analysis of copy number variants in attention deficit hyperactivity disorder: the role of rare variants and duplications at 15q13. 3. Am J Psychiatry. 2012;169:195–204.
59. Williams NM, Zaharieva I, Martin A, Langley K, Mantripragada K, Fossdal R, et al. Rare chromosomal deletions and duplications in attention-deficit hyperactivity disorder: a genome-wide analysis. Lancet. 2010;376:1401–8.
60. Davis NO, Kollins SH. Treatment for co-occurring attention deficit/hyperactivity disorder and autism spectrum disorder. Neurotherapeutics. 2012;9:518–30. https://doi.org/10.1007/s13311-012-0126-9.
61. Ghirardi L, Brikell I, Kuja-Halkola R, Freitag CM, Franke B, Asherson P, et al. The familial co-aggregation of ASD and ADHD: a register-based cohort study. Mol Psychiatry. 2017;23:257–62.
62. Mason J, Scior K. 'Diagnostic Overshadowing' amongst clinicians working with people with intellectual disabilities in the UK. JARID. 2004;17:85–90. https://doi.org/10.1111/j.1360-2322.2004.00184.x.
63. Thapar A, Cooper M, Eyre O, Langley K. What have we learnt about the causes of ADHD? J Child Psychol Psychiatry. 2013;54:3–16.
64. Oerlemans AM, Burmanje MJ, Franke B, Buitelaar JK, Hartman CA, Rommelse NN. Identifying unique versus shared pre- and perinatal risk factors for ASD and ADHD using a simplex-multiplex stratification. J Abnorm Child Psychol. 2015;44(5):923–35.
65. Hoogman M, Bralten J, Hibar DP, Mennes M, Zwiers MP, Schweren LSJ, van Hulzen KJE, Medland SE, Shumskaya E, Jahanshad N, Zeeuw P, Szekely E, Sudre G, Wolfers T, Onnink AMH, Dammers JT, Mostert JC, Vives-Gilabert Y, Kohls G, Oberwelland E, Seitz J, Schulte-Rüther M, Ambrosino S, Doyle AE, Høvik MF, Dramsdahl M, Tamm L, van Erp TGM, Dale A, Schork A, Conzelmann A, Zierhut K, Baur R, McCarthy H, Yoncheva YN, Cubillo A, Chantiluke K, Mehta MA, Paloyelis Y, Hohmann S, Baumeister S, Bramati I, Mattos P, Tovar-Moll F, Douglas P, Banaschewski T, Brandeis D, Kuntsi J, Asherson P, Rubia K, Kelly C, Martino AD, Milham MP, Castellanos FX, Frodl T, Zentis M, Lesch KP, Reif A, Pauli P, Jernigan TL, Haavik J, Plessen KJ, Lundervold AJ, Hugdahl K, Seidman LJ, Biederman J, Rommelse N, Heslenfeld DJ, Hartman CA, Hoekstra PJ, Oosterlaan J, Polier GV, Konrad K, Vilarroya O, Ramos-Quiroga JA, Soliva JC, Durston S, Buitelaar JK, Faraone SV, Shaw P, Thompson PM, Franke B. Subcortical brain volume differences in participants with attention deficit hyperactivity disorder in children and adults: a cross-sectional mega-analysis. Lancet Psychiatry. 2017;4(4):310–9.
66. Antshel KM, Zhang-James Y, Faraone SV. The comorbidity of ADHD and autism spectrum disorder. Expert Rev Neurother. 2013;13(10):1117–28.
67. Sudre G, Szekely E, Sharp W, Kasparek S, Shaw P. Multimodal mapping of the brain's functional connectivity and the adult outcome of attention deficit hyperactivity disorder. Proc Natl Acad Sci U S A. 2017;114(44):11787–92.
68. Shaw P, Eckstrand K, Sharp W, Blumenthal J, Lerch JP, Greenstein D, et al. Attention-deficit/hyperactivity disorder is characterized by a delay in cortical maturation. Proc Natl Acad Sci U S A. 2007;104:19649–54. https://doi.org/10.1073/pnas.0707741104.
69. Shaw P, Malek M, Watson B, Sharp W, Evans A, Greenstein D. Development of cortical surface area and gyrification in attention-deficit/hyperactivity disorder. Biol Psychiatry. 2012;72:191–7. https://doi.org/10.1016/j.biopsych.2012.01.031.
70. Adamo N, Huo L, Adelsberg S, Petkova E, Castellanos FX, Di Martino A. Response time intra-subject variability: commonalities between children with autism spectrum disorders and children with ADHD. Eur Child Adolesc Psychiatry. 2014b;23(2):69–79.
71. Flehming HC, Steinborn M, Langner R, Scholz A, Westhoff K. Assessing intraindividual variability in sustained attention: reliability, relation to speed and accuracy, and practice effects. Psychol Sci. 2007;49(2):132–49.
72. Johnson KA, Robertson IH, Kelly SP, Silk TJ, Barry E, et al. Dissociation in performance of children with ADHD and high-functioning autism on a task of sustained attention. Neuropsychologia. 2007;45:2234–45.

73. Saville CWN, Pawling R, Trullinger M, Daley D, Intriligator J, Klein C. On the stability of instability: optimising the reliability of intra-subject variability of reaction times. Personal Individ Differ. 2011;51(2):148–53.
74. Kuntsi J, Stevenson J. Psychological mechanisms in hyperactivity: II. The role of genetic factors. J Child Psychol Psychiatry. 2001;42(2):211–9.
75. Wood AC, Asherson P, van der Meere JJ, Kuntsi J. Separation of genetic influences on attention deficit hyperactivity disorder symptoms and reaction time performance from those in IQ. Psychol Med. 2010;40(6):1027–37.
76. Kuntsi J, Wood AC, Rijsdijk F, Johnson KA, Andreou P, Albrecht B, Arias- Vasquez A, et al. Separation of cognitive impairments in attention-deficit/hyperactivity disorder into 2 familial factors. Arch Gen Psychiatry. 2010;67(11):1159–67.
77. Rommelse NN, Altink ME, Oosterlaan J, Beem L, Buschgens CJ, Buitelaar J, Sergeant JA. Speed, variability, and timing of motor output in ADHD: which measures are useful for endophenotypic research? Behav Genet. 2008;38(2):121–32.
78. Kofler MJ, Alderson RM, Raiker JS, Bolden J, Sarver DE, Rapport MD. Working memory and intraindividual variability as neurocognitive indicators in ADHD: examining competing model predictions. Neuropsychology. 2014;28(3):459–71.
79. Castellanos FX, Sonuga-Barke EJ, Scheres A, Di Martino A, Hyde C, Walters JR. Varieties of attention-deficit/hyperactivity disorder-related intra-individual variability. Biol Psychiatry. 2005;57:1416–23.
80. Epstein JN, Langberg JM, Rosen PJ, Graham A, Narad ME, Antonini TN, et al. Evidence for higher reaction time variability for children with ADHD on a range of cognitive tasks including reward and event rate manipulations. [Research Support, N.I.H., Extramural]. Neuropsychology. 2011;25:427–41. https://doi.org/10.1037/a0022155.
81. Adamo N, Di Martino A, Esu L, Petkova E, Johnson K, Kelly S, Castellanos FX, Zuddas A. Increased response-time variability across different cognitive tasks in children with ADHD. J Atten Disord. 2014a;18(5):434–46. https://doi.org/10.1177/1087054712439419. Epub 2012 Apr 16.
82. Lundervold AJ, et al. Attention deficits in children with combined autism and ADHD: a CPT study. J Atten Disord. 2016;20:599–609.
83. Tye C, Asherson P, Ashwood KL, Azadi B, Bolton P, McLoughlin G. Attention and inhibition in children with ASD, ADHD and co-morbid ASD + ADHD: an event- related potential study. Psychol Med. 2013;44(5):1101–16.
84. Anholt GE, Cath DC, van Oppen P, Eikelenboom M, Smit JH, van Megen H, van Balkom AJ. Autism and ADHD symptoms in patients with OCD: are they associated with specific OC symptom dimensions or OC symptom severity? J Autism Dev Disord. 2010;40(5):580–9.
85. Craig F, Lamanna AL, Margari F, Matera E, Simone M, Margari L. Overlap between autism spectrum disorders and attention deficit hyperactivity disorder: searching for distinctive/common clinical features. Autism Res. 2015;8(3):328–37. https://doi.org/10.1002/aur.1449.
86. Sinzig J, Morsch D, Bruning N, Schmidt MH, Lehmkuhl G. Inhibition, flexibility, working memory and planning in autism spectrum disorders with and without comorbid ADHD-symptoms. Child Adolesc Psychiatry Ment Health. 2008;2:4.
87. Lawson RA, Papadakis AA, Higginson CI, Barnett JE, Wills MC, Strang JF, Wallace GL, Kenworthy L. Everyday executive function impairments predict comorbid psychopathology in autism spectrum and attention deficit hyperactivity disorders. Neuropsychology. 2015;29(3):445–53.
88. Kerekes N, Brandstrom S, Lundstrom S, Rastam M, Nilsson T, Anckarsater H. ADHD, autism spectrum disorder, temperament, and character: phenotypical associations and etiology in a Swedish childhood twin study. Compr Psychiatry. 2013;54:1140–7. https://doi.org/10.1016/j.comppsych.2013.05.009.
89. Yerys BE, Wallace GL, Sokoloff JL, Shook DA, James JD, Kenworthy L. Attention deficit/hyperactivity disorder symptoms moderate cogni tion and behavior in children with autism spectrum disorders. Autism Res. 2009;2:322–33. https://doi.org/10.1002/aur.103.

90. Wilens TE, Upadhyaya HP. Impact of substance use disorder on ADHD and its treatment. J Clin Psychiatry. 2007;68(8):e20.
91. van Emmerik van Oortmerssen K, Van de Glind G, Van den Brink B, Smit F, Crunelle CL, Swetsa M, Schoevers RA. Prevalence of attention-deficit hyperactivity disorder in substance use disorder patients: a meta-analysis and meta-regression analysis. Drug Alcohol Depend. 2012;122:11–9.
92. Rengit AC, McKowen JW, O'Brien J, Howe YJ, McDougle CJ. Brief report: autism spectrum disorder and substance use disorder: a review and case study. J Autism Dev Disord. 2016;46(7):2514–9.
93. Hofvander B, Delorme R, Chaste P, Agneta Nydén A, Wentz E, Stahlberg O, Herbrecht E, Stopin A, Anckarsäter H, Gillberg C, Rastam M, Leboyer M. Psychiatric and psychosocial problems in adults with normal-intelligence autism spectrum disorders. BMC Psychiatry. 2009;9:35.
94. Lugnegard T, Hallerback MU, Gillberg C. Psychiatric comorbidity in young adults with a clinical diagnosis of Asperger syndrome. Res Dev Disabil. 2011;32:1910–7.
95. Sizoo B, Van den Brink W, Koeter M, Gorissen van Eenigee M, Van Wijngaarden-Cremers P, Van der Gaag RJ. Treatment seeking adults with autism or ADHD and co-morbid substance use disorder: prevalence, risk factors and functional disability. Drug Alcohol Depend. 2010;107:44–50.
96. De Alwis D, Agrawal A, Reiersen AM, Constantino JN, Henders A, Martin NG, Lynskey MT. ADHD symptoms, autistic traits, and substance use and misuse in adult Australian twins. J Stud Alcohol Drugs. 2014;75(2):211–21.
97. Antshel KM, Polacek C, McMahon M, Dygert K, Spenceley L, Dygert L, Miller L, Faisal F. Comorbid ADHD and anxiety affect social skills group intervention treatment efficacy in children with autism spectrum disorders. J Dev Behav Pediatr. 2011;32(6):439–46.
98. Zablotsky B, Bradshaw CP, Anderson C, Law PA. The association between bullying and the psychological functioning of children with autism spectrum disorders. J Dev Behav Pediatr. 2013;34(1):1–8.
99. Sterzing PR, Shattuck PT, Narendorf SC, Wagner M, Cooper BP. Bullying involvement and autism spectrum disorders: prevalence and correlates of bullying involvement among adolescents with an autism spectrum disorder. Arch Pediatr Adolesc Med. 2012;166(11):1058–64.
100. Goodheart CD. A primer for ICD-10-CM users: psychological and behavioural conditions. Washington, DC: American Psychological Association; 2014.
101. Goodman D. ADHD in adults: update for clinicians on diagnosis and assessment. Prim Psychiatry. 2009;16(11):38–47.
102. Kooij JJS, Francken MH. Diagnostic interview of ADHD in Adults. Version 2.0 (DIVA). Hague: DIVA Foundation; 2010.
103. Pettersson R, Soderstrom S, Nilsson KW. Diagnosing ADHD in adults: an examination of the discriminative validity of neuropsychological tests and diagnostic assessment instruments. J Atten Disord. 2018;22:1019–31.
104. Ramos-Quiroga JA, Bosch R, Richarte V, Valero S, Gomez-Barros N, Nogueira M, et al. Criterion and concurrent validity of Conners Adult ADHD Diagnostic Interview for DSM-IV (CAADID) Spanish version. [Spanish] Validez de criterio y concurrente de la version espanola de la Conners Adult ADHD Diagnostic Interview for DSM-IV. Rev Psiquiatr Salud Ment. 2012;5(4):229–35.
105. Adler LA, Kessler RC, Spencer T. Adult Self Report Scale. ASRS-V1.1. New York: World Health Organization; 2003.
106. Barkley RA. Barkley Adult ADHD Rating Scale-IV (BAARS-IV). New York: Guilford Press; 2011.
107. Conners CK, Erhardt D, Sparrow E. Conners' Adult ADHD Rating Scales: technical manual. North Tonawanda: Multi-Health Systems; 1999.
108. Brown TE. Brown attention-deficit disorder scales. San Antonio: The Psychological Corporation; 1996.
109. Epstein J, Johnson DE, Conners CK. Conners' adult ADHD diagnostic interview for DSM-IV. North Tonawanda: Multi-Health Systems; 2001.

110. Wasserman T, Wasserman LD. The sensitivity and specificity of neuropsychological tests in the diagnosis of attention deficit hyperactivity disorder. Appl Neuropsychol Child. 2012;1(2):90–9. https://doi.org/10.1080/21622965.2012.702025. Epub 2012 Jul 10.
111. Kooij JJS, Boonstra MA, Swinkels SHN, Bekker EM, de Noord I, Buitelaar JK. Reliability, validity, and utility of instruments for self-report and informant report concerning symptoms of ADHD in adult patients. J Atten Disord. 2008;11(4):445–58. https://doi.org/10.1177/1087054707299367.
112. De Crescenzo F, Cortese S, Adamo N, et al. Pharmacological and non-pharmacological treatment of adults with ADHD: a meta-review. Evid Based Ment Health. 2017;20:4–11.
113. Faraone SV, Glatt SJ. A comparison of the efficacy of medications for adult attention-deficit/hyperactivity disorder using meta-analysis of effect sizes. J Clin Psychiatry. 2010;71:754–63.
114. Cortese S, Adamo N, Del Giovane C, Mohr-Jensen C, Hayes AJ, Carucci S, Atkinson LZ, Tessari L, Banaschewski T, Coghill D, Hollis C, Simonoff E, Zuddas A, Barbui C, Purgato M, Steinhausen HC, Shokraneh F, Xia J, Cipriani A. Comparative efficacy and tolerability of medications for attention-deficit hyperactivity disorder in children, adolescents, and adults: a systematic review and network meta-analysis. Lancet Psychiatry. 2018;5(9):727–38.
115. Wietecha LA, Clemow DB, Buchanan AS, Young JL, Sarkis EH, Findling RL. Atomoxetine increased effect over time in adults with attention-deficit/hyperactivity disorder treated for up to 6 months: pooled analysis of two double-blind, placebo-controlled, randomized trials. CNS Neurosci Ther. 2016;22(7):546–57.
116. Maneeton N, Maneeton B, Intaprasert S, Woottiluk P. A systematic review of randomized controlled trials of bupropion versus methylphenidate in the treatment of attention-deficit/hyperactivity disorder. Neuropsychiatr Dis Treat. 2014;10:1439–49.
117. Hamedi M, Mohammdi M, Ghaleiha A, Keshavarzi Z, Jafarnia M, Keramatfar R, et al. Bupropion in adults with attention-deficit/hyperactivity disorder: a randomized, double-blind study. Acta Med Iran. 2014;52(9):675–80.
118. Turner D. A review of the use of modafinil for attention-deficit hyperactivity disorder. Expert Rev Neurother. 2006;6(4):455–68.
119. Arnold VK, Feifel D, Earl CQ, Yang R, Adler LA. A 9-week, randomized, double-blind, placebo-controlled, parallel-group, dose-finding study to evaluate the efficacy and safety of modafinil as treatment for adults with ADHD. J Atten Disord. 2014;18(2):133–44.
120. Wernicke JF, Faries D, Girod D, et al. Cardiovascular effects of atomoxetine in children, adolescents, and adults. Drug Saf. 2003;26(10):729–40.
121. Dean L. Atomoxetine therapy and CYP2D6 genotype. In: Pratt V, McLeod H, Rubinstein W, et al., editors. Medical genetics summaries [Internet]. Bethesda, MD: National Center for Biotechnology Information (US); 2015. https://www.ncbi.nlm.nih.gov/books/NBK315951/.
122. Mészáros A, Czobor P, Bálint S, Komlósi S, Simon V, Bitter I. Pharmacotherapy of adult attention deficit hyperactivity disorder (ADHD): a meta-analysis. Int J Neuropsychopharmacol. 2009;12(8):1137–47. https://doi.org/10.1017/S1461145709990198.
123. Hirvikoski T, Waaler E, Alfredsson J, Pihlgren C, Holmstrom A, Johnson A, et al. Reduced ADHD symptoms in adults with ADHD after structured skills training group: results from a randomized controlled trial. Behav Res Ther. 2011;49(3):175–85.
124. Mongia M, Hechtman L. Cognitive behavior therapy for adults with attention deficit/hyperactivity disorder: a review of recent randomized controlled trials. Curr Psychiatry Rep. 2012;14(5):561–7.
125. Emilsson B, Gudjonsson G, Sigurdsson JF, Baldursson G, Einarsson E, Olafsdottir H, et al. Cognitive behaviour therapy in medication-treated adults with ADHD and persistent Symptoms: a randomized controlled trial. BMC Psychiatry. 2011;11:116.
126. Seixas M, Weiss M, Muller U. Systematic review of national and international guidelines on attention-deficit hyperactivity disorder. J Psychopharmacol (Oxf). 2012;26(6):753–65.
127. Arnold LE, Hodgkins P, Caci H, Kahle J, Young S. Effect of treatment modality on long-term outcomes in attention-deficit/hyperactivity disorder: a systematic review. PLoS One. 2015;10(2):e0116407. https://doi.org/10.1371/journal.pone.eCollection.2015.
128. Philipsen A. Psychotherapy in adult attention deficit hyperactivity disorder: implications for treatment and research. Expert Rev. 2012;12(10):1217–25.

129. Young S, Bramham J. Cognitive-behavioural therapy for ADHD in adolescents and adults: a psychological guide to practice. 2nd ed. Chichester: Wiley; 2012.
130. Kubik JA. Efficacy of ADHD coaching for adults with ADHD. J Atten Disord. 2010;13(5):442–53. https://doi.org/10.1177/1087054708329960.
131. Prevatt F, Yelland S. An empirical evaluation of ADHD coaching in college students. J Atten Disord. 2015;19(8):666–77. https://doi.org/10.1177/1087054713480036.
132. Pearson DA, Santos CW, Aman MG, Arnold LE, Casat CD, Mansour R, Lane DM, Loveland KA, Bukstein OG, Jerger SW, Factor P, Vanwoerden S, Perez E, et al. Effects of extended release methylphenidate treatment on ratings of attention-deficit/hyperactivity disorder (ADHD) and associated behavior in children with autism spectrum disorders and ADHD symptoms. J Child Adolesc Psychopharmacol. 2013;23(5):337–51.
133. Reichow B, Volkmar FR, Bloch MH. Systematic review and meta-analysis of pharmacological treatment of the symptoms of attention-deficit/hyperactivity disorder in children with pervasive developmental disorders. J Autism Dev Disord. 2013;43(10):2435–41.
134. Kilincaslan A, Mutluer TD, Pasabeyoglu B, Tutkunkardas MD, Mukaddes NM. Effects of atomoxetine in individuals with attention-deficit/hyperactivity disorder and low-functioning autism spectrum disorder. J Child Adolesc Psychopharmacol. 2016;26(9):798–806.
135. Ghanizadeh A. Atomoxetine for treating ADHD symptoms in autism: a systematic review. J Atten Disord. 2013;17(8):635–40. https://doi.org/10.1177/1087054712443154. Epub 2012 Apr 27.
136. Gajria K, Lu M, Sikirica V, Greven P, Zhong Y, Qin P, Xie J. Adherence, persistence, and medication discontinuation in patients with attention-deficit/hyperactivity disorder - a systematic literature review. Neuropsychiatr Dis Treat. 2014;10:1543–69. https://doi.org/10.2147/NDT.S65721.
137. Barkley RA, Guevremont DC, Anastopoulos AD, DuPaul GJ, Shelton TL. Driving-related risks and outcomes of attention deficit/hyper-activity disorder in adolescents and young adults: a 3-5 year follow-up survey. Pediatrics. 1993;92:212–8.
138. Baeyens D, Moniquet A, Danckaerts M, van der Oord S. A comparative study of the structural stigmatisation of ADHD and autism spectrum disorder in Flemish newspapers. Tijdschr Psychiatr. 2017;59(5):269–77.
139. Mueller AK, Fuermaier ABM, Koerts J, Tucha L. Stigma in attention deficit hyperactivity disorder. Atten Defic Hyperact Disord. 2012;4(3):101–14.
140. Geffen J, Forster K. Treatment of adult ADHD: a clinical perspective. Ther Adv Psychopharmacol. 2018;8:25–32.
141. Gargaro BA, Rinehart NJ, Bradshaw JL, Tonge BJ, Sheppard DM. Autism and ADHD: how far have we come in the comorbidity debate? Neurosci Biobehav Rev. 2011;35(5):1081–8.

Behavioural Interventions in Challenging Behaviours

12

Serafino Corti, Roberto Cavagnola, Giovanni Miselli, Francesco Fioriti, Mauro Leoni, Davide Carnevali, Laura Galli, Giovanni Michelini, and Giuseppe Chiodelli

12.1 Differential Diagnosis of Challenging Behaviour, Psychopathology or Other Health Problems

People with ASD have a very high prevalence of challenging behaviour and psychopathological problems. Several scientific studies demonstrate that the severity and intensity of these states are directly correlated to the severity of the patients' autism, their communication and social difficulties, and adaptive skills [1]. However, some psychoeducational treatments may significantly decrease the frequency, duration or intensity of challenging behaviour. The choice of a suitable treatment for challenging behaviour means identifying a clear methodology for the analysis of the problem and finding the most appropriate psychoeducational and behavioural treatments [2].

The first step of this methodological approach is to make a correct differential diagnosis of challenging behaviour, psychopathologies or other health problems. In the autism spectrum, these phenomena may very often be either overlapping or confused. It is therefore crucial to understand the condition of the individual in order to identify the best treatment.

A brief summary of the threefold differential analysis follows:

1. *The observed behaviour is challenging behaviour.*

   In this case, it means that the learning history of the person with ASD is the "cause" of the observed behaviour. In this situation, it is necessary to proceed as indicated in the following pages:

S. Corti (✉) · R. Cavagnola · G. Miselli · F. Fioriti · M. Leoni · D. Carnevali · L. Galli
G. Michelini · G. Chiodelli
Department of Disability, Fondazione Istituto Ospedaliero di Sospiro, Sospiro, Italy
e-mail: serafino.corti@fondazionesospiro.it; roberto.cavagnola@fondazionesospiro.it; giovanni.miselli@fondazionesospiro.it; francesco.fioriti@fondazionesospiro.it; mauro.leoni@fondazionesospiro.it; davide.carnevali@fondazionesospiro.it; maria_laura.galli@fondazionesospiro.it; giovanni.michelini@fondazionesospiro.it; chiodelli.giuseppe@fondazionesospiro.it

R. Keller (ed.), *Psychopathology in Adolescents and Adults with Autism Spectrum Disorders*, https://doi.org/10.1007/978-3-030-26276-1_12

- By defining in operational terms the challenging behaviour
- By measuring its intensity, duration, frequency and latency in order to establish a baseline
- By carrying out a functional analysis in order to identify the function of the challenging behaviour
- By implementing behavioural strategies both to increase skills in the person with ASD and decrease their challenging behaviour

When the observed behaviour is clearly defined as challenging, the main treatment strategy should be behavioural, whereas pharmacological therapy should only be used as a second-choice approach [2].

2. *The observed behaviour is not challenging behaviour, but it is the expression of a form of psychopathology or other health problems.*

   In this case, psychopathologies (such as depression, anxiety disorder, obsessive-compulsive behaviour and psychosis) or other health problems (such as pain) are co-morbid with ASD. These conditions are often expressed in very different forms in people with ASD as opposed to the neurotypical population. The communicative and social deficits of people with autism and the condition of intellectual disability, often associated with ASD, may in fact mask (diagnostic overshadowing) the presence of psychopathologies or other health problems, chief among them pain. In this case, it is necessary to understand whether the observed behaviours are the behavioural equivalents of some forms of psychopathologies or the atypical expression of pain. This differential diagnosis is carried out both by applying a functional analysis (i.e. verifying the relationship between the observed behaviour and the changes in its context) and by using tools for the assessment of pain and specific psychopathologies for this population, such as the Diagnostic manual—Intellectual Disability (DM-ID-2) [3], Diagnostic Criteria for Psychiatric Disorders for Use with Adults with Learning Disabilities (DC-LD) [4], SPAIID-G [5], Pain and Discomfort Scale (PADS) [6]. In this latter case, pharmacological treatment is no longer a second choice, but it is an option that should be used from the beginning of treatment, in addition to psychoeducational and psychotherapeutic treatments. The present chapter will not address the treatments related to this second case.

3. *The observed behaviour is a form of challenging behaviour in co-morbidity with a psychopathological problem.*

   In this third case, the observed behaviour derives both from a learning history and from a psychopathological problem. It is not of paramount importance to understand whether the challenging behaviour is secondary to the psychopathological problems or the psychopathological problem is secondary to the challenging behaviour. In both cases, it is necessary to apply multi-component strategies for the treatment of the psychopathological problem and the lessening of the challenging behaviour. The present chapter will not address the treatments for this third case.

12.2 Operationalisation of Challenging Behaviour and Problem-Solving

The first operational step towards decreasing challenging behaviour is the definition and description of challenging behaviour [7].

When challenging behaviours are described, usually general terms such as the following are employed: agitated, aggressive, nervous, etc.

However, this type of language creates difficulties because not only does it not allow for a common vision of the observed behaviour and treatment, but also because it prevents the use of a precise measurement system of the behaviour.

Behaviour can be said to be well described if it can be measured. Measurement is the cornerstone of the evidence-based philosophy. Operationalisation is therefore also a prerequisite for the subsequent observation and measurement. Operationalising behaviour means describing it very precisely by separating the phase of interpretation of the behaviour with that of its description and measurement. Behaviour generally described as "aggressive" can thus be operationalised in different ways according to the actual form of behaviour; for example: (a) "they punched people's back"; (b) other people's hair pulling; (c) "they bite people's arms"; (d) "they spit in other people's faces"; (e) "they shout insults such as 'I hate you, I'll beat you up'".

Once behaviour has been operationalised, an assessment of how problematic it may be should be carried out in order to start the treatment of more severe behaviours. Evans and Meyer identify a series of indexes for the categorisation of behaviour as excessive, and aiding problem-solving decisions:

1. Does the behaviour represent a life threat?
2. Does the behaviour put the person's health at risk?
3. Is the behaviour dangerous for others?
4. Does the behaviour cause damage to property?
5. Does the behaviour interfere with learning?
6. Could the extinction of the behaviour lead to the improvement of other behaviours?
7. Is there no positive evolution in the course of the behaviour, and/or is it worsening?
8. Could the behaviour deteriorate in the near future if not treated?
9. Is the behaviour of major concern to family members and educators?
10. Has the behaviour been a problem for some time now?
11. Does this behaviour interfere with community acceptance?

These indexes can be evaluated on a dichotomous scale of absence/presence which helps to identify an index of problematicity for each form of challenging behaviour.

12.3 Observation and Measurement of Challenging Behaviour

The key to understanding the functions of behaviour is the measure of variability of behaviour itself. In which context does it increase its frequency? In which others does it decrease? Each variation of a behaviour parameter is a valuable source of information about the variables that control and maintain it.

In the observation and measurement of the same individual's behaviour, therefore, there is an opportunity to verify both how this "moves" at different times and in different contexts, thus shedding light on the functions that govern it, and on the appropriateness of the interventions that have been implemented [7].

When approaching challenging behaviour, the first step is understanding how present and pervasive it is in the patient's life, from the point of view its frequency, duration and intensity. This type of measurement is called "baseline". The baseline thus represents a condition of control which allows for the verification of the efficacy of the interventions which have been designed at the same time as they are being applied. It is worth mentioning that not only do the recorded results represent a benefit for the patient receiving treatment, but they are also an important source of reinforcement for all the people involved in the treatment process. In this sense, monitoring the intervention represents the highest degree of flexibility. Appropriate and necessary changes to the intervention plan can only be put into action when there is full understanding of the progress of the intervention [7].

Continuously gathering and recording the occurrences of behaviour, especially if it is a prolonged phase and the behaviour is particularly pervasive, may be a costly practice. Alternative forms, such as auto-monitoring procedures, may be of great help from this point of view; however, the use of such a technique can only be carried out by people who are able to distinguish their own behaviours. For all these reasons, the frequent use of sampling observation and behaviour measurement procedures represent a far more economic approach.

As far as observation systems are concerned, there is a broad array of methods for collecting assessment data. The following is not a comprehensive analysis of such procedures, an in-depth review would go far beyond the purposes of this chapter, but it is only a simple overview to understand how, starting from the different characteristics of certain challenging behaviours, specific procedures could be identified.

A distinction can be made between continuous and sample recording [7]. Continuous recording registers all occurrences of behaviour. In other words, behaviour is measured by continuous recording when its entire frequency is recorded for a given time of observation, or when within a set time frame, all the behaviour's duration is measured. For example, data can be collected and observed for the entire period of wakefulness, and either during attendance at the day centre or during the activity hours. This procedure, as mentioned above, may represent a problem both for the observational load and for the human resources available to conduct such an observation.

The main alternatives to continuous recording are sampling techniques which divide the observation period in time intervals, or the recordings of the permanent products of behaviour.

The observation period in the sampling techniques is divided into intervals and the observers record whether the behaviour occurs during each interval [7]. For this reason, these procedures provide an estimate of the behaviour.

The most common sampling observation procedures are:

(a) whole interval
(b) partial interval
(c) momentary time sampling

The whole interval procedure consists in dividing the observation period into equal short intervals and record when and if the behaviour occurs for the whole duration of the interval. It is used when the behaviour denotes continuity or duration (cooperative game; or behaviours such as rocking back and forth, verbal or motor stereotypies). It provides a better estimate of brief behaviours with shorter intervals and it is possible to improve the estimate of the behaviour by shortening the interval.

The partial interval procedure is similar to the previous one, but the recording only takes place if the behaviour occurs during any part of the interval. It requires the observer's attention only until the behaviour is observed in that interval. It works well for momentary behaviours (such as punching someone sitting at the table, swearing and spitting) or actions of short duration.

During the momentary time sampling, in the same way as in the previous procedures, the observation period is divided into equal intervals and the behaviour is recorded only at the end of the interval. When the time interval expires, the observer records the presence or absence of the behaviour at that precise moment. It is particularly easy as it greatly reduces the observational load. It is also useful when recording multiple individuals of a same group engaged in particular behaviours, as well as recording different behaviours of a single individual. It is suitable for the observation of high-frequency (i.e. very frequent self-injury) and continuous behaviours (i.e. sleeping) [7].

12.4 Assessment and Functional Analysis

The essential and important skills for the successful and evidence-based treatment of challenging behaviour are knowing how to measure a behaviour's baseline and verifying the effectiveness of an ongoing intervention. However, another fundamental professional skill is needed and it should be put into practice in the intervention on challenging behaviours: isolating the behaviour's functions. Functional analysis represents, from this perspective, the set of useful procedures for understanding the reasons why specific challenging behaviour, following a learning history, has arisen and is maintained within the behavioural repertoire of an individual [8–10].

A truly effective intervention must necessarily focus on carrying out a functional analysis and identifying the hypothesis of the functional value of behaviour [11, 12].

For this reason, there are different methodologies of functional assessment that aim to help us provide answers to fundamental questions: why does a certain behaviour continue to manifest itself? What are the functions it performs? What are its motivations? What kind of relationship exists between the challenging behaviour and the context in which it manifests itself?

The ABC analysis (Antecedent, Behaviour, Consequence), through the three contingency terms, is what ultimately allows us to comprehend how the context affects the behaviour and vice versa.

Understanding or identifying the hypothesis of functional value of behaviour will not only enable the selection of effective psychoeducational procedures for decreasing challenging behaviour, but also and most importantly it will indicate which new behaviours should be taught, increased, or which new opportunities should be provided to the individual.

The functional analysis' systems can be classified in different ways. Here, we will limit the description to two different, though heterogeneous, categories of procedures:

Indirect functional assessment procedures in which the hypotheses regarding the functional value of behaviour are formulated through interviews, questionnaires, checklists or interviews with the parents, operators, people who know the patient with autism well. However effective these indirect tools may be, they should be considered as the first step towards the functional assessment process.

A few examples of functional assessment tools are:

- ***Motivation Assessment Scale*** (M.A.S., [13–16])
- ***Functional Analysis Screening Tool*** [17, 18]
- ***Setting Events Checklist*** [19]
- ***Open-Ended Functional Assessment Interview*** developed by Gregory P. Hanley, (Developed August, 2002; Revised: August, 2009)

In the **direct** procedures, unlike the previous ones, the observation and recording of the behaviour take place during, or immediately close to, the occurrence of the behaviour itself. In other words, the operators or parents themselves are the direct observers of the challenging behaviour in what may be called "real time" [7].

The direct measures of behaviour clearly require more time and precision from the users, but they concurrently guarantee a greater abundance of information than indirect measurements.

The descriptive ABC is the most common form of functional assessment of behaviour. This type of analysis requires a precise description of the antecedent event of the challenging behaviour, within which it will be possible to identify the discriminative stimuli that control the behaviour and all the motivational events that favour its manifestation. Then, a description of the behaviour's consequence is required. Such consequences contain the main function of the behaviour itself. In particular, the description may provide correlations between the behaviours and consequences which may reinforce, positively or negatively, the challenging behaviour.

The compilation of different cards according to the scheme of the three contingency terms enables the identification of those contextual variables which activate and maintain the behaviour.

The direct functional assessment procedure (ABC) has several advantages; the main one is that the observer witnesses and records the antecedent events and consequences of the challenging behaviour immediately after its manifestation, thus contributing to increasing the objectivity and accuracy of the recording. However, the downside of this procedure is related to the large amount of time needed in comparison with the indirect methods.

Within direct functional analysis, in the last 30 years an important role has been taken on by experimental functional analysis. Experimental functional analysis implies, unlike the previous one which merely recorded the events in a naturalistic way, the manipulation of the antecedent events and consequences of the behaviour in order to identify a functional relationship between the behaviour and the context variables.

In the early 1980s, B. Iwata proposed an experimental model to evaluate the sensitivity of target behaviours to positive, negative, and automatic reinforcement contingencies [20].

This type of functional analysis involves direct observations and repeated measurements in some test situations intentionally constructed and manipulated by the operator (usually four experimental and one control situation) [21–23].

The experimental conditions that are generally implemented are the following:

1. Alone, the person is observed in the absence of stimuli or other people (it is useful to identify systems of automatic reinforcement).
2. The condition of attention provided contingently to the manifestation of the challenging behaviour (positive social reinforcement).
3. The condition of control (or more commonly defined as game for the youngest) in which reinforcements are provided continuously and not contingently.
4. The condition of request offered by the opportunity of escape contingent to the manifestation of the challenging behaviour (negative reinforcement).
5. The "tangible" conditions in which reinforcements, tangible ones, are given as a contingency to the manifestation of the challenging behaviour.

These and other forms of experimental functional analysis such as the one summarised above [24] have proved to be valuable tools for conducting functional analysis. This is mainly due to their ability to bring under experimental control those variables that in the indirect systems or in the descriptive functional assessments are only hypothetical or correlational.

12.5 The Psychoeducational Intervention

The use of functional assessment tools is a very useful support to identify the hypothesis of functional value of challenging behaviour. This phase of the intervention, besides being the most important, is certainly also the most complex because it requires the operator to analyse the collected data and construct hypotheses on the adaptive meaning of behaviour.

We know that it is not the form of the behaviour that explains its function [25]. It is therefore necessary that the clinician proceeds with the specific analysis of the antecedent events and consequences of the behaviour and its context. In this phase, the clinician is called upon to identify a hypothesis which, if correct, will be confirmed only after the intervention.

Challenging behaviours may be related to the consequences of behaviour observable in the outside world (e.g. in the form of situations experienced as adversive, the avoidance of tasks which are too difficult, or in the form of enrichment, such as the search for physical contact or attention or environmental control on things, people, etc.), rather than producing consequences on the inside world, on one's own belief systems, values and symbolic systems.

The next step towards the identification of the functional value of challenging behaviour is the choice of psychoeducational procedures and the continuation of data collection to verify the treatments' effectiveness. Cooper et al. [7, 26, 27] exhaustively list all the behavioural procedures that may be used for the constructions of new behaviours and reduction of maladaptive ones [2, 28]. The team will therefore work towards producing not only different hypotheses of functional value, but also identifying the psychoeducational treatment procedures coherent with the functional value attributed to the behaviour [29]. In short, it could be said that if the main objective of the intervention on the challenging behaviours is their reduction, the priority will be supporting and changing the person and/or their context so that they may increase or create new behaviours that will replace the challenging ones [30]. In other words, it will be necessary to identify those adaptive behaviours that share the same functional value.

In the choice of interventions, which are often multi-component, it is equally important to remember to maintain a balanced relationship between pro-active and reactive procedures. Indeed, even if the opposite is often true in clinical practice, an effective and respectful treatment of the quality of life and the person's context should tend towards more pro-active interventions rather than reactive ones [31–33].

A balanced ratio between pro-active and reactive procedures should amount to 80% and 20% respectively [34]. Pro-active interventions work on the antecedents and consequences to teach the person a replacement behaviour, whereas the reactive ones only manipulate the consequences of the challenging behaviour by minimising the possibility to reinforce it [35].

For these reasons, the first interventional steps to reduce the challenging behaviour should be anticipated by a precise study of the person's abilities, strengths and weaknesses, and by an in-depth evaluation of the preferences and values of the person [36, 37].

References

1. Murphy O, Healy O, Leader G. Risk factors for challenging behaviors among 157 children with autism spectrum disorder in Ireland. Res Autism Spectr Disord. 2009;3:474–82. https://doi.org/10.1016/j.rasd.2008.09.008.
2. Ministero della Salute. Sistema Nazionale per le linee guida. "Il trattamento dei disturbi dello spettro autistico nei bambini e negli adolescenti". Linea guida 21. Ottobre 2011; 2011.
3. Fletcher RJ, Barnhill J, Cooper S-A. Diagnostic manual—intellectual disability (DM-ID-2): a textbook of diagnosis of mental disorders in persons with intellectual disability. Kingston, NY: NADD Press; 2016.
4. Royal College of Psychiatrists. DC-LD (diagnostic criteria for psychiatric disorders for use with adults with learning disabilities/mental retardation). London: Gaskell Press; 2001.
5. Bertelli M, Cavagnola R, et al. II. SPAIDD-G (Valutazione Psicopatologica Sistematica per le Persone con Disabilità Intellettiva o dello Sviluppo: screening Generale). Firenze: Edizione Giunti; in press.
6. Bodfish JW, Harper VN, Deacon JR, Symons FJ. Identifying and measuring pain in persons with developmental disabilities: a manual for the Pain and Discomfort Scale (PADS). Western Carolina Center Research Reports; 2001.
7. Cooper JO, Heron TE, Heward WL. Applied behavior analysis. 2nd ed. Upper Saddle River, NJ: Pearson Prentice Hall; 2007.
8. Betz A, Fisher WW. Functional analysis: history and methods. In: Fisher WW, Piazza CC, Roane HS, editors. Handbook of applied behavior analysis. New York: Guilford; 2011. p. 206–25.
9. Fisher WW, Adelinis JD, Thompson RH, Worsdell AS, Zarcone JR. Functional analysis and treatment of destructive behavior maintained by termination of "don't" (and symmetrical "do") requests. J Appl Behav Anal. 1998a;31:339–56. https://doi.org/10.1901/jaba.1998.31-339.
10. Hanley GP, Iwata BA, McCord BE. Functional analysis of problem behavior: a review. J Appl Behav Anal. 2003;36:147–85. https://doi.org/10.1901/jaba.2003.36-147.
11. Hagopian LP, Fisher WW, Thompson RH, Owen-DeSchryver J, Iwata BA, Wacker DP. Toward the development of structured criteria for interpretation of functional analysis data. J Appl Behav Anal. 1997;30:313–26. https://doi.org/10.1901/jaba.1997.30-313.
12. Hagopian LP, Rooker GW, Jessel J, DeLeon IG. Initial functional analysis outcomes and modifications in pursuit of differentiation: a summary of 176 inpatient cases. J Appl Behav Anal. 2013;46:88–100. https://doi.org/10.1002/jaba.25.
13. Durand V, Crimmins D. Identifying the variable maintaining self-injurious behaviors. J Autism Dev Disord. 1988;18:99–117.
14. Newton JT, Sturmey P. The motivation assessment scale: inter-rater reliability and internal consistency in a British sample. J Intellect Disabil Res. 1991;35:472–4. https://doi.org/10.1111/j.1365-2788.1991.tb00429.x.
15. Shogren KA, Rojahn J. Convergent reliability and validity of the questions about behavioral function and the motivation assessment scale: a replication study. J Dev Phys Disabil. 2003;15:367–75. https://doi.org/10.1023/A:1026314316977.
16. Zarcone JR, Rodgers TA, Iwata BA, Rourke DA, Dorsey MF. Reliability analysis of the motivation assessment scale: a failure to replicate. Res Dev Disabil. 1991;12:349–60. https://doi.org/10.1016/0891-4222(91)90031-M. Received 14 Jun 2013, Final acceptance November 17, 2013 Action Editor, Wayne Fisher.
17. Iwata BA, DeLeon IG. The functional analysis screening tool (FAST). Gainesville, FL: University of Florida; 1995.
18. Iwata BA, DeLeon IG, Roscoe EM. Reliability and validity of the functional analysis screening tool. J Appl Behav Anal. 2013;46:271–84. https://doi.org/10.1002/jaba.31.
19. Gardner WI, Cole CL, Davidson DP, Karan OC. Reducing aggression in individuals with developmental disabilities: an expanded stimulus control, assessment, and intervention model. Educ Training Mental Retard. 1986;21:3–12.

20. Thompson RH, Iwata BA. A comparison of outcomes from descriptive and functional analyses of problem behavior. J Appl Behav Anal. 2007;40:333–8. https://doi.org/10.1901/jaba.2007.56-06.
21. Iwata BA, Dorsey MF, Slifer KJ, Bauman KE, Richman GS. Toward a functional analysis of self-injury. J Appl Behav Anal. 1994a;27:197–209. https://doi.org/10.1901/jaba.1994.27-197. (Reprinted from Analysis and Intervention in Developmental Disabilities, 2, 3–20, 1982).
22. Iwata BA, Dozier CL. Clinical application of functional analysis methodology. Behav Anal Pract. 2008;1:3–9.
23. Iwata BA, Pace GM, Dorsey MF, Zarcone JR, Vollmer TR, Smith RG, et al. The functions of self-injurious behavior: an experimental-epidemiological analysis. J Appl Behav Anal. 1994c;27:215–40. https://doi.org/10.1901/jaba.1994.27-215.
24. Hanley GP, Jin CS, Vanselow NR, Hanratty LA. Producing meaningful improvements in problem behavior of children with autism via synthesized analyses and treatments. J Appl Behav Anal. 2014;47:16–36.
25. Thompson RH, Fisher WW, Piazza CC, Kuhn DE. The evaluation and treatment of aggression maintained by attention and automatic reinforcement. J Appl Behav Anal. 1998;31:103–16. https://doi.org/10.1901/jaba.1998.31-103.
26. Campbell JM. Efficacy of behavioral interven- tions for reducing problem behavior in persons with autism: a quantitative synthesis of single-subject research. Res Dev Disabil. 2003;24:120–38. https://doi.org/10.1016/S0891-4222(03)00014-3.
27. Carr EG, Durand VM. Reducing behavior problems through functional communication training. J Appl Behav Anal. 1985;18:111–26. https://doi.org/10.1901/jaba.1985.18-111.
28. Fisher W, Piazza C, Cataldo M, Harrell R, Jefferson G, Conner R. Functional communication training with and without extinction and punishment. J Appl Behav Anal. 1993;26:23–36. https://doi.org/10.1901/jaba.1993.26-23.
29. Scotti JR, Evans IM, Meyer LH, Walker P. A meta-analysis of intervention research with problem behavior: treatment validity and standards of practice. Am J Ment Retard. 1991;96:233–56.
30. Fisher WW, Thompson RH, Hagopian LP, Bowman LG, Krug A. Facilitating tolerance of delayed reinforcement during functional communication training. Behav Modif. 2000;24:3–29. https://doi.org/10.1177/0145445500241001.
31. Kahng S, Iwata BA, DeLeon IG, Worsdell AS. Evaluation of the "control over reinforcement" component in functional communication training. J Appl Behav Anal. 1997;30:267–77. https://doi.org/10.1901/jaba.1997.30-267.
32. Kahng S, Iwata BA, Lewin AB. Behavioral treatment of self-injury, 1964 to 2000. Am J Ment Retard. 2002;107:212–21.
33. Luczynski KC, Hanley GP. Prevention of problem behavior by teaching functional communication and self-control skills to preschoolers. J Appl Behav Anal. 2013;46:355–68. https://doi.org/10.1002/jaba.44.
34. Meazzini P. Handicap passi verso l'autonomia. Presupposti teorici e tecniche d'intervento. Firenze: Giunti; 1997.
35. Northup J, Wacker D, Sasso G, Steege M, Cigrand K, Cook J, DeRaad A. A brief functional analysis of aggressive and alternative behavior in an outclinic setting. J Appl Behav Anal. 1991;24:509–22. https://doi.org/10.1901/jaba.1991.24-509.
36. Beavers GA, Iwata BA, Lerman DC. Thirty years of research on the functional analysis of problem behavior. J Appl Behav Anal. 2013;46:1–21. https://doi.org/10.1002/jaba.30.
37. Jin CS, Hanley GP, Beaulieu L. An individualized and comprehensive approach to treating sleep problems in young children. J Appl Behav Anal. 2013;46:161–80. https://doi.org/10.1002/jaba.16.

MIX
Papier aus verantwortungsvollen Quellen
Paper from responsible sources
FSC® C105338

If you have any concerns about our products,
you can contact us on
ProductSafety@springernature.com

In case Publisher is established outside the EU,
the EU authorized representative is:
Springer Nature Customer Service Center GmbH
Europaplatz 3, 69115 Heidelberg, Germany

Printed by Libri Plureos GmbH
in Hamburg, Germany